The Creation of Health

The Creation of Health

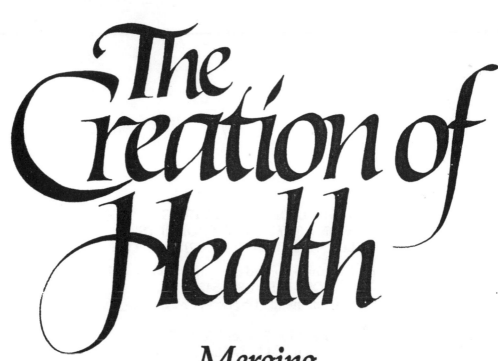

Merging

Traditional Medicine

with

Intuitive Diagnosis

C. NORMAN SHEALY M.D. Ph.D.
CAROLINE M. MYSS, M.A.

STILLPOINT

STILLPOINT PUBLISHING
BOOKS, TAPES AND PRODUCTS
FOR LIVING THE EXTRAORDINARY LIFE

For a free catalog or ordering information, call
TOLL-FREE 1-800-847-4014
(Continental US, except NH)
or
1-603-756-3508 or 756-4225
(Foreign and New Hampshire)
or write Stillpoint Publishing, Box 640,
Walpole, NH 03608 U.S.A.

First Edition
Copyright 1988 © C. Norman Shealy, M.D., and Caroline M. Myss, M.A.

This book is manufactured in the United States of America.
Cover and text design by Rostislav Eismont Design, Richmond, NH
Published by Stillpoint Publishing, a division of
Stillpoint International, Inc.
Box 640, Meetinghouse Road, Walpole, NH 03608, U.S.A.

Published simultaneously in Canada by
Fitzhenry & Whiteside Ltd., Toronto

Library of Congress Card Catalog Number 88-062555
ISBN 0-913299-40-5

9 8 7 6 5 4 3 2 1

A Stillpoint CREATION OF HEALTH Series Book

To my parents,
who were my first and finest teachers.
With all my love.
CMM

To all intuitive physicians
who use their gifts to help humanity.
CNS

Table of Contents

FOREWORD by Bernard S. Siegel, M.D.
and Barbara H. Siegel, B.S.

AUTHORS' PREFACES
ACKNOWLEDGEMENTS

S E C T I O N   I
SHIFTING TO THE DIMENSION OF ENERGY

**CHAPTER ONE: ENTERING THE AGE
OF CO-CREATION**

(M y s s)

CHAPTER TWO: TOWARD MEDICINE OF THE TWENTY-FIRST CENTURY

(S h e a l y)

CHAPTER THREE: THE PROOF OF THE PUDDING

(S h e a l y)

CHAPTER FOUR: INTUITIVE DIAGNOSIS AND THE HUMAN ENERGY SYSTEM

(Myss)

CHAPTER FIVE: THE JOURNEY OF HEALING

(Myss)

SECTION II
UNDERSTANDING THE ORIGIN OF DISEASE

CHAPTER SIX: THE POPULAR WAY TO DIE:
THE BIG THREE—HEART DISEASE,
CANCER AND STROKE

(Shealy and Myss)

CHAPTER SEVEN: ACUTE DISEASES AND
INJURIES: INFECTIONS AND ACCIDENTS

(Shealy and Myss)

CHAPTER EIGHT: CHRONIC DISEASES— THE LONG WAY HOME

(S h e a l y a n d M y s s)

CHAPTER NINE: CHRONIC PAIN

(Shealy and Myss)

CHAPTER TEN: PRIMARY MENTAL AND
EMOTIONAL DISORDERS

(Shealy and Myss)

SECTION III
STRESS: THE COMMON DENOMINATOR

CHAPTER ELEVEN: CONFLICTS OF SEX AND SEXUALITY: THE ROOTS OF LOW SELF-ESTEEM

(S h e a l y)

CHAPTER TWELVE: PSYCHOSOMATIC HEALTH

(S h e a l y)

CHAPTER THIRTEEN: SELF-TESTING

(S h e a l y a n d M y s s)

SECTION IV
CREATING HEALTH

CHAPTER FOURTEEN: CREATING HEALTH AND STAYING HEALTHY

(Shealy and Myss)

CHAPTER FIFTEEN: THE WAY OF THE ELEGANT SPIRIT

(Myss)

||||||||||||||||||||||||||||||||||||||||||||||||||||||||||||||||||||||||||||||||||||||||||||||||||||||||||||

FOREWORD

By Bernard S. Siegel, M.D.

The concepts presented in *The Creation of Health* are very appropriate to healing in our time. We are now faced with the threats of nuclear warfare and AIDS, which have no simple, intellectual solutions. A rebirth of the techniques of healing or perhaps a relearning of what our ancestors already knew is required. If there is to be a twenty-first century, it will need to reflect a new level of spiritual wisdom and intuitive insight.

There may be a vocabulary in this book that seems strange to some, but remember, all healing is "scientific." We are just beginning to explore areas of mind-body interactions and measure what emotional states (such as depression or love) do to the body.

We have struggled endlessly to gain acceptance of the fact that the health of the psyche and spirit are manifested on a cellular level, as physical health or disease. We are the soil in which the disease can take root. We are not simply attacked by "nice" or "nasty" diseases. We have a lot to say about our health and healing. *The Creation of Health* helps one look at this total picture to help one successfully live one's life.

I am still a surgeon, despite what I know about healing . . . and Norm started as a neurosurgeon. We are grounded people but we also have seen the true nature of healing.

Every day, I see what love and peace of mind do to help people heal. I also know the resistance to learning what is not taught in medical school.

One of my subversive acts was to post a double-blind study of the effectiveness of prayer in avoiding post-myocardial infarction complications on the bulletin board of the Doctors' Lounge at Yale-New Haven Hospital. In twenty-four hours, someone had written "bullshit" across it. One cannot change the closed-minded with statistics. Beliefs are a matter of faith, not logic. As the Quakers say, "Speak truth to power."

My wife Bobbie and I, originally skeptics, have both personally experienced healings of physical problems. These healings were viewed by physicians who were also altered by what they "saw."

One of my patients is a medium. She regularly gives me information about the living and messages from the dead that she could not possibly "know" intellectually. I do not reject it. I stay open and accept it.

I know I use my intuition as I evaluate patients. I "know" when people are "sick." They give off a different feeling, vibration, aura . . . call it what you will; it is obvious to me. I don't give up my diagnostic tools but combine intuition, symbolism and medicine in treating people.

The issue isn't to cure all illnesses. Everyone dies, someday. The issue is to love and live an authentic life and to understand that healing and curing may be two different entities. A quadriplegic painter, who holds a brush in his mouth, loves and beautifies the world and is closer to his wholeness than many of us who are without physical limitations.

What is our responsibility to ourselves and the cosmos? I believe it is all related to the role of love. Self-love and self-esteem are required. We must start with self-love and self-healing in order to be able to extend it to others. Free will is the key ingredient to making it meaningful.

What, despite all my scientific training keeps me open to the seemingly mystical and unconscious awareness? Life! To me it is mystical how a wound "knows" how to heal. How a fertilized egg carries all the knowledge to grow up to be a human being is mystical. Where in the DNA is the blueprint for our quadrants . . . psychological, intellectual, physical and spiritual? All the information for us to be whole individuals is there. If we listen to our four quadrants, we will stay on our path. Illness is a reset button . . . a redirector of one's life. It says "change your life pattern." It is not a matter of blame or guilt but *the courage to grow and change.* Is it scientific? Yes! Teach type-A post-myocardial infarct patients to love and you halve the reinfarction rate. Psychotherapy can reduce the psychological and *physical* side effects of radiation and chemotherapy. DNA repair mechanisms are enhanced in stable individuals. This is all scientific, all measurable.

The greatest reason to live the message is that it feels good. No one will live forever . . . the longer one lives, the more loss one experiences. *It is what you choose to do with the pain that is the choice.*

Love is a difficult problem for many of us. As discussed in *The Creation of Health*, the sexual or romantic and spiritual love have been separated. This separation leads to difficulties on all planes. At this point in our development, we must see the need for achieving spiritual, unconditional love as a means of healing ourselves and our fellow travelers on this planet.

The Creation of Health carries within it the seeds to help us grow and bloom, to utilize our innate abilities and take on the challenge of life. The process is the product.

Open your eyes and mind to see, and you will believe. Do not let others tell you what you can see and believe. They will create defects in your visual fields that will lead you to deny what your collective unconscious has always known.

Listen to that inner voice and be born again and healed in the only true sense of the word. Let the creation of health begin in you.

Bernard S. Siegel, M.D., FACS
Author, *Love, Medicine & Miracles* with
Barbara H. Siegel, B.S.

AUTHOR'S PREFACE

(M y s s)

There is a spiritual renaissance at work on our planet. This is a most extraordinary time to be alive. We are discovering the power of the human spirit and thus, we are bracing ourselves to learn about an entirely new dimension of what it means to be human.

We are living at a time when human beings all over the planet are gathering together to meditate, to work for peace, to heal the earth, to reach out beyond national borders and embrace their neighbors. Never before have so many genuinely planetary activities occurred on this globe.

Again and again, these groups gathering from Mt. Shasta, California to Moscow, carry the same message: we want to be and to live differently tomorrow than we did yesterday. We want to live in this world as one species, sharing one home, one sky, one planet. *WE WANT TO HEAL.*

This book is about the human spirit and its potential to create and to heal. Had it been written with case studies from the people of Mt. Shasta, or case studies from the people of Moscow, it would not have made any difference. We are all alike. We all need love. We all need people. We all want to live and be healthy.

I believe it is possible to create a healthy planet, with healthy people and healthy politics. Though I know we are many years, maybe even centuries away from living on such a holy planet, I nonetheless know that we *potentially have the power to create such a place.*

I know this because I have learned that we do indeed create our realities, from the health of our bodies, to the health of our relationships to the health of our planet. That is the message of this book.

We are changing rapidly now. We are changing our ways

of thinking, eating, living and working. We are waking up and in that process, though it is a painful process, we are learning that many forms of pain and disease are optional. The more we learn about the power of our emotions and thoughts to affect what we experience, the more we learn about our power of choice and the need to choose wisely the words and emotions we hold in our bodies.

Years ago, I heard a man quote a spiritual teacher who said, "The greatest gift we can give each other is to be fully healthy." My reaction to that comment was that it sounded to be the *least* powerful gift we could give. I have since learned that this spiritual teacher spoke the truth.

It is my hope that this book will generate health in all who read it.

Caroline M. Myss
Walpole, New Hampshire
July 1988

AUTHOR'S PREFACE

(Shealy)

In 1970, I developed an intense interest in the possibility of intuitive diagnosis as an assistance to medical practice. In the ensuing years, I have had the opportunity to evaluate a wide variety of intuitive individuals and to work very closely with a small number of them. I have become aware of the numerous instances in which intuition has allowed me to make a diagnosis or to get a therapeutic message through to a patient. I have observed a number of geniuses who have used intuition to invent practical tools to help humanity. I am equally convinced that artists and writers function primarily through proper focus of their intuitive abilities. Indeed, I am convinced that intuition is the essential ingredient in the growth of human consciousness and that all inventions and progress in every aspect of human life, from interpersonal relationships to the development of great scientific breakthroughs, is the result of intuition.

Animals have a different type of intuition, one that is more instinctive, and many human beings seem to have lost large aspects of instinctive intuition, the type that allows one to find one's way home when lost at a great distance. On the other hand, we human beings have used intuition to create great beauty in music, art and literature and to provide comfort to billions of our fellow citizens with scientific innovations.

There are many purposes in writing a book. The major reason for me is to provide a stimulus to other physicians to develop their intuitive powers more completely and to provide to all individuals the opportunity to use their own intuition to assist them in an ever-increasing fulfillment of the potential for total health.

C. Norman Shealy, M.D., Ph.D.
Springfield, Missouri
July 1988

ACKNOWLEDGMENTS

Caroline M. Myss, M.A.

My thanks and gratitude to the staff of Stillpoint International: First, to my partners and colleagues, Meredith Young and Errol Sowers, for their continual support of this project, both editorially and emotionally and, most especially, during the darker months of the creative process; and to the rest of the staff: Susan Kryger, for her editorial and proofreading skills; Kathi Tacy, for her patience at doing endless computer input of the manuscript; Marsha Passoja, for organizing me and the continual mailing of material to Norm; Clare Innes, for her care at overseeing the production process and Joe Murphy, for his good-natured presence in the office—my deepest appreciation to each of you; Beverly Beane, for superb proofreading, my thanks for your "finishing touches" and to Rostislav Eismont for all his care and attention in designing this book.

I also wish to extend my love and gratitude for the support of my friends and family whose encouragement in this work, and in my life, has never ceased to warm my heart: Gary Zukav, Marjorie P. Allen, Gerry Paddock, Sally Ember, Jean Sowers, Nina Lynn, Ray and Karol Fenner and, of course, my dear friend, Norm Shealy, a man of deep courage and vision, without whom I would not have had the confidence to do this work.

ACKNOWLEDGMENTS

C. Norman Shealy, M.D., Ph.D.

As one develops one's purpose in life, it is obvious that the way has been blessed by numerous individuals. My mother first introduced me to the concept of intuitive knowing. In medical school, two individuals particularly stimulated my thinking: Talmage L. Peele, M.D. and Eugene A. Stead, Jr., M.D. In my years of residency, Carl A. Moyer, M.D. was perhaps the most intellectually challenging and exciting teacher that I met.

In 1972 Genevieve Haller, D.C., and Jeffrey Furst introduced me to an ever-broadening concept of consciousness, and they were responsible for my meeting Rev. Henry Rucker, one of the greatest intuitives that I have known. Robert Leichtman, M.D. further strengthened my enthusiasm for the benefits of intuitive diagnosis and has served as counselor and friend for many years. Elmer Green, Ph.D. has also provided me with more opportunities to expand my own consciousness than any other teacher or friend. My wife and family have allowed me the opportunity to pursue these interests. Roger K. Cady, M.D. and Robert G. Wilkie, M.D., my partners, have allowed me the freedom to pursue the writing of our experiences. Caroline Myss, M.A. has provided a far greater share of this work than have I, and without her intuitive abilities, this book would not even have been begun. Finally, Jody Trotter has done a Herculean job in typing and retyping and retyping and helping us to keep it straight. My thanks to all of you.

SHIFTING TO THE DIMENSION OF ENERGY

CHAPTER ONE

Entering the Age of Co-Creation

(M y s s)

T he time has come to assert one primal fact: The human spirit is real. Beyond the chemical, physical and physiological study of disease, there comes a point, as we search for the cause of illness, when we are led directly to the core of a person's soul. This is a bold notion with which to begin a book on health. It is not, however, original. In recent decades, numerous health professionals have suggested that the cause of illness is ultimately connected to inner stresses present in a person's life.

The language used to describe this connection between illness and stress varies from source to source. Some use psychological terms, others use the language of stress. Still others emphasize the body-mind-spirit connection. In combining the significance of all of this research, it becomes apparent that something of great value is being universally introduced into our world. Our "spirits" are longing to be recognized as legitimate, meaning they are every bit as real as our physical selves. Beyond the religious and poetic acceptance of the human spirit, our spiritual natures are breaking through the barriers of our psychological and emotional language, demanding to be identified as the underlying force of life from which all else flows.

Were this book to be written twenty-five or perhaps even fifteen years from now, we would undoubtedly begin by listing the causes of illness in language that describes the basic crises of the spirit: loss of meaning in one's life, grief, guilt, an unforgiving heart, contamination through hatred, loss of self-esteem and personal dignity, and all forms of fear. Once these crises were identified, the physical dysfunction being manifested by the body would be understood as a reflection of these deeper spiritual issues.

Most of us are not yet ready to accept fully this analysis of illness. We are all products of a complex technological society in which we have grown up to think of ourselves in technological terms. In order even to consider the human experience in spiritual language, much less recognize disease as a spiritual crisis, we have to bring a reverence for Life into the forefront of what it means to be a human being.

For all of the many explanations considered as to why Life exists, few people have on the tips of their tongues the notion that Life might be, in and of itself, *sacred*. Indeed, for many people, the notion of "holiness" is not present in their understanding of what it means to be human, alive and a part of the vast continuum of life that exists on this planet and beyond. Our system for appreciating life is essentially an economic one in which the value we ascribe to people and to other life forms is based upon earning capabilities and the acquisition of earthly power. This value system is transculturally applied to individuals, nations and to the earth itself, and serves as strong evidence that the human society finds it difficult to honor Life for Life's sake.

Thus, as a result of what our value system has done to the quality of life, we have in our midst a wide variety of epidemics, many of which are virus-associated. The other "epidemics," such as drug and alcohol addiction, are purely emotional and spiritual in nature. The human experience, except for occasional pockets of enlightenment, is diminished in dignity. People in countless numbers are lost within the very fabric of their lives. Whether financially, politically or socially persecuted, millions and millions of people's lives have been reduced to little or no value because of the economic scale upon which we measure the worth of life.

We now face an epidemic of the fragmentation of the human spiritual condition. Out of this epidemic, physical disease arises in the form of AIDS, cancer, depression, anxiety, nervous breakdowns, alcoholism and drug addiction as well as environmental toxic poisoning and pollution. If this book were being written in the year 2,000, we would be writing a purely spiritual text on how to heal these illnesses. But our world is now only slightly open to considering the possibility that the human spirit needs serious attention, much less genuine healing. It is appropriate, therefore, that this book represent the traditional medical model of health and disease alongside the emerging voice of the human spirit.

We have a substantial journey ahead of us. This book represents one step, hopefully a major one, in that direction.

FORMING OUR PARTNERSHIP

Norm Shealy and I have worked together since 1985 in a partnership that combines our perceptions and training to help people understand why they have become ill. He is a physician, neurosurgeon and expert on pain and stress management.

I am a publisher of books, a former journalist and I earned a Master's Degree in Religious Studies, specializing in the Psychological Dimensions of Spirituality. During the years I spent studying spirituality, I realized that the skill of intuition is a natural attribute of the human spirit that can be developed and disciplined to benefit one's life. I specifically focused the development of my intuition on learning to do intuitive diagnosis.

This skill enables me to perceive a person's energy, or life force, to such an exact degree that I can intuitively identify and locate the presence of a physical disease within a person's body. More importantly, however, I am able to recognize and identify the patterns of emotional, psychological and spiritual stress within a person's life. This information provides Norm and his patients, as well as me and my clients, with a perspective more inclusive of the total stress-related circumstances of a patient's life.

In addition to the physical data that is determined through a physician's medical examination and laboratory tests, the information acquired through an intuitive reading uncovers the fears, emotional stresses, deeply rooted insecurities and personal traumas that exist as a very real part of each person's life. When all of this data is compiled, a comprehensive profile of a patient's life emerges. Then it is possible to understand how a person, consciously or unconsciously, participated in the creation of disease.

Through the years of our work together, Norm and I have dealt with hundreds of patients. We work together with people who have cancer, arthritis, chronic pain, accidental injury, brain injuries, coma, AIDS, heart problems, strokes and many other diseases. We have consistently noted that illness tends to follow certain patterns of stress or trauma that emerge organically out of the day-to-day business of living. How well our inner resources serve us in terms of helping us to cope with the ordinary events of life, such as disappointment or frustration over our personal or professional relationships, the experience of loss, financial traumas, to name just a few, is intimately linked with one's quality of health.

THE STRESS FACTOR

In recent years, we have, as a society, turned our attention toward studying the effects of stress upon health. There is general agreement between both the medical community and the public that stress is indeed a major contributor to diseases such as heart attacks, high blood pressure, ulcers and nervous disorders.

The medical trend of looking seriously at the varied influences of stress marks a major turning point in the diagnosis and understanding of disease because it introduces the factor that emotional tension is, in fact, disruptive to the physical body. Even though the influence of stress is still viewed as only a partial contributor to physical dysfunction, nevertheless this recognition that human emotions do indeed affect physical health has brought the traditional medical world face to face with *the fundamental principle of holistic health*: The majority of physical illnesses result from an overload of emotional, psychological and spiritual crises.

Because the study of stress continues to produce hard evidence that emotions influence health, it is now inevitable that the findings of traditional medical research in this area will eventually merge with the principles of holistic health because both fields are discovering the same reality: Emotions exert the controlling influence upon the physical body. Even though the traditional medical community takes a more cautious approach in forming conclusions on this matter, the door, nevertheless, has been opened.

The use of the term "stress" itself contributes to this merger of the two medical worlds because it is a bridge term—a safe word that describes what traditional physicians are nervous about describing. Without having officially to recognize emotional, psychological or spiritual crises, the use of the word "stress" provides a legitimate and non-threatening term to describe what holistically minded physicians and health care practitioners are comfortable discussing in detail, namely, the human response to the difficulties of life.

The work that Norm and I do together serves much the same function as does the general term "stress"—it's bridge work. Our research with people includes the study of their "disease" and extends into the study of who they are, what they believe and how well they provide for their emotional needs within the environment of their lives.

SIGNIFICANT STRESS PATTERNS

In general, we have learned that people who become ill identify consistently with one or more of the following eight dysfunctional patterns.

The first pattern involves the presence of *unresolved or deeply consuming* emotional, psychological or spiritual stress within a person's life. This stress may be either a long-running pattern reaching as far back as childhood, such as a feeling of rejection or inadequacy, or it may be the result of some recent event within his or her life, such as the death of a spouse. Whatever the type of stress, it need not be dramatic or even obvious to be real. Inevitably, however, unresolved or consuming inner stress is present in larger measure in a person who becomes ill.

The second consistent pattern relates to the degree of control that negative belief patterns have upon a person's reality. Each of us is a complex system of positive and negative beliefs, attitudes and experiences.

What a person believes to be true about life, about God, about other people, about fate or luck, for instance, plays a very powerful role in determining how a person lives. Because what we believe is intimately connected to our emotions, our beliefs influence our emotional response to life. The empowering belief patterns and positive mental attitudes that we possess are, therefore, essential to creating a healthy body as well as a healthy life.

People who become ill, however, tend to have belief patterns that are disempowering in such an effective way that these patterns override the influence of whatever positive attitudes exist. For example, an individual may be educated and talented and give the appearance of having all things working in his or her favor. And yet, underneath that illusion, that person may have such low self-esteem that he or she feels unworthy of success. That belief most assuredly guarantees failure, and failure guarantees anger and bitterness which, in turn, result in physical distress.

The third consistent pattern that plays a major role in our becoming ill is the inability to give and/or receive love. People's lives revolve around love, and when stressful experiences in relationships exist, the physical body can easily break down in response. A person who lives a life devoid of love or of any degree of human warmth is a prime candidate for disease.

The fourth consistent pattern that is central to creating illness is lack of humor and the inability to distinguish serious concerns from the lesser issues of life. Certainly there are those situations in life that merit a strong emotional response. Many upsets, however, are not earth-shattering; they are simply the day-to-day "stuff" of life. It is worth learning how to let go of the lesser "stuff" in order to avoid problems such as high blood pressure, migraines or ulcers. Laughter is extremely healing. Finding humor in our struggles does not mean we do not take them seriously. Rather, it is an indication of the natural transcendent qualities of the human being.

The fifth consistent pattern that influences the quality of health is how effectively one exercises the power of choice in terms of holding dominion over the movement and activities of their own life. "Holding dominion over" has a substantially different and far healthier meaning than does the common attitude of thinking of yourself as in control of all of the parts and all of the people in your life. A person can maintain control over his or her life and have a heart attack in the process, due to the anxiety and stress that accompany the effort to control the events of the outside world.

"Holding dominion over" refers to our capacity to maintain the controlling influence in terms of the flow of our own lives, even if the flow includes compromise or altering our plans. Holding dominion does not mean always getting one's own way. It means being able to participate in the natural give and take of life, to be flexible, to respond to the needs of others and to reach for what you need from a position of inner strength and confidence. It means being able to have an effective voice in making your own choices.

Every person must feel that he or she has a choice in the matters of his or her own life. When the dynamic of choice is violated or interfered with, a person's emotional response can often lead to the development of disease. This is because the individual's response to a violation of choice will be filled with anger, hostility, fear and rage.

In people who are ill, there is often a history of experiences in which they either have abdicated their power of choice to a more dominant personality or have felt that their choices have not been respected.

The sixth consistent pattern concerns how well a person has attended to the needs of the physical body itself. Nutrition, exercise, the impact of drugs or alcohol, as well as a person's genetic makeup, provide the foundation for the quality of health. How well an individual attends to the emotional, physical and chemical stresses of life is very strongly connected to the degree of vigor and stamina in the physical body itself.

The seventh consistent pattern relates to the "existential vacuum" or the suffering that accompanies the absence or loss of meaning in one's life. The lost soul, or wandering person, is very susceptible to illness, primarily because a life devoid of meaning often leads to despair, depression and feelings of worthlessness. The physical body is strongly affected when one's state of mind and emotions are consumed with the suffering that comes from feelings of emptiness. This is a frequent condition reported by people who are ill.

The eighth pattern that is characteristic of people who become ill is the tendency toward denial. Tremendous inner stress is created from the inability to face the challenges of one's life and neither to acknowledge nor consciously recognize what it is that is not working in one's life. Much of this stress is created as a result of *choosing* to block one's own intuition or awareness

in order to allow certain situations to continue without address-
ing the deeper problems that exist.

Situations arise in everyone's life that are difficult to acknowledge—for example, a child on drugs or a marriage that is
in great difficulty. Acknowledging the situation, which means
discussing it, makes it real in such a way that one can no longer
deny the problem. Denying the presence of difficulty by avoiding conversations about it does not make it evaporate. Rather,
the stress that is generated through keeping denial alive becomes
extremely destructive to the human body.

Many of our patients who are working through an illness
have commented that they simply could not face a particular
stressful issue in their lives. Once the illness surfaced, however,
denial of that particular situation became impossible, and facing
the stress frequently produced a calm they had previously not
known.

These patterns have led Norm and me to develop significant
conclusions that form the basis of this book. We believe that
each person directly participates, either consciously or unconsciously, in the creation of his or her own reality, including the
reality of their health. The tools that we use in this process of
creation reside within us. They are our attitudes, emotions and
belief patterns as well as an awareness of our spiritual self.

By expanding an appreciation of the power of the inner
self, two things happen. First, the individual becomes receptive
to learning *how* emotions, attitudes and belief patterns contribute
in very specific ways to the creation of health or of disease.
Secondly, the individual develops the capacity to keep healthy
through being aware that *negative attitudes create negative responses
within the physical body*. It becomes difficult to allow negativity
to go unchallenged in one's life once this level of awareness is
attained, since the consequences of disease are understood to
be a very real potential outcome of negative emotions.

Throughout this book, Norm and I explore the emotional,

psychological, physical and spiritual patterns that create health and those dysfunctional patterns that create illness. We have come to recognize that all negative patterns essentially break down into four basic areas of human challenges. These are issues of power, responsibility, wisdom and love.

Regardless of the specific circumstances present in every human dilemma, the actual cause of anguish for every person has to do with that circumstance generating feelings of insecurity rooted in issues of power, responsibility, wisdom and love. To be specific about how we understand these four areas, I describe our working definitions of these terms.

POWER/RESPONSIBILITY/WISDOM/LOVE

POWER

Every human being must find an inner road to self-empowerment. Struggles with becoming empowered are present in every person's life. The forms they take are varied, but their root is similar. Early in our development, we learn to associate power with external symbols: money, political or social status, the ability to control others, an endless desire for approval and attention, material goods, and professional and academic titles. We strive for these goals because they communicate powerful messages to the outside world: we are invulnerable; we cannot be victimized; we are successful; we have *control* over our lives.

The attainment of earthly power is ultimately tied to the desire to have and to exert control over all of the aspects of one's life. It is a substitute for a well-developed human spirit whose strength is based upon a deep regard for one's own self-esteem, personal dignity, spiritual principles and self-love. This quality of power cannot be bought. It is earned through the development of inner strength and the qualities of the spirit.

When an individual is focused upon the acquisition of any form of external power, it is indicative of what is absent internally in that person. The stronger the obsession, the greater the lack of authentic power.

Struggles for power occur constantly and in innumerable different forms. From out of balance male-female relationships to power plays at the office to needing always to be first in line— these are just minor examples of the continual interaction of power struggles in our everyday situations. Characteristics such as always having to get one's way, always having to be right, never acknowledging the value of another's opinion and needing to criticize other people occur because a person is lacking in personal power.

Ulcers and high blood pressure are always evidence that the individual is seeking self-empowerment through external gratification with no satisfaction. Migraines frequently indicate a reaction of rage, a frustration that a person is experiencing due to feelings of not being able to control either another individual or a situation that he or she perceives as threatening.

The fear of being victimized by the outside world, or of being used or taken advantage of develops because a person has little or no personal power. The world becomes a threatening place and feelings of intimidation are always present in that person's emotions. This type of stress, in its extreme, produces cancer.

RESPONSIBILITY

Learning to take responsibility for ourselves is a massive challenge. It is very tempting and attractive to find a stronger person who seems able enough to take charge of one's life and all of the responsibilities that go along with living in this world. The reality is, however, that we are each responsible for ourselves, for the quality of our lives, for our attitudes, for our failures and successes and for our health. There is *no getting around this reality*.

Yet we are constantly confronted with wanting others to pick up our loose ends, or blaming others for situations gone sour. If there is one point that healing a disease brings home loud and clear, it is that each person must ultimately take full responsibility for the quality of his or her own life.

When we are motivated through fear to create situations in which we either want to relinquish personal responsibility or we find others are threatened by our desire to take more responsibility for our lives, stresses result that produce illness. Diabetes (as explored in Chapter Eight) is a prime example of a disease that develops over issues of responsibility.

WISDOM

Wisdom is the capacity to seek the learning present in all of the situations of our lives. It is the ability to accept, as the prayer of Reinhold Neibuhr states, what we cannot change and to have the courage to change what we need to change.

Life is a learning experience. As such, there is not one situation in which, painful as it might be, learning in some form does not exist. It is not always easy to accept this perception, especially because we expect life to be fair. We expect somehow that if we do everything right, nothing wrong will ever happen. Life just does not work out that way, not for any of us.

We will all face circumstances during our lifetimes that seem unfair, unjust or unnecessarily painful. And we will all continue to experience situations that seem to repeat themselves, as is often the case with a series of relationships that have the same problems. It is a challenge to all of us to break the cycles of repeated difficult experiences or to transcend the unfair circumstances of our lives. Remaining angry or clinging to a feeling that something is unfair is not only unproductive, it is unhealthy. The only way to take the sting out of life's "unfair" or "repeatedly painful" situations is to seek the learning present in the challenge. For those who can do this, their lives move forward. For those who cannot, their lives become embittered experiences. And it is that feeling that lies at the root of many chronic illnesses.

LOVE

We all need love. We thrive on love and we disintegrate without it. Unfortunately, we fill our lives with many substitutes for love. We become involved in relationships where we hope to find love but are disappointed. We manipulate for love. We are capable of developing illnesses in order to receive even the slightest amount of loving attention. In short, we find it extremely difficult to establish emotional satisfaction and security in our relationships.

At the source of many of our stresses are issues related to love. These include, among others, loneliness, resentment over rejection, fear of being loved or of not being loved, disappointments in personal relationships and guilt over not fulfilling the expectations of another. Diseases of the heart are always connected to issues relating to love.

Regardless of the particular disease or the specific patterns of emotional stress which create that disease, Norm and I emphasize that life presents us all with challenges so that we can become increasingly empowered human beings. This is the nature of life itself, and it is impossible to separate our quality of health from our capacity to respond appropriately and effectively to the challenges we create in our lives.

MERGING TRADITIONAL MEDICINE WITH
INTUITIVE DIAGNOSIS

Traditional medicine and holistic health represent more than just two different approaches to healing disease. They illustrate two essentially different paradigms of reality.

The model of traditional medicine is a scientifically constructed one. The type of knowledge and data that is considered valid and trustworthy by a physician must fit scientifically acceptable criteria. This means that what is considered "real" must be measurable, usable and reliable through scientific methodology.

Disease and the causes of disease are studied and treated within this physically oriented reality system. As a result, both the causes identified for the breakdown of the human body and the treatments applied to heal them are physical.

Moreover, because of the physical orientation of science and medicine, the perception is widely held that illnesses such as viruses, infections and cancer occur as a result of an invasion by an outside source, such as germs and bacteria. The difficulty with this perception is not that it is inaccurate but that it is *incomplete* and leads to the further assumption that every cause for every disease comes only from the outside world.

The result of this perception is that the inner world of emotions is not valued in terms of having any real power or influence over the workings of the physical body because these attributes are not scientifically quantifiable. Emotions, of course, do not fit into the exacting language of science. The paradigm of traditional medicine, developed with serious regard to scientific (i.e., unemotional) terminology, therefore embraces the premise that it is the physical world that contains the forces which exert the strongest influence on the body.

The holistic paradigm is almost the exact opposite of the traditional medicinal model. While traditional medicine can be said to work from the "outside in," holistic medicine approaches disease from the "inside out." That is, the fundamental principle of holistic philosophy is that illness results when emotional, psychological or spiritual stresses become overwhelming and thus cause a weakening of the body.

In other words, the body reflects or manifests the deeper struggles of the person's entire life. To the extent that an individual becomes unable to process emotional, psychological or spiritual stresses, the individual becomes "receptive" or "susceptible" to the viruses, bacteria or germs present in the atmosphere.

What the holistic paradigm suggests—and this is the central difference between these two views of disease—is that the "energy" level of the human being, meaning the inner emotional and spiritual world, precedes, and in fact determines, all that is experienced at the physical level of life.

What this means is that the traditional medical model and the holistic model are both based upon fundamentally different reality systems that challenge the relationship of energy to matter, or mind to body. The question becomes, "What comes first— the energy of the mind and spirit or the physical world of the body and matter?" This challenge is so significant that it has implications not just for the future of medicine and health care, but for the future of science and technology as well. It is this fundamental difference, more than any of the specific therapies and health technologies, that has created the division which exists between these two paradigms of health.

The response that has arisen from the traditional medical community toward the emergence of a second model of health care has been to discredit and disregard its validity. Even some of the language that is used by both groups of professionals is the language of opposition in that the holistic approach to health considers itself to be an "alternative" to traditional medicine. "Alternative" suggests a better, more effective, more compassionate, more humane approach to healing, and it implies that the traditional system is lacking in all of these qualities.

In point of fact, the use of the term "alternative" actually applies to the various therapeutic techniques available in the holistic field. "Holistic" is not a technique. Rather, it is a way of approaching healing through which a person incorporates several different therapies, including traditional medicine. Indeed, holistic medicine should *include* traditional approaches in order to be considered truly "holistic."

Norm and I represent voices from both of these paradigms. It is our strong belief that these two paradigms of health care are not meant to compete with each other, but to complement one another and become integrated. The experience, knowledge and technologies of both traditional medicine and holistic health care are valid, substantial and potent.

Metaphorically speaking, traditional medicine represents the "mind" of health care and the holistic approach represents the "heart" of health care. In the merger of these two systems, a third and more integrated health care system will emerge that honors the validity of the full spectrum of the human being. It is, after all, impossible to separate our emotions from what it means to be a living, breathing human being who gives and receives love and strives to fulfill dreams and ambitions. Given the degree to which emotions affect every move and choice we make, it would seem an act against our own nature to separate the emotional part of ourselves from our understanding of why we become ill. We are, by design, mental, emotional, psychological, spiritual and physical creatures.

At the same time, the merger of these two approaches to healing presents an entirely new challenge. As Norm and I have discovered, emotions are not quantifiable in the same way as is a white blood cell count. The emotional makeup of every person is like a moving object in that it is a complex weave of relationships, experiences, fulfilled and unfulfilled needs, fears, strengths and unique characteristics that are always in motion. The only aspect that is consistent about our emotional nature is that it is inconsistent—one day up and the next day down. Science demands consistency.

The body and mind form one unit. Psychoneuroimmunology, the scientific study of how psychological and emotional imbalances affect the immune system, is beginning to provide scientific proof of this relationship. The scientific community now needs to move beyond the limitations of the technological model of health diagnosis that prevent us from studying the power of the human mind and its incredibly intimate relationship to the physical body.

Toward that end, there are several central issues that need to be addressed as they represent legitimate roadblocks to the creation of a SYNTHESIZED paradigm of health.

WHY HAVE ALTERNATIVE THERAPIES
BECOME A THREAT
TO TRADITIONAL MEDICINE?

Because the holistic paradigm lacks the respect and authority of the traditional medical community, it exists in a position of having to "prove" its own validity. That is both a disadvantage and a necessary challenge toward its own process of maturation.

At present, the hesitancy of the traditional medical community to trust holistic health methodologies is very understandable. For one thing, you cannot really "prove" why and how someone healed a disease. While people have successfully healed their illnesses through the use of holistic practices such as nutrition and visualization, people also have been healed through the assistance of drugs and surgery. Arguments based upon the experiences of people who have healed themselves through the holistic approach, therefore, do not necessarily sway an opinion or prove the validity of the system.

The reasons for the lack of regard on the part of the traditional medical community for the holistic field are both obvious and not so obvious. Some of the criticisms are valid and some exist because of a lack of appreciation and open-mindedness on the part of the traditional medical community for any approaches other than hard-core medical ones.

It is important to clarify to whom we are referring when we use the general terms of the traditional medical community and the holistic field. By traditional medical community, we are referring mainly to the commentary and opinions expressed by the majority of allopathic physicians (M.D.'s), especially in publications that are accepted as the "standards" by those who control publications and licensure. Certainly at the level of individual opinion, there are exceptions to the positions we are discussing. Likewise, in referring to the holistic field, we are once again referring to commentary and opinions that are generally expressed. We realize that there are professionals in both areas who represent more synergistic positions.

Let's begin, then, with looking into the obvious reasons

why the traditional medical community is cautious about the holistic health care approach to healing.

EMOTIONAL REALITY VERSUS
MEDICAL REALITY

The first reason concerns the need to prove the authenticity of the relationship of emotional stress to physical disease, and the need to treat both the emotions and the body in order to heal. Because this is the foundation of the holistic approach to determining how and why an illness develops, the emphasis placed on the influence of emotions has resulted in what the traditional medical community sees as an exaggerated underplay of the physical factors involved in a disease.

This position is doubly complicated because of the reputation the traditional medical world has gained in recent years for being insensitive to the emotional needs of patients and the tendency of physicians to rely upon drugs (which may or may not be necessary) and/or surgery for treatment. Many people who have turned to alternative practices have done so in response to that position, often with hostility and anger directed at the medical profession. The problem is that they have thrown the proverbial baby out with the bath water by shutting out not only medical treatment, which may well be effective, but also the medical perspective.

Viruses, germs, bacteria and infections are real. Genetic patterning is real. Tumors are real. The effects of working and/ or living in a contaminated environment are real. The effects these elements have upon the physical body are real. In order to heal any disease, it is necessary to acknowledge the reality of the illness and its activity in the physical body. Acknowledgment does not mean accepting the illness as a permanent condition. It does mean recognizing that one's body has produced a very real dysfunction that needs the right kind of attention in order to heal. There are numerous holistic practitioners who recognize and work with the physical level of illness.

The following case history is that of a woman with whom

I worked five years ago. Her story effectively illustrates this discussion.

LORI'S STORY

Lori developed cancer in her cervix that spread to her uterus and intestines. It was suggested by her physician that to save her life, she should have the diseased organs, plus the surrounding tissue, surgically removed. She was told that this would mean that the major organs from the waist down would be removed.

This prognosis sent Lori on a desperate search for alternative treatments. She investigated numerous holistic treatments, from Oriental herbs to following a macrobiotic diet to homeopathy to shiatsu, and on and on. She threw herself into her healing with great intent, convinced that she could, and in fact would, heal the cancer in her body.

In the process, she gave the appearance of someone who had taken charge of her healing process successfully. She removed herself completely from any medical care that was not her concept of holistic. I met with Lori several times during this experience, and I came to realize that the appearance she was projecting to the outside world—as well as to herself—was a massive cover-up for fear—fear both of the cancer and of making the cancer "real" by going through surgery.

The difficult pattern that Lori had entered was one of creating distraction through following alternative treatments that allowed her to believe that the tumor had no "reality" in her body. The focus and intention of her consciousness were more involved with the *denial* of the disease than the acknowledgment of its presence in order that the fears she felt so deeply could be dealt with. Her efforts to avoid contact with the cancer on any physical level caused her to cut off contact with her physicians and to focus only on the treatments she adapted for her healing. These were mainly emotional therapy and a macrobiotic nutritional program.

In reality, all of the benefits that could have come into her mind, body and spirit through the holistic approach were tremendously hampered because her focus shifted from healing herself to denial of the physical presence of cancer. Rather than learning how to acknowledge the condition of cancer from an empowered emotional position, Lori could only feel secure through denying that the cancer was having any effect on her body whatsoever.

Lori also set herself up for a lonely healing journey because her pattern of denial resulted in the creation of very high expectations about her ability to heal herself. She found herself in the position of having to heal as a testimony to others of the power inherent in the holistic system. This was a multi-headed dragon for Lori; not only did the positive support of other people give her the type of external feedback she required in order to keep the denial pattern working (such as, "you're looking great"), but it also increased the distance inside of her between her fears and her capacity to get in touch with them.

Lori died almost two years after her odyssey began. Following her death, several people expressed their disappointment that Lori had not succeeded in her healing, as if she had been running a race for them. They needed to see some proof that healing emotions resulted in the healing of the physical body, and she had failed. Therefore, the holistic system lost a tremendous amount of credibility in their eyes. They never knew that, all along, Lori had been emotionally paralyzed with her fears and that what looked like healing was, in actuality, the activity of denial.

Could Lori have changed the outcome of events had she been able to deal more effectively with the physical reality of her cancer or to confront her emotional/spiritual vacuum? Who knows? I am convinced, however, that the denial of the physical reality of her cancer was probably as contaminating to her body and mind as she feared the surgery and chemotherapy would be.

HOLISTIC EVALUATION OF
THE ORIGIN OF DISEASE

A basic premise in the holistic field is that *illness does not happen randomly*. Every illness or dysfunction a person develops is an indication of a specific type of emotional, psychological or spiritual stress. Each of the characteristics of an illness, such as its location in the physical body, is symbolically important. A tumor found in the colon, for example, has a different meaning than does a tumor located on the knee.

A strong criticism frequently directed toward the holistic field is that holistic practitioners tend to reduce even the most complex of physical disorders to simplistic, symbolic language. This seems to ignore the reality of the seriousness of the physical problem. The complexity of the gradual loss of eyesight through a neurological disorder, when expressed in symbolic terms, for example, becomes a serious difficulty that the person is having with "wanting to see the problems in life clearly."

Understanding the emotional, psychological and spiritual stresses that underlie the creation of illness is a complex process. It is not like a game of connecting the dots in which eye problems connect to a desire not to see clearly, ear problems connect to a desire to tune something or someone out of a person's life, and leg problems signify difficulty standing on one's own. Symbolic analysis is not that simple and not that obvious. People are complicated and their personal histories and emotional patterns are highly individual and complex.

An oversimplification of the significance of a disease can cause someone to feel that the holistic interpretation of illness is nonsense because it is difficult to appreciate the connection between complex disorders and simplistic explanations. The impression often projected to the traditional medical community is that this simplistic reduction of the complex condition of disease represents the most sophisticated level of holistic thinking.

EDUCATIONAL STANDARDS

The traditional medical community, which includes physicians, nurses, psychiatrists and psychologists, has specific professional standards and academic requirements. Within the holistic field, there are numerous forms of therapy that do not require the same intense periods of education.

The training needed to become a massage, color or polarity therapist, for instance, is not as formal a process as is medical or nursing school training. That is not to say that the work therapists do in these alternative fields is not of immense value nor that the training they receive is inadequate. The training involved for several categories of holistic therapies, however, is not as formally organized in traditional academia, and that difference is cause for much of the lack of appreciation for the work of holistic practitioners.

It is difficult for a physician to appreciate the advice of a therapist when the educational process in each field is so different. It is not easy for the traditionally trained individual to understand why the softer, more emotional approach of a massage therapist, for instance, might be of value to someone facing cancer.

In addition to that, the casualness that exists within the holistic field in terms of attaining qualifications for certain skills, as well as the fog around what it means to be "qualified," needs to be examined from both perspectives. By that, I mean that both traditionally trained medical people and trained alternative therapists need to become open to appreciating the language, skills and approaches of each other's perspectives.

One strong criticism on the subject of language that has been expressed to me on several occasions by people in the traditional field has to do with the use of the term "healer." Many alternative therapists use the term "healer" in describing themselves. That is a potent word and it *implies* that these practitioners have the skill to heal a disease. The argument presented by traditionally educated medical people is that the use of the term "healer" to describe one's work is misleading. The more accurate description is that alternative therapists help to facilitate an individual's healing process. While many, if not most, of these therapists would agree with the interpretation that they facilitate healing, the impression given by the use of the title "healer" misrepresents the actual "physiological" effectiveness of their skills.

The position held by traditional professionals is that during an illness, the patient is extremely vulnerable. As such, patients are always desperately seeking the positive feedback that their disease is disappearing. While working with any therapist, the patient is inclined to ask questions about how to proceed with his or her healing process as well as questions about the nature of the illness. The training of many alternative therapies does not necessarily include knowledge about the physiological or psychological characteristics of a disease. Therefore, questions often arise that the therapist is unqualified to answer, but nevertheless, he or she may attempt to do so.

My own experience is filled with conversations with people who are facing major decisions, such as surgery or chemotherapy. I have come to realize that while these people are aware of the nature of my profession, that is, that I am giving them very specific counsel on how their emotions led to the development of an illness, the advice they are seeking frequently has to do with whether or not they should go through surgery. In their minds, they do not clearly differentiate between the advice they feel I am qualified to give and the advice that should come from a physician or other health professional. Always, at that point, I refer them either to their own physician or to Norm, even though I often have strong feelings as to how they should proceed.

While this may seem to be an argument in favor of all authority resting with the traditional medical community, *it is not*. Rather, this is an evaluation of the present climate that exists between the traditional medical community and the holistic field as a result of the gap in educational standards and the lack of appreciation for alternative practices and where they fit legitimately into the process of healing. On the other hand, in matters of the spirit, I am both trained and qualified to give advice that most physicians would not be qualified to give.

This existing situation, however, does represent an argument in favor of the need to merge the skills of both approaches to healing, because the reality is that many traditionally trained physicians are not necessarily qualified to respond to specific emotional, psychological or spiritual crises. Based upon the enormous numbers of people who are seeking therapeutic assistance, these skills are very much a reflection of the changing needs of our society in general.

EXPECTATIONS OF ALTERNATIVE THERAPIES

In addition to the educational gap that exists between the two fields, alternative therapies are questionable in general because their effectiveness is mistrusted in terms of contributing any measurable physiological assistance to the healing of a disease. The therapeutic approaches most often cited as examples are visualization, meditation, acupuncture, massage, color and polarity therapies, rebirthing and various forms of alternative counseling, such as bereavement counseling.

Part of the difficulty in proving that these technologies are valid has to do with a much larger issue, and that is proving that emotional, psychological and spiritual crises lie at the core of the breakdown of the physical body.

The other part of the difficulty of proving the effectiveness of these alternative technologies has to do with understanding what makes these technologies work. This issue brings us back to the major difference that exists between the paradigm of traditional medicine and the paradigm of the holistic approach as illustrated in the question: Does the mind (energy) influence the formation of the body (matter) or does it not?

Alternative therapies and technologies operate on the premise that through healing the mind, emotions and spirit, the body is healed. This does not mean that treatment of the body is ignored until such time as the rest of a person's reality is in order. It means that *simultaneously* with appropriately treating the body, a person must also heal that part of him or herself that drugs or surgery is not able to touch, such as traumatic emotional memories or negative attitudes.

The difficulty with the effectiveness of these technologies has more to do with not understanding how and why they work than with a limitation in terms of the quality of any of the therapeutic techniques themselves. The reason is this: people enter into the holistic field through two doors—curiosity or crisis. By far, however, the majority enter through the experience of a health crisis. They are people seeking every level of information possible on how to work with their health dilemma.

In turning to the holistic field for assistance, what needs to be appreciated is that a person is not just reaching for a new type of tool but rather an *entirely new way of thinking about reality itself.* In many cases, this amounts to learning the skills of relaxation, visualization and the disciplined use of the mind, not to mention much-needed information about nutrition and vitamins. To understand the depth of this challenge, we need to explore how and why alternative therapies work.

UNDERSTANDING THE HEART OF
ALTERNATIVE TECHNOLOGIES

For all of the many and varied approaches that are available to people within the field of holistic health, they all share three basic premises. First—the body breaks down in response to emotional, psychological and spiritual stress; second—in order to heal completely, these unresolved areas of stress need to be dealt with effectively; and third—the patient is responsible for his or her own healing process. It is this third perception, more than the other two, that determines the effectiveness of any of the alternative technologies.

The position that it is the patient who is responsible for his or her healing process challenges the very core of the traditional medical paradigm and, in particular, the doctor-patient relationship. In the traditional model, patients look to physicians to find a way of healing their illness. Because of the nature of this relationship, the patient becomes dependent upon the physician for the majority of the decisions central to the healing process. As a result, the element of choice—so necessary to human self-esteem and dignity—is frequently abdicated to such a degree that deep feelings of helplessness often develop in the patient.

Within the holistic model, the responsibility for the process of healing rests with the patient. Drugs cannot remove emotional pain and surgery cannot accomplish the removal of fear, guilt or resentments that might be raging within a person's being. This is work that the patient alone must do.

The alternative therapies available—from counseling to acupuncture to every level of body work, such as massage, to meditation and visualization—are all focused on assisting the patient in releasing the very stresses that are causing the destruction of the physical body. Therapists, practitioners and holistic physicians serve more in the capacity of facilitators for the healing process than as the person in charge. When a *comprehensive* integration of these therapies is offered, the approach to healing becomes truly *holistic*.

The success of any of the available holistic tools rests on two critical points: the patient's courage to evaluate honestly his or her life, and the patient's ability to make choices that authentically empower the inner "Self." The term "Self" refers to the core of one's inner resources. Many people identify this core as one's spirit.

This process of evaluation is stressful, in its own way, because it frequently brings a person face to face with the very aspects of life that he or she has been trying to avoid confronting. While the characteristic of denial is treated as a negative behavioral pattern within the traditional world, from the holistic perspective, denial is recognized as a serious blockage to the healing process because it allows the stresses that exist as the source of the illness to remain unresolved.

This level of inner work is very intense and, for that reason, it can be quite intimidating for many people. Because there is so little encouragement in our society to foster skills of introspection and self-examination, people do not know how to begin to "go to work on themselves." Moreover, they are unprepared for the nature of the process of inner work itself; that is, self-examination is a catalyst for change. Once a person begins to make a conscious evaluation of his or her life, it becomes no longer possible to hide or to deny what is not working. Regardless of what the cause of stress is in one's life, once the problem is unearthed, it demands attention. Attention means choice and choice means change.

Equally important to personal honesty is learning how to activate and empower the natural healing resources of the mind and the inner Self. This is what is meant by the phrase, "the body-mind-spirit connection." This is also the area that requires the most attention to re-educate because a person must learn to relate to their thoughts, emotions and imagination as power tools that have the force to rebuild the body.

For most people, the difficulty in accepting that thoughts, emotions and imagination actually have power presents the greatest stumbling block to working with the holistic paradigm. We are not accustomed to appreciating that "thoughts are things" that actually influence our physical realities.

This perspective—that we create our own realities through the power of our emotions, attitudes and beliefs—is only now appearing upon the general public's horizon, even though it has been an area of discussion in humanistic psychology for thirty years. Though this perspective is finding its way into the minds of people through every available avenue—quantum physics, holistic health and eastern philosophy, to name just a few—it is not enough for an idea to engage just the power of the mind. What releases the power of an idea is belief in that idea and not just intellectual understanding. The heart must work in agreement and in harmony with the mind, or a person cannot au-

thentically empower any of the work being done—particularly
if that work is healing. Getting the "heart" involved, then, is a
much deeper challenge than is attracting the mind.

Even under the best of circumstances, this shift in perspective is a tough one to manage because it challenges how we
have been conditioned to understand the relationship of energy
to matter or, more specifically in the area of health, the relationship of the mind to the body.

Learning to work with visualization, for instance, is a perfect illustration of the stumbling block that occurs frequently in
learning to work with energy and with the "thoughts are things"
reality. Though the following section is focused on the technology of visualization, the information presented can be applied to holistic therapies in general.

VISUALIZATION AND THE CHALLENGE OF
WORKING WITH THE MIND

Visualization is the discipline of using mental imagery (or energy) for a specific purpose, such as to rebuild a healthy physical
body. The premise of visualization is that the body responds to
what the mind tells it to do. The mind feeds information to the
body in words, in emotions and in images.

When people who are ill decide to work with a tool such
as visualization, the necessary foundation has to be put into
place carefully and thoroughly. First, individuals have to be
introduced to the concept behind the tool and "re-educated" to
think in terms of using their thoughts and emotions to rebuild
the body. It takes time and experience to learn to trust a new
method of doing something, and because time becomes a very
precious commodity in relation to disease, a competent instruc-
tor in the beginning stages is highly recommended and often
essential.

Secondly, people have to be totally reprogrammed *not* to
approach the use of visualization with the same attitude with
which they have always approached traditional medicine. This

means that people need to be alerted to the probability that they will assume that visualization works in the same way that a drug does, that is, automatically and without the need for conscious attention. A drug does the work for the patient. With visualization, the patient does the work.

Drugs also have a time factor, meaning that a patient can expect to feel the effects of a drug within a given period of time. It is extremely important to understand that the effects of visualization are not as readily obvious as are the effects of drug therapy, and that the factor of time is somewhat meaningless when applied to visualization. How well visualization "works" is dependent upon factors that vary from individual to individual. Not everyone is able to engage his or her mental and emotional skills with the same degree of clarity and focus. People are not identical in their aptitude to do inner work. Some are skilled at introspective processes while others may have deliberately avoided such internal activity all of their lives.

The intensity of what a person is confronting in terms of the type of illness as well as the underlying stresses involved are also significant variables. These differences are important to note, as each one contributes a major factor toward how successful visualization is to an individual's healing process.

Even for a healthy person, learning to work with a new skill that requires so much background understanding is a sizable challenge. For a person facing the dilemma of a serious disease, the task of learning an entirely new system of thinking and mental discipline becomes a mountain that may be almost too high to climb. The old ways of thinking and acting are not easily changed. Add to that the fact that many illnesses cause high pain and anxiety, and then imagine trying to learn something new in this vulnerable condition.

I worked with one man, for instance, who had developed stomach cancer. Dan wanted to work with visualization because it intellectually made sense to him. I shared with him the need to reprogram his thinking and challenge the old tendency to approach holistic techniques as if they worked in the same way as drugs. I also recommended that he work with visualizations that had been recorded on cassette tapes, because listening to someone guiding the activity of the mind helps to keep the mind focused more intently.

Dan responded with enthusiasm and immediately created a visualization program of exercises to be done for twenty minutes in the morning and twenty minutes in the evening.

Two weeks later, Dan came to see me. He pulled the cassette tapes out of his pocket and said, "These aren't working." At first, I thought he meant that the tape itself was broken. However, he quickly pointed out that he had diligently used the tape for two weeks and "it" (referring to the tape itself and not the act of visualization) had failed to heal the cancer.

I reminded Dan of our earlier conversation in which I explained that the tapes themselves did not have any "power" to heal anything. Tapes serve as tools to help strengthen one's own inner focus, because that is the part of oneself that does the healing.

This conversation left a very strong impression with me because, in spite of my repeated and careful explanation of visualization and the purpose of using cassette tapes to guide the mind, Dan wanted visualization to work just the way drugs work. Though he intellectually understood the principle of visualization, what became apparent in our discussion was that Dan's expectations (and therefore all of his emotional energy) were still invested in the traditional model of medical healing.

His situation also brought to light my understanding of the difficulty people have with appreciating the fact that the human mind *never stops visualizing*. Visualization, as a human skill, is not something new. We are constantly visualizing, from imagining how we want to dress, to imagining what we are going to say to someone, to imagining what might happen in all of our tomorrows.

What is new, however, is that we finally are beginning to

realize that *our thoughts influence physical reality*. We have been using our minds to create our realities for centuries, only we have not been in a position, either intellectually or spiritually, even to consider such a possibility.

The most overwhelming fact about visualization that needs careful explanation is that every thought and feeling that one has is an act of visualization. People with whom I have worked, such as Dan, may participate in visualization exercises every morning, afternoon and evening with total dedication, focusing on the mental model of a completely healthy body, and yet this does not seem to influence the course of the disease. Why?

In between those visualization exercises may be hours filled with fear and attention given to the disease. Focusing on the disease and worrying about whether or not it is spreading *is also a visualization*. For many people, their healing routine becomes one hour spent on positive visualization and twenty-three hours spent visualizing (through worry) the disease spreading throughout the body. Imaging the disease through worry promotes its strength in one's body. Imaging health creates health. One hour of positive mental imagining is simply not enough effort to undo the negative reinforcement of the condition of disease through twenty-three hours of hard-core, focused worry.

Before any substantial evaluations of the effectiveness of alternative technologies can be made, these educational concerns and realistic limitations need to be appreciated fully. People in pain do not make the best students, even with the most sincere of efforts.

Fair evaluation of skills, such as visualization, must wait until such time as these skills are taught within normal educational settings, not primarily as healing techniques but from the perspective that because we create our realities through the use of our minds and our beliefs, it is necessary to learn during childhood, or in situations free of the stress of disease, to pay attention to what and how we think. Eventually we will come to value the skill as the activity of "conscious creation." A skill

learned under normal educational circumstances stands a much
better chance of taking root than it does during the onset of a
serious illness.

The differences between traditional and holistic approaches
to healing mentioned in this chapter all represent significant
challenges to both areas: the gap in education, the softer healing
technologies of the holistic field and the appreciation of emotions
in relationship to disease. Beyond these obvious areas of concern
is an even more subtle, not so obvious current of change that
is invisibly present in all of the challenges facing modern medicine.

All of the different concepts and approaches within the
field of holistic health serve as very strong indications that we
human beings are undergoing fundamental changes at our core.
We are redefining our understanding of the nature of power
and, in particular, of our relationship to and command of power
as applied to the process of creation itself.

A SHIFT IN THE BALANCE OF POWER

What causes a change, such as the emergence of a second paradigm of health care, to occur within a society? Certainly, the
process of change in life is constant; yet, there is ordinary change
and then there is evolutionary change. Evolutionary change represents a shift in the thinking of the group mind of a society
that is so complete that the known social order is re-built.

The emergence of the holistic model of health is an evolutionary change. The rapid growth and development of the
holistic health field indicates that our needs are changing in
fundamental ways and that the model of traditional medicine
and health care cannot adequately meet these needs. Fundamental change means that movement is taking place at the very
core of human nature itself.

What is the nature of this evolutionary change now taking
place? A transformation is occurring in terms of how the concept
of "responsibility" is understood and then applied to every aspect of one's life, from relationships to personal needs to plan-

etary ecological problems to responding to another nation's hunger problems to taking responsibility for the quality of one's health.

The human being, in essence, is in the process of discovering self-responsibility and personal empowerment. These two newly emerging characteristics contain the necessary seeds for creating an entirely new global society. The reason is that self-responsibility and personal empowerment are potent internal mechanisms of change, signaling that a shift in awareness is occurring in terms of how individuals perceive the balance of power that exists between themselves and the outside world.

This shift in the balance of power is illustrated perfectly within the changing dynamics of the doctor-patient relationship. The strongest message of the holistic health movement is that physicians are *not* responsible for the quality of a patient's health, nor for how successfully a patient heals. A physician is only responsible for providing the best technology and treatment available in the traditional field, as well as the best counsel he or she is able to provide. But the *responsibility* for implementing the technologies that are available, as well as working to heal one's inner stresses, belongs rightfully to the *patient*.

As a result of this shift in power, the "patient's role" is changing radically. Rather than accepting without question the treatments and medication prescribed by the physician, patients are assuming a more central role in their own treatment program, beginning with wanting to know the full extent of their illness and the risks of drugs or surgery. In the traditional medical model, withholding serious or terminal diagnosis has been seen as—and sometimes still is—an acceptable practice. This is not an acceptable practice for any patient who desires to participate fully in his or her own recovery program, even if that program is the preparation for death.

Since what I am describing represents changes that are beginning to occur within patients and physicians involved in the healing process, it must be stated clearly that *not every patient is ready or able to accept what the holistic field has to offer*. Moreover, the premise that a patient has created his or her own disease through negative emotional, psychological or physical patterns can frequently contribute feelings of guilt, fear and defensiveness to the patient's general attitude. It is highly significant, therefore, that patients be afforded the choice to proceed with their healing process according to what suits their needs and capabilities as well as what they trust to work most effectively for them.

The advent of the holistic approach to healing offers options to patients in terms of how they can best proceed with their healing program, and these options are important to present to a patient. Patients facing cancer are no longer limited to receiving chemotherapy, radiation or surgery. The choice on how to proceed now includes several alternative options such as nutritional programs, the use of visualization and positive affirmations, and extensive counseling.

It is important to recognize that the many options for treatment of illnesses that now exist because of the expanding nature of traditional and holistic health care can generate a conflict for the patient who chooses to proceed with a path that is not in agreement with particular beliefs of that patient's family. In several instances, I have been a part of discussions in which a patient elects to follow a holistic approach, and this choice has resulted in the loss of support from his or her family members because of their lack of faith in alternative treatments. I also have been a part of the exact opposite situation in which a person who is part of a family unit that is supportive of only alternative methods chooses, nevertheless, to follow a more traditional course of treatment.

Ultimately, it is the patient who knows best what he or she can have faith in and, no matter what choices are made, it is of the utmost importance that family members and friends support those choices, regardless of personal preferences.

Certainly, this factor of choice on the part of the patient represents the empowerment of the patient and, as such, the disempowerment of the traditional medical approach to healing.

The traditional medical community is losing its strongly held position of authority as more and more patients recognize that their own life stresses have contributed to the creation of their illness. It is this shift in the balance of power that is ultimately the greatest threat to the traditional medical community.

THE LARGER QUESTION: WHO IS RESPONSIBLE FOR CREATION?

The action of reaching for choice and personal power within the framework of illness is symbolic of a process of human empowerment that extends well beyond the issues of health and disease. As patients begin to grapple with how their emotional and psychological life stresses affect the quality of health in their physical body, they come to realize, even if it is in small doses, that somehow they have a degree of power in terms of the process of creation itself.

Like a small string that has the power to unravel one's entire reality, the realization that one's own emotional currents have the force to influence one's body does not stop with the boundaries of the physical body. Little by little, the realization of the creative influence of emotions extends beyond the physical body and into a person's life environment, the quality of one's relationships, and the quality of one's living and working environment.

After all, where does one draw the line in terms of the question of creation? Can we allow ourselves to acknowledge that we possess the dominant creative influence in terms of the health of our physical body, but then deny that this same energy has any influence over the activity in the rest of our lives?

Ultimately, the tiny thread that is attached to the question of how much influence we have over the creation of health or disease in our bodies also is attached to the largest cosmological question we are capable of asking, and that is, "Who or what is responsible for creation? Is it us or random chance or a Universal Force?" Just as Copernicus's single realization that the earth revolves around the sun eventually unraveled the entire scientific and astronomical reality of its day, so also does the realization that we create our health represent a challenge to our concept of reality itself.

It is this question regarding the responsibility for creation that is emerging now into the collective mind of the human species. It is symbolically present in every global crisis, whether it be nuclear issues, acid rain or planetary hunger. These crises are generating the realization in thousands of people that we—each of us—share the responsibility for what is created in this world. If we do not want our lives to end in a nuclear holocaust, then we ourselves must be willing to do something on behalf of peace. Like the creation of one's health, peace will not come into being in our world without conscious attention and choices made by each and every one of us toward that goal.

The question of creation is also symbolically present in every personal crisis we experience. Whether we are in a difficult relationship situation or an unfulfilling occupation or in the midst of a financial crisis, ultimately what we are confronting in ourselves as we struggle with these difficulties is the challenge of not settling for less than what we need to make our lives healthy and fulfilling—which means learning to *create consciously* our realities.

We need to recognize, too, that while none of the major areas of human crisis has substantially changed throughout the centuries of life (i.e., relationships, disease, love, death, sex, money and power), the recognition of ourselves as holding the power of choice and of creation within our grasp indicates that perhaps we—as a species—are changing in deeply fundamental ways. It may not be an exaggeration, in fact, to consider the possibility that we may be stepping forward into a new cycle of human evolution itself.

THE AGE OF CO-CREATION

Once you notice something for the first time, then, it seems, you see it everywhere. The shift in the balance of power taking place in the world of traditional medicine is but one area of life in which the rebalancing of the dynamics of power is occurring. Like a grand cosmic blueprint replacing the former archetype of power, this new blueprint of "the empowered individual" is initiating dramatic changes that are reaching across the boundaries of nations, economics, politics and religion, and touching the lives of every person on this planet.

Whether one focuses on global-political occurrences, such as the recent movement for free expression in the Soviet Union, or global-spiritual occurrences, such as the massive movement away from traditional religion to a more personalized spirituality, or whether one focuses on life at the more personal level, such as the shifting roles of men and women in relationships, the core issue is the same: the renegotiation of the shifting balance of power in order that individuals can assume a greater degree of self-responsibility.

These two new currents of thought—that we create our own reality and that we are headed on a path toward becoming more empowered individuals—are occurring simultaneously in order that an entirely new paradigm of reality can be born upon this planet.

Given the highly critical situation that we face as a global community—specifically, the possibility of nuclear war, planetary destruction, depletion of all natural resources and the total destruction of the earth's ecological system—it is also possible that the natural intelligence of our species' survival mechanism is fostering an alternative and more highly evolved plan for living that is based upon the realization that we must assume more responsibility for the creation and maintenance of life itself.

This single notion—that we create our realities—is a truth that will inevitably cause us to rethink every one of our actions, both at the individual level and at the level of global interaction. We have entered a new cycle of life. In spite of the fact that we are being forced through this passageway via the route of personal and global crises, we are nonetheless heading toward a time in which we must learn to merge our energies as people and as nations in order to heal the impending disasters on this planet. The truth is that without the merger of our intelligence, resources and cooperation, none of us will survive the consequences that await us. The message of cooperation and co-creation is remarkably clear.

This book also carries the message of cooperation, co-creation and merger. The two paradigms of health that now co-exist in this world are here to stay. Holistic health is not a temporary fad. It represents an alternative lifestyle and system of reality that offers individuals self-empowering perceptions about how to take responsibility for the quality of their health and the quality of their lives. The holistic philosophy is essentially a path that teaches the principles of co-creation, first within your individual physical body, and then within and for the larger body of life on the planet itself. For ultimately, what is in one is indeed found in the whole.

This message is also true for the technological world of nuclear power. We must advance the wisdom of the heart into our technological decision-making bodies of knowledge lest we perish as a result of a war created out of the minds of humanity. The technology and knowledge of traditional medicine is also a part of us. It's in our bones, philosophically speaking. Yet, what is clear is that our technological knowledge must proceed forward with the assistance of the knowledge of the heart.

This new cycle of life that is emerging—this age of co-creation—is our hope for the future. May we proceed with wisdom and with openness, prepared to learn from all that we have to give to one another.

CHAPTER TWO

Toward Medicine of the Twenty-First Century

(Shealy)

Scientific principles became the major motivating moral, spiritual, intellectual and philosophical power of our country as a result of the technological demands of World War II. World War II initiated the social transformation not only of America but of the entire planet. Technology provided us with a quality of power that struck at the roots of our social fabric. Prior to World War II, most Americans lived within fifty to one hundred miles of their homes, their families, their social system, their churches and their communities. Until the early 1940s, 95% of all food was grown within fifty miles of the consumer; almost all food was grown using only natural fertilizers; and our soils were neither highly polluted and toxic, nor depleted in essential minerals.

As this emerging technological model gained in power, it put to rest the age-old battle between naturalists and the mechanists. Naturalists have always insisted that there is an ultimate limit to the creativity of human beings, that only God can create life, that there is a natural order, and that natural order has intelligence and spirit, divine direction and evolutionary purpose.

Mechanists, on the other hand, have maintained that human beings view the universe and life itself mechanically, believing that we can understand the function of every cell and every organ and ultimately replace those or create new ones. Within the strictures of the mechanical world view, the human being is a chemical, physical structure, chemically or physically manipulated, including the mind, emotions and spirit, with no input from the invisible realm.

Prior to the 1940s, physicians were naturalists and almost all physicians were generalists or general practitioners. They worked from the heart and soul because medicine had yet to become a science. Physicians were healers. They often worked with herbs, mustard plasters, the laying on of hands and counseling. Each physician knew the entire family and most of the social problems of that family. They were often the closest family friend and confidant.

As a result of the technological explosion of the 1940s, medicine was converted from an art of the heart to the technological power of the mind. Technology provided such a rapid expansion of knowledge that no one individual could learn all of the rapidly emerging facts. Thus, we entered the age of superspecialization and, within less than twenty years, a majority of physicians were no longer generalists but were specialists, treating not the whole patient and the family but only the individual diseased organ. In addition to shifting the balance of power between the naturalists and the mechanists, the quality and quantity of technological power that was unlocked as a result of World War II gave the technological world an authoritative lead over the religious and moral voice. Technology provided the scientific community, for the first time, sufficient authority to challenge social and moral limitations. With moral limitations no longer empowered, physicians and scientists were permitted to begin research—without restrictions—into genetics, and ultimately into the forces of creation itself. Moral issues and the belief in divine design had previously placed limits upon scientific exploration, challenging the power of science to proceed with genetic experimentation, for example.

During the last forty-five years, science has introduced into medicine antibiotics, tranquilizers, organ transplants, laser treatment, artificial ventilation for maintaining life in comatose patients, chemotherapy, effective radiation therapy for some types of cancer, and a remarkable variety of pharmaceutical agents for "treating" virtually every human symptom. As we look at the number of sophisticated therapeutic advances, it is easy to see how this type of power could challenge the unmeasurable, invisible power of the spirit.

In further assessing the remarkable medical accomplishments of the past forty years, we can expect that the next forty years will bring similar and extraordinary innovations such as:

- More sophisticated organ transplants and, perhaps, virtually total body transplants.
- More genetic experiments with attempts to prevent the manifestations of genetic defects.
- The creation of life in a test tube.
- More pharmaceutical controls for the treatment of disease.
- Chemical and other artificial means for increasing longevity but without necessarily increasing the quality of life.
- Creating new drugs in outer space, a technology we haven't even considered yet which is just beginning.

Can we afford to enter this next forty years with the same scientific preoccupation with power while ignoring the human dimension, the spiritual nature of human beings and of life itself? Before we accept unlimited technology, let us look at what has been ignored in the past forty years: feelings, intuition and spirit.

Is it possible to create a morality transcendent of religion, inclusive of science and embracing a reverence for life?

The most fundamental questions facing us as we proceed into the twenty-first century are: Does the human spirit exist and, if so, what is the nature of its power? What are the limits of its power? If it exists, how does the reality of that fact become a part of our technological, scientific world? Can science accommodate both morality and spirituality? Once science acknowledges the critical nature of the spiritual dimension and intuition as the foundation for scientific creativity, we can introduce the concept of the sacred into our world view.

Questions such as these are threatening to the scientific world because they imply that the scientific model does not have all the answers and that science is not the only system of research that is of value. Science has been riding a wave of authority that has not been effectively challenged in the last forty years. Questions such as these challenge the very foundations of the scientific balance of power. If, for example, science is willing to recognize the validity of the human spirit, it must begin to question its right to do genetic experimentation, abortions, euthanasia, organ transplants and artificial prolongation of life. The door is also open for discussions about the quality of life and the source of disease. Does the spirit affect physical and chemical health? What is the relationship between the human spirit and the physical form we call the body?

It is considerations such as these that are leading us to the potential creation of a new paradigm of health care and medicine, a paradigm that will take us well into the twenty-first century by combining technology, science and spirit, while humanizing the practice of medicine.

Little did I realize when I began neurosurgery that my studies of the brain would ultimately lead me to the spirit. In fact, when I entered my residency, I recognized fairly early that neurosurgeons were interested in the physical aspects of the brain but had paid very little attention to the mind itself. As I began to observe nonphysical influences upon health and disease, basic philosophical questions had to be asked, questions that I had not addressed since I was a teenager. What is the purpose of life? Is there a lesson to be learned from disease? If the mind can create a physical illness, such as a peptic ulcer, can it also reach outside its apparent physical boundaries and influence the environment around us? Traditionally, these questions have been primarily the province of philosophy and theology. In this century, they have also been examined by parapsychologists. It is considerations such as these, of mind and spirit, that eventually led me to rediscover an interest in the possibility of intuitive diagnosis.

In the 1970s, a small number of physicians began to question the morality of technology without spirit. We began to recognize that illness had an attitudinal and emotional component. Out of this complex social format, and recognition of the dehumanizing aspects of technology, has emerged holistic medicine.

These questions are so significant that they have also spawned the development of a new field of scientific research—psychoneuroimmunology, "interactions between the central nervous system and the immune system." Psychoneuroimmunology, one of the most exciting and innovative fields today, includes the study of the effect of attitudes, thoughts and social stress upon all aspects of the immune system and, ultimately, of health. In addition to the effects of attitudes upon the immune system, we are increasingly discovering neurochemical correlates of anger, hostility, guilt and depression.

The fundamental principles of holistic medicine—that emotional, psychological and spiritual stress affect the body—are gaining critical proof and validity. It is increasingly evident that holistic concepts are not a fad—that we are, as a society, undergoing another major transformation, rebalancing from forty years of unbridled technology without the spirit.

I grew up in this age of technological medicine and was educated at some of our most respected and prestigious scientific institutions—Duke University, Washington University, Harvard

University and Massachusetts General Hospital. My own background in scientific research includes over one hundred articles published in scientific journals. Even in undergraduate school, I was fascinated with the possibility of scientific research in parapsychology. While at Duke University, I was asked to investigate Dr. J. B. Rhine's work. He seemed, beyond any reasonable doubt, to have demonstrated the power of the mind to identify remote objects. It seemed to me that it should be applicable to medicine itself. It seemed natural to me that there would be an interconnection of mind, body and spirit.

However, when I entered medical school, such thoughts were dismissed by the scientific community and I became distracted with scientific inquiry. My interest in matters of the spirit was reawakened unexpectedly in 1970 when I made a trip to Colorado to look at horses. When the wife of the rancher opened the door, she and I felt an intuitive recognition of each other that sparked an immediate conversation, not about horses but about coincidence, serendipity and intuitive knowing. She provided me with two books that excited my curiosity. These were *Psychic Discoveries Behind the Iron Curtain* and *Breakthrough to Creativity*. I was particularly intrigued by Shaffiga Karagula's book, *Breakthrough to Creativity*, in which she discussed intuitive diagnosis and related techniques. Fortuitously, Paul Dudley White, President Eisenhower's physician and the grand cardiologist who brought us the idea of exercise to help prevent heart disease, provided the opportunity for me to explore my reawakened interest in the dimensions of the mind.

In January 1973, Janet Travell, President Kennedy's physician, in an interview in the *Wall Street Journal*, stated that the sudden interest of the American media in acupuncture was of less importance than the work of a young, midwestern neurosurgeon, C. Norman Shealy, who had discovered a "western form of acupuncture." Because of that interview, Dr. Paul Dudley White invited me to Boston to discuss my "western acupuncture." This actually referred to my work with transcutaneous electrical nerve stimulation, the application of electricity to the surface of the body for control of pain. One month after a personal interview with Dr. White, I was asked to replace him as a speaker at Stanford University at a symposium on acupuncture attended by twelve hundred physicians. At that meeting, I met Olga Worrall, America's most tested spiritual healer, Bill Tiller, Ph.D., a Stanford physicist who has explored scientifically the concepts of the human aura, and Bill McGarey, M.D., of the A.R.E. (Association for Research and Enlightenment) Clinic in Phoenix.

Dr. McGarey had already spent at least fifteen years applying the principles of Edgar Cayce (the famous "sleeping prophet") to clinical medicine. He suggested that my interest in a wide variety of healing techniques would be shared by another surgeon, Dr. Robert Brewer, who was planning a meeting at the A.R.E. in Virginia Beach that fall. Each of these individuals contributed to the development of my own attitude that disease is more than a physical-chemical reaction and that there is far more to life than what is physically obvious. Ultimately this allowed me to pursue my interest in intuitive diagnosis that had emerged in 1970. I was open to considering intuitive diagnosis as a potential legitimate tool, because most physicians arrive at a diagnosis through their use of intuition. Irvine Page, the great Cleveland Clinic physician, wrote a wonderful article on intuition and medical diagnosis in *Postgraduate Medicine*. He stated,

> Intuition in medicine is crucial . . . More than half of medical practice requires decisions which have little or no technologic basis. There are no absolute rights or wrongs; there are only decisions of the head and heart, of wisdom and compassion. The magic of medicine is disdained by us at our peril. No society has ever thrived for centuries without a transcendent belief in something greater than self. Each must choose and accept the responsibilities that accompany choice. The good physician is able to combine . . . intuition and common sense.

I am clearly not alone in my belief that intuition plays a crucial role in diagnosis.

My studies in intuitive diagnosis, which will be discussed later, opened me to explore a wide variety of other approaches to life and health including: biofeedback, autogenic training, nutrition, physical exercise, homeopathy, osteopathy, the use of visualization and meditation, the potential for music and sound therapy, past-life therapy, massage and even some herbs. Many of these techniques have been ignored or disparaged by traditional medicine.

Before we consider these components of holistic medicine, let us first discuss the allopathic (M.D.) concepts of disease and health.

ALLOPATHIC MEDICINE

Allopathic medicine, that is, medicine as it is commonly practiced by M.D.'s today, generally looks at disease as an externally induced problem, and therapy is often aimed at removing that external cause. In the concept of allopathic medicine, diseases are generally considered the result of:

Congenital genetic predisposition

Congenital (in utero injuries, i.e., German measles, smoking, alcohol or narcotic abuse, poor nutrition, etc.)

Trauma

Infection

Neoplasm

Degeneration

Circulation disorders

Hematological disorders

Emotions

Immunological disorders

Stress and psychosomatic contributions to illness are given rather short attention in the traditional medical model. Many physicians don't want to admit that 85% or more of all illness is psychosomatic, as I was taught in medical school; they tend to consider such patients "crocks." In the last few years, however, psychoneuroimmunology is increasingly demonstrating, from a very scientific point of view, that mood is perhaps the most critical factor in maintaining the integrity of the body, especially of the immune system. Depression essentially clobbers the ability of the immune system to be healthy. On the other hand, positive thinking and a cheerful outlook can go a long way toward helping us become, and remain, healthy. THINK RIGHT to *BE RIGHT*.

In discussing individual disease processes, allopathy increasingly considers multiple causes, including nutritional contributions, such as excess fat, inadequate fiber and excess salt. Medicine is also rapidly recognizing that both lack of physical exercise and having a driven, "Type A" personality contribute to illness. And, of course, cigarette smoking is acknowledged as the number one "measurable" cause of illness and death. Smokers average 1.8 times as much illness as non-smokers. They have a marked increase in incidence of cancer of the lung, bladder and cervix, as well as pneumonia, coronary artery disease (heart attacks), Alzheimer's disease, peptic ulcers, back pain and disc disease, influenza, emphysema and giving premature birth at a low birth weight. Also, it is now recognized that chemical pollution is a major contributor to illness, especially to cancer. Slow viruses are also being accepted as potential factors and have been strongly suspected, although not unequivocally proven, in cancer, leukemia, Alzheimer's disease and many of the so-called autoimmune disorders, or degenerative central nervous system diseases, such as amyotrophic lateral sclerosis and multiple sclerosis.

Allopathic, conventional or "traditional" medicine lacks a unified concept of health and disease but, in general, considers disease an *external* attack upon the body more than a failure of normal homeostasis (the relatively stable state of equilibrium). Allopathically, and in order of importance, the major causes of illness and death are:

Cigarette Smoking

Alcohol

Obesity

Excess consumption of fat, salt and sugar

Inadequate exercise

Failure to wear seat belts and/or to observe speed limits

Please note that all of these are the result of personal attitudes and choices.

But the nagging questions remain. Why doesn't *every* smoker develop heart disease, cancer or emphysema? Why doesn't *every* alcoholic die of cirrhosis or an accident? Why doesn't *every* obese person have cancer, heart trouble, diabetes or stroke? Why do some people die of hepatitis while others develop antibodies to the virus without ever being aware they've had the infection? Why doesn't *every* depressed person die of cancer or commit suicide? Why do some individuals survive unbelievably serious injuries with no apparent permanent damage, while others die or have various types and degrees of permanent malfunction from minor injuries?

PERSONALITY AND ILLNESS:
Dr. Caroline Thomas

Why, why, why? These questions are among the most serious and most important facing science today. A few scientists have investigated these problems. Perhaps the best work in this field has been done by Dr. Caroline Thomas of John Hopkins Medical School. Her prospective studies of medical students have shown a high correlation with personality. Relatively specific personality quirks or defects predispose one to high blood pressure, tuberculosis, heart attack, cancer or suicide. These traits are present twenty to thirty or more years *before* the onset of disease. It appears that our "life script," meaning our unconscious decisions regarding how our life will play itself out, provides a long-term attitudinal precursor of illness.

FREUD AND ERIC BERNE

Psychiatrists, although grudgingly accepted by allopathy, also have attempted answering the basic questions of mental causality.

Freud attracted a huge following with his victorian age, revolutionary theory that the cause of neurosis (psychosomatic illnesses) is a repressed Oedipal complex—a desire to have sex with the parent of the opposite sex. His inner circle of supporters began to break apart when he later decided that one of the most basic human drives is a desire to die. We all recognize that depressed individuals may want to die, or even to commit suicide, but a "death wish" in "normal" people?

Eric Berne, the great psychiatrist whose textbook for therapists, *Games People Play*, became a bestseller, reported that we not only play games but we have a "life script." He demonstrated that a majority of us decide at an early age both the age and cause of our death. Years before he died of a heart attack at age sixty, he told his friends that his life script called for him to die at age sixty of a heart attack. Elvis Presley's preoccupation with death when he reached the same age his mother was when she died may have contributed to his fulfilling such a script.

If we "choose" the cause of death, do we also "choose" illnesses? Or do we choose parents, personality, attitudes and/or lifestyles that predispose us to a specific illness? If it is true that we choose a lifescript, can we also choose to change it? And how late in the play can we reverse the process?

PREVENTIVE AND BEHAVIORAL MEDICINE

None of the allopathic discussion has approached the broader question of health itself. From a pragmatic point of view, health is most often defined as the absence of illness. But what *is* illness? Is it the presence of a *single* symptom of malfunction or of certain *clusters* of symptoms? Does it have to include *measurable* abnormalities of chemical, electrical or physical function?

Preventive medicine provided a first attempt to answer these questions. Preventive medicine, a recognized specialty for over forty years, still has only about three thousand practitioners. The techniques used are largely aimed at studying habits such as smoking, alcohol, obesity, nutrition and physical exercise. Nowhere in modern, mainline, allopathic medicine is either spiritual distress or basic mental attitude deemed a significant consideration. Science simply ignores these two factors that are basic and crucial to an understanding of health.

The major diseases in American society are heart attacks, stroke, cancer, accidents and infectious diseases. These account for the vast majority of deaths and illnesses. In general, there is no unified theory in allopathic medicine to explain why one individual will develop a given illness in a given society and another will not. Why, in an Orlon producing factory, where the incidence of cancer among workers is several times higher than it is in people not working in an Orlon factory, do certain individuals develop cancer while others, equally exposed to the same chemicals, do not?

In the asbestos industry, there is no question that scientific medicine has made an association between cigarette smoking and the exposure to asbestos in the development of lung cancer. The same is true of coal miners: those who smoke and are exposed to asbestos or coal dust have a much higher incidence of lung disease. But even then, there are some smokers who do not develop brown lung, emphysema or cancer. There obviously are many factors other than smoking cigarettes, or working in an asbestos factory, that have a great impact upon the development of disease. In other words, the physical factors seem to provide but one level of influence in a person's life. If cigarette smoking were *the* cause of lung cancer, then one would theorize that everyone who smokes will develop lung cancer without exception. In fact, a majority of smokers do not develop lung cancer, even though smokers are seventeen times as likely to develop lung cancer as are non-smokers, and the majority of people who do develop lung cancer are smokers. The point is that smoking is not the only cause of lung cancer. What are the unknowns that lead to lung cancer in one smoker while other individuals may live to be ninety years of age as cigarette smokers? These questions have not been addressed adequately by allopathic medicine because they imply that the missing factors are related to the subjective life of each individual and the unmeasurable area of emotions, mental attitudes and spiritual distress.

Although Preventive Medicine and Psychiatry are considered part of contemporary allopathic medicine, these two recognized specialties are not understood well by most physicians, and psychiatry is looked at with suspicion. In the last twenty-five years, another field, Behavioral Medicine, has emerged, spawned largely by psychologists who work with biofeedback training. The groundwork for behavioral theory was begun by Ivan Petrovich Pavlov, the Russian scientist who demonstrated that animals and people are "conditioned" to respond in a given way. For instance, if you electrically shock a dog at the same time that you give it meat, the dog quickly adapts to wagging its tail and salivating when shocked! B. F. Skinner gave behavioral concepts a cold and impersonal image with his idea of raising children in isolated boxes!

In the late 1960s, Dr. Elmer Green incorporated the self-hypnotic technique of autogenic training with feedback, visually and/or audibly, of changes taking place inside the body with mental images and words. Over twelve thousand scientific papers have been published in the field of self-regulation, reporting personal control of every function from blood pressure to pulse to pressure inside the eyes. Despite this information, the medical profession has largely ignored biofeedback and Behavioral Medicine, which is not a recognized specialty. And most medical insurance companies refuse to pay for behavioral therapy, even though it is often the most effective treatment possible. Although part of "contemporary" scientific research, all these well-thought-out attempts by traditional scientists are ignored. And none of them has addressed the question of the spirit. This lack of integration of spirit with all other aspects of health and disease along with the need for a unifying theory have led to the development of Holistic Medicine.

THE HOLISTIC PERSPECTIVE

From a holistic perspective, disease is generally considered the integrated result of all cosmic, environmental, chemical, electrical, mental, physical, emotional, attitudinal and spiritual stress. Thus, there is no single "cause." Similarly, any given cause may produce either no illness or any conceivable illness, depending upon the weakest spot in an individual's constitution.

Constitution, or *resistance* to disease, is the result of genes (heredity), maternal habits, nutrition and emotional stability combined with all post-birth environmental conditioning and exposure. Thus, all illness is the result of *all* stress with varying degrees of relevance. Theoretically, any individual could develop any illness under the right (or wrong!) total stress. Each disease would potentially involve all the possible causes listed earlier, plus many others.

Most often ignored in allopathic medicine is spiritual, attitudinal and emotional stress. The root of spiritual stress is the fear of loss of life, health, money, love or moral values. This fear leads to anger, guilt, depression and frustration or anxiety. Another way of defining spiritual stress is that it is a lack of conscious unity with all of creation. Spiritual deficits leading to illness are lack of forgiveness, tolerance, serenity, love, reason, wisdom, will, faith, hope, charity, courage, joy, motivation, confidence and compassion. Theoretically, *perfect* practice and expression of these attitudes should result in perfect health. While most individuals consider a perfect body essential for health, the fact is that that definition lacks consideration of the significance of a healthy attitude. Individuals should choose healthy habits and treat the body as the Holy Temple of the Soul. Cigarette smoking and most unhealthy habits represent defects at least in love, wisdom, reason and will. Health *begins*, from the holistic perspective, with a conscious determination to grow optimally in expressing these spiritual goals.

VALID CRITICISMS OF HOLISTIC MEDICINE

Without a doubt, the concepts of holistic medicine are valid and will form the basis for twenty-first century medicine. Some of the criticisms by traditional physicians are equally valid and worth discussing briefly.

There are two major areas that generate legitimate criticism: lack of legitimate training and lack of adequate research. Lay persons often accept enthusiastically individuals who refer to themselves as holistic health "practitioners" or "healers." These individuals lack the type of academic training that gives credibility to their work. Caroline mentioned this earlier, but I feel it is important to cite some additional concerns.

Not only is certification casual, but many of the techniques themselves have been overrated in terms of the contribution they make to physical healing.

First of all, holism is a philosophical concept, not a technique. It is inappropriate to consider massage or any other technique holistic!! In California, we first heard of holistic massage, which implies to me a massage parlor that massages the whole person.

Similarly, kinesiology and many herbal therapies cannot be considered holistic therapies. Rather, they are alternative therapies available within the holistic model.

Many of the therapies offered by non-credentialed or casually credentialed therapists have no clinical validation whatsoever. Often these techniques are based upon intuition without evaluation of their actual physical or physiological influence upon health. Intuition is often useful, but it should not be accepted without critical analysis. Although we recognize that healing of emotions and spirit is essential to the healing of physical disease, all too often enthusiasts claim that their techniques can produce a physical healing simply because patients temporarily report feeling better.

There are, of course, naturally gifted individuals, such as Olga and Ambrose Worrall, who have no formal "credentials" but who attain respect through the integrity and results of their work. This may appear to challenge our earlier statements, but the Worralls freely allowed scientists to test their abilities.

Holistic physicians most often use techniques that have centuries of acceptance in some cultures—such as acupuncture and homeopathy. More importantly, these physicians have a philosophy that embraces the patient's responsibility as a participant in the choice of therapy and in the healing process. Patients are encouraged to be responsible for their lifestyle, habits and wellness. Finally, they value the human spirit above all techniques. Any physician who denies the patient the right to choose or who pushes a given therapy is, by definition, not holistic.

The holistic "world" includes such unusual techniques as healing with pyramids, crystals, color and sound, to name a few. We need to emphasize that *people* empower these techniques. Crystals in and of themselves do not have the power to heal. Indeed, from the scientific perspective, objects or devices such as these are preposterous healing tools. Traditional medicine, however, could well benefit from recognizing the power of the mind and spirit to be channeled positively through the use of symbolic tools. Almost any object may be used as a mantric device to focus the patient's faith, hope, belief and attention. As Dr. Albert Schweitzer said, "It is more important for the doctor to know the patient who has the disease than to know the disease that has the patient."

Traditionalists and holistic practitioners have much to learn from one another. The holistic world view is not a fad; it marks a major turning point in the evolution of our understanding.

Ultimately we need to recognize the importance of empowering the human spirit.

Indeed, this unified concept is much more scientific, even though we do not yet have all the facts to support the interrelationships. Bringing in intuitive influence leads one to accept that there is a capacity to perceive electromagnetic influence of consciousness. That "energy" has to be considered along with data from the physical and chemical planes. We reported earlier the recognition of intuition by Irvin Page, a great allopathic physician.

Allopathic medicine stands to gain a great deal from expanding its definition and understanding of the disease state to include the fullness of human life in its diagnostic range of thinking. Actually, most psychological influences tend to be ignored and are still separated in allopathic thinking and teaching into an either/or phenomena. That is, it has to be *either* psychological *or* chemical/physical. The facts presented in the next chapter serve as an initial report of physical, measurable data that indicates that wider-ranging, intuitive diagnostic tools have to be considered in a most serious manner. A statistical reality is no less real because we do not understand the origins of the information.

In fact, *once science acknowledges adequately the crucial nature of intuition as the basis for invention and discovery*, it will become possible to include, in medical school, courses in development of intuitive skills. Physicians will benefit from the expansion of personal ability, and the quality of medical practice will take a quantum leap forward.

Although intuition has been emphasized in this chapter, a truly holistic perspective, as outlined later in quotes from Edgar Cayce, requires a broader, comprehensive attitude. As we move toward a medical paradigm for the twenty-first century, physicians and other health care professionals will work as teams. The days of the solo practitioner are passing, as is the extraordinary awe and blind faith accorded physicians. No one person can learn and integrate all the facts. A minimum team will consist of physician (M.D. or D.O.), nurse, physical therapist and psychotherapist, working with the patient to reach a consensus. Patients will be recognized as part of the healing team.

Manipulation of the spine (by D.O., D.C. or a specially trained physical therapist) will be an integral part of evolution and treatment, as well as massage. Acupuncture and various forms of electrical and electromagnetic therapy will be coupled with the use of music and sound to assist in balancing the electromagnetic energy system. Nutrition and a healthy lifestyle will be taught and exemplified by all the team members. Relaxation techniques will be essential components, as will a comprehensive exercise program, including aerobic exercise and hatha yoga. The concepts of naturopathy will become a standard part of medicine. Holistic health education will begin in kindergarten and continue throughout life, emphasizing physical exercise, nutrition and healthy habits and attitudes. Parents will attend special preparatory courses and embark upon the sacred path of parenthood with reverence and a combination of a healthy lifestyle and attitudinal awareness. Pragmatic reality will force patients to confront their stubborn, unhealthy attitudes. Society simply cannot afford to condone and support unhealthy behavior. Smoking and use of tobacco will vanish. Healthy nutrition will become more important than fast junk food. Exercise will become more important than watching TV.

The subtle energy benefits of homeopathy will be discovered to be of use especially in individuals who are choosing a healthy lifestyle. And I suspect that empirical research will ultimately reveal the power of crystals to *magnify* consciousness and balance subtle energy.

All team members will work to maximize their own intuition and to use that intuitive power to guide them and the patient in reaching a consensus on the plan to follow for each patient. They will use the talents of one or more qualified intuitives as needed. Techniques for certifying intuitive competency will be developed.

Spiritual healing will provide the conscious framework for all the related physical, chemical and behavioral approaches. Therapeutic touch and other forms of "laying on of hands" will be as accepted as aspirin. More importantly, the staff and patients will be working on their individual and collective spiritual transformation, accepting wisely and responsibly their power to choose healthy attitudes, knowing that a perfect expression of love is the ultimate healer. Drugs and surgery will remain as adjuncts, to be used as giant band-aids in acute situations, to tide patients over until they can develop the strength to enter consciously the path to their own spiritual transformation, to express fully the light of the Soul.

CHAPTER THREE

The Proof of the Pudding

(S h e a l y)

No one can claim infallibility; and physicians, even with remarkably elaborate and expensive diagnostic tests, are never 100% accurate. Part of the diagnostic dilemma is the basic question: what is wrong? There are several dozen organ systems, and the number of symptoms of dysfunction are limited to only about one hundred and sixty. A symptom is a feeling that something is wrong.

SYMPTOMATOLOGY

Physicians who understand symptomatology can make a diagnosis with 80% accuracy when they review the total list of current symptoms, plus past history and family history. Although there are less than two hundred symptoms, there are thousands of illnesses categorized by Western science. A 1950 *Textbook of Bacteriology* listed well over one hundred individual infectious agents capable of creating specific infectious illnesses. And remember, those don't include the additions in recent years, such as AIDS and Legionnaire's Disease.

There is at least an equal number of parasites that can create specific disease states. Add to that hundreds of drugs that create their own toxic problems and thousands of chemicals that can poison the body. Combine these with the *external* causes of diseases, such as smog or other environmental poisons. Then there are accidents and diseases of internal origins, such as inadequate digestion, malnutrition, vitamin deficiency, diseases of over or under excretion, over or under metabolism, congenital abnormalities, wear and tear and psychological maladjustment. You begin to have a picture of the complexity of the diagnostic dilemma. It's a miracle that any accurate diagnosis is ever made! Keep in mind that we have only about one hundred and sixty symptoms to alert the patient and physician that something is wrong. My average patient has forty-nine current symptoms. Obviously the same symptom occurs in many different diseases.

A SIMPLE HEADACHE . . .

Consider headache for a moment. This very common symptom may be the result of eye strain; meningitis (many different infectious agents); hemorrhage (from several dozen causes); toxicity (from hundreds of causes); increased intracranial pressure (from many types of tumor or an overdose of Vitamin A; a head injury with bleeding, a blood clot, failure to absorb fluid, excess production of fluid); vascular irritation (dilated blood vessels such as in migraine); or muscle tension—among others! Just knowing the symptoms is not an adequate basis on which to make a diagnosis. There are thousands of laboratory tests that physicians use to assist in making diagnoses, many of which involve analysis of blood or urine chemistry and include, as well, a wide variety of x-rays, special measurements, a thorough physical examination and various psychological tests.

Understanding the phenomenal breadth of illness and the variety of diagnostic tools available to physicians, I find even more startling the accuracy that Caroline and a few other talented intuitives have shown. Of course, most thinking physicians are aware that, ultimately, it is their own intuition that allows them to "guess" which tests to order to make a "suspected" diagnosis. As traditional medicine becomes more and more open to recognizing the effects of environmental, emotional and spiritual stresses on our health, our society may begin to realize the potential that a combined medical and intuitive perspective can offer.

CREATIVE GENIUS AND INTUITION

Creativity includes the broad realm of art, music, mathematics, science and inventions. These are the result of inspiration, intuition, premonition, insight, illumination or gifts from God or the Soul. Virtually every scientific discovery, every musical masterpiece, every great novel is "created" in a brief overview—often after poorly productive days or years of logical study or deductive reasoning.

The gifts to society of Brahms, Newton, Gauss, Einstein, Tesla, Goethe, Shelley, Keats, Bohr (structure of the atom), Thackeray, Wordsworth, Kipling, Longfellow, Schubert, Mozart, Wagner, Elias Howe (sewing machine), Robert Louis Stevenson, Otto Loewi (the duality of electrical and chemical aspects of nerve conduction), Tchaikovsky, Strauss, Puccini, Mendeleyev (the atomic table), Tartini (the modern violin bow), Beethoven and Kekule (the benzene ring) were all gifts from the "unconscious", "superconscious", "ever-conscious", intuitive spectrum of the mind. The inventor of hydraulic brakes and engines, holder of eighty-eight patents, made his discoveries in this same way. The founders of our country were intuitive visionaries, just as were the founders of every religion in history. Personal stories of sudden genius or inspiration abound.

Intuition is so *natural*, so ever-present, that it is accepted without question when it comes in the form of a symphony or a great painting; it is, however, often somewhat grudgingly acknowledged by non-intuitives when a great scientific invention or theory is the result of intuition. The list of examples of intuitive creativity is only the "tip of the iceberg." Very little of value has resulted exclusively from simple deductive reasoning. Logic and hard work are used to verify great insights, to polish and perfect musical or literary masterpieces. The inspiration that gave that illumination, often with the entire symphony or invention presented to the "originator" in a brief flash, is usually received in a dream, in a state of reverie or in a sudden insight while the conscious mind is engaged in some more mundane activity.

Almost every description of creative genius includes examples of errors or corrections made during later verification of the intuitively received image, words, numbers or musical notes. Thus it is not surprising that individuals with "pure" creative intuition would not be perfectly accurate. Even Einstein was not *always* right! Few artists can create constantly. Accuracy of intuition can be expected to follow a typical bell distribution curve. Geniuses are often genius only in one narrow area; Brahms was not a genius in the broader field of physics, even though music involves principles of physics. Intuition, then, can be expected to follow the same principle. Some individuals are aware of an "insight" occasionally; others are flooded with a steady stream of consciousness such as Thomas Wolfe in his book *Look Homeward, Angel*. Still others can tune in and intuit the medical diagnosis of a complicated patient. Exceptionally accurate physical diagnosticians are on one end of the bell curve; students who flunk Physical Diagnosis are on the opposite end of this curve.

Throughout history there are examples of uneducated geniuses, great mathematicians who "knew" complicated math and who discovered new principles, and great musical composers who had no training. Edgar Cayce is perhaps the best known of these. Olga Worrall, whose primary work was spiritual healing, was an outstanding diagnostician. She would often "intuit" that a person in a distant room was a smoker and then name the specific problem. Henry Rucker first confirmed my belief in intuitive diagnosis. Robert Leichtman, M.D., internist and superb intuitive diagnostician, and Henry proved to me that these talents could be highly accurate and practical. And, of course, John Elliotson, M.D., and James Esdaile, M.D. both reported almost one hundred and fifty years ago that some mesmerized individuals "became" intuitive diagnosticians.

Caroline Myss, a theologian, writer and publisher, "happens" to be on that most accurate part of the intuitive diagnosis curve. Though without medical training, she is much more intuitively accurate than I am. Hers is a talent that is *usually* available at any time. Occasionally it falters; her talent can be exhausted fairly easily. Just as Edgar Cayce was able to do justice only to a limited number of "readings," Caroline, during a single session, begins to err after eight to ten back-to-back patient presentations. At times she needs to allow the problem to incubate overnight, to access her higher resources more slowly and deliberately. Just as a great musician or writer cannot *always* compose on the spot, a great intuitive is still first and foremost a living human being, not a machine. Within this framework, intuitive diagnosis is presented as one manifestation of creative genius.

THE HISTORY OF INTUITIVE DIAGNOSIS

The use of intuitive diagnosis is probably as old as medicine, and it almost certainly goes back to the days of Hippocrates. Many famous physicians throughout the history of the world seem to have been involved in things that today we would call parapsychology, and many of them were probably outstanding intuitives. Paracelsus is one example of such an individual; Franz Anton Mesmer, who some two hundred years ago laid the foundations of psychiatry and psychology, is another. To my knowledge, however, the first formal study of intuitive diagnosis occurred about one hundred and thirty years ago when a British physician, John Elliotson, began to work with mesmerism.

Dr. Elliotson had introduced to England the stethoscope, the use of narcotics and a variety of other medical techniques. He was the leading internist in London and a professor of medicine at University Hospital, University College, London. But suddenly he became bored with what was going on in medicine and got involved in mesmerism. Although most hypnotists believed that mesmerism was "just hypnosis," the technique of mesmerism was quite different. Introduced by Franz Anton Mesmer, mesmerism requires the therapist to make silent "passes" of the hands over the patient's body for fifteen to one hundred and eighty minutes. Patients can safely become totally entranced and anesthetized in this way. Elliotson then learned that patients who were mesmerized could properly diagnose difficult medical cases. He would accompany one of his mesmerized patients through the wards and have them diagnose patients whose illnesses had confounded the faculty. He even staged public demonstrations with Charles Dickens and William Thackeray. (Thackeray later dedicated one of his books to Elliotson, who in the book is called Dr. Goodenough.)

As anyone acquainted with the history of medicine might expect, Elliotson's innovative ideas were not well received among his conservative colleagues. They finally suggested that if he wished to continue to practice medicine, he should give up that mesmerism nonsense. His reaction was: "Gentlemen, I resign." He then went into private practice and continued to practice mesmerism, demonstrating, among other things, that mesmerized patients could be successfully operated on, apparently without feeling any pain. Elliotson, because of his tilting at the windmill of traditional medicine, is not well known today, and no serious scientific study of intuitive diagnosis has been done since that time. Esdaile, another British physician who practiced mesmerism, published a book on the subject of mesmeric-induced intuition in 1850. His work was also ignored.

MODERN SCIENCE STUDIES
INTUITIVE DIAGNOSIS

As I mentioned earlier, thanks to Dr. Paul Dudley White, who asked me to speak at a meeting of the Academy of Parapsychology and Medicine at Stanford in 1972, I came into contact with individuals who eventually led me to meet my first known intuitive, the Reverend Henry Rucker of Chicago. I was so intrigued by Henry's analysis of me, whom he had never met before, that I invited him and his colleagues to come to La Crosse, Wisconsin so that I might see how good they would be at doing intuitive diagnosis. Henry and seven other intuitives proved to be remarkably accurate. Each individual saw the patient but was not allowed to ask questions or discuss the case with anyone. Each wrote his or her diagnostic impression on a separate piece of paper presented to me. In eleven of seventeen patients, all eight intuitives were in agreement, and in all seventeen patients, at least two intuitives gave the correct medical diagnosis. For three patients who were paralyzed, they correctly gave the cause of the paralysis.

These results led me to seek a research grant to study intuitive diagnosis. I obtained $50,000 from one of the Fortune 500 companies which has asked to remain anonymous.

In 1973, this formal research project was carried out with fifty-four different questions. Each patient to be studied was known to me, had been examined by me and had taken an elaborate personality test, the Minnesota Multi-Phasic Personality Inventory. A color Polaroid photograph of each patient was taken by my research assistant, and the patient's name and birthdate were written on the back of the photograph. Standard handwriting samples were obtained from each patient, and palm prints were taken.

Intuitives were supplied with the photographs, names and birthdates of each patient. A numerologist used only the patient's name and birthdate. The graphologist was given the handwriting sample, and the palmist evaluated the palm prints. Each sensitive was asked to fill out the same questionnaire, having had no other contact with the patient.

The control measure consisted of my filling out the same questionnaire to serve as the "correct" answer sheet. In addition, random choices were made by two psychology students who filled out questionnaires. A professor of psychology, with no known intuitive ability, did his own "guessing" of the answers, using the patients' photographs.

Unfortunately, I could not be certain of a number of the answers on the personality test, and so the master sheet had to be shortened. We settled on retaining two categories of questions: (1) Where does the patient have difficulty or pain? and (2) What is the major and primary cause of the patient's illness? In answering these questions, the sensitives showed a significant rate of accuracy as determined by computerized evaluation of the various answer sheets.

Seventy-eight patients were "diagnosed" by at least ten intuitives. In two hundred other patients, one or two intuitives evaluated the patient. Two of the intuitives were 74% accurate and a third was 70% accurate in locating the site of the pain. A numerologist was 60% accurate, an astrologer 35%, and the palmist and graphologist 25%—not much better than chance. In determining the cause of the pain, the intuitives ranged from 65% accuracy down to 30%. There was only a 10% probability of obtaining the correct diagnosis by chance.

In a separate study of personality, one outstanding intuitive, Dr. Robert Leichtman, an internist and one of the most talented intuitives in the country today, was 96% accurate in giving very lengthy and elaborate descriptions of the patients' personalities. He used only photographs, the patients' names and birthdates to do his intuitive interpretation.

These statistics show that intuitive diagnosis not only is possible but can be highly successful. The real question is where it fits into the scheme of healing and medicine today.

Although we physicians are generally about 80% accurate in our primary diagnostic attempts, we are frustrated in determining the *exact* diagnoses for a variety of illnesses. Furthermore, many of the diagnostic tests carry a significant risk of damage to the patient. In instances such as these, it seems most obvious that the opinion of two or three talented intuitives could help us avoid risky diagnostic tests and help both physician and patient rest more comfortably in the knowledge that everything reasonable has been done to make the proper diagnosis.

We mentioned earlier the work with intuitive diagnosis

done by Elliotson and Esdaile in the nineteenth century. The most famous intuitive diagnostician of all time lived in this century. It might be said that the work of Edgar Cayce has laid the groundwork for all intuitive diagnosticians to follow.

EDGAR CAYCE

Edgar Cayce suggested in *The Edgar Cayce Encyclopedia of Healing*, by Reba and Karp, that causes of disease included poor assimilation, poor elimination, inadequate diet, improper acid-alkaline balance, spinal subluxation and other spinal abnormalities, imbalance-incoordination of the nervous system, imbalance-incoordination of the circulatory system, glandular malfunction, stress, over-taxation and over-exertion, karma, attitude and infection. Certainly a number of these were not considered primarily psychological, psychosomatic or attitudinal.

Cayce considered each individual "entity" as a being consisting of body, mind, and spirit or soul. In many metaphysical discussions, he used spirit and soul interchangeably, and he frequently called the body the "temple of the Living God." He held that the body and mind come into being for the purpose of manifesting the soul in the realm of materiality. According to Cayce's concepts, until the complete entity "achieves full attunement with God, the principle of karma operates." Cayce firmly believed the biblical statement that "for whatsoever a man soweth, that shall he reap."

Edgar Cayce gave extensive readings on the effects of attitudes and emotions and stated, for instance, that anger creates headaches or indigestion, depression results in weariness, emotional turbulence triggers asthmatic conditions and so on. He said "no one can hate his neighbor and not have stomach or liver trouble" and "one cannot be jealous and allow anger of same and not have upset digestion or heart disorder." He emphasized that anger, resentment, hate, self-condemnation, animosity and related attitudinal problems release poisons from the glandular system, deplete body energy, block elimination and generally predispose people to disease. Frequently describing emotions as "electronics" that act as vibratory communication among body, mind and soul, Cayce stated that "any illness involves all three aspects of an entity in a meeting of self."

Even a cold requires mental and emotional change and spiritual lessons to be learned, according to Cayce; a cold could come from becoming angry or "chewing someone out." He often emphasized the interrelationship of various stress factors in creating illness. For instance, in the common cold, he mentioned that a poor diet in combination with over-exertion leads to fatigue; that negative attitudes and emotions further deplete total energy; that acid-alkaline balance becomes disturbed; and that the body becomes over-acid and a cold results. Similarly, more serious complications such as pneumonia could result if the general weakening is bad enough.

DR. ROBERT LEICHTMAN

Dr. Robert Leichtman, the M.D. internist mentioned earlier and the only other intuitive diagnostician I have met who is as accurate as Caroline, has emphasized that "to appreciate the nature of health, we must start with an understanding of the nature of consciousness, not with an awareness of how the physical body feels . . . It is in consciousness, not sensation, that health begins." He believes the human personality is composed of body, mind and emotions but that even these three are not "the source of our life and vitality." He emphasizes that the consciousness behind body, mind and emotions is a "center of life essence that created the three vehicles of the personality, animates them, and maintains the health according to its own ideals, plans and purposes. This life center can be called the soul, the inner being, the higher self, the superconscious or the human spirit." Leichtman looks upon the soul as "pure consciousness" and feels that the soul "cannot be healthy—it is the origin of health" and contains "all the ideal patterns of health for mind, emotions and body." The purpose of the body, according to Leichtman, is to express the light of the soul.

Ill health, then, is a condition in which the soul is blocked by the personality—body, mind and emotions. Individuals who become overly content and complacent, who lack motivation to search deeper than the superficial, those who fail to recognize and invite the soul to participate in their life and those who do not make constructive contributions to life become unhealthy. The physical body that is able to work to help others and to "bear witness to the reality of the soul" must be considered healthy even if there are minor or serious defects. Leichtman states that "if the individual is able to transcend these defects and carry on, the body is healthy." An individual who is "lazy, unproductive and lethargic is not physically healthy."

With regard to emotions, the healthy purpose of the soul is "to provide a vehicle for expressing benevolent and compassionate ideals for qualities of life . . . The measure of emotional health, therefore, is the capacity to act with good will." As stated in his book, *The Way to Health*, Leichtman feels that

> as long as the emotions are basically free of selfishness, harmfulness, and malcontent, and are used to inspire others, help others, and treat others kindly, they can be considered healthy . . . The purpose of the mind is to be a channel through which the soul can condense its wisdom and intent, thus enlighten the life of the personality. The measure of the health of the mind, consequently, is the clarity of thought. Whenever there is confusion, misunderstanding of the guidance of the soul, immature thinking, or distortion of ideals, the health of the mind is poor.

A disciplined mind, "responsive to inspiration of the soul, stable and aware of its connections and purposes, is basically healthy."

Ultimately, it is a commitment to purity and inner morality that creates health. Healthy individuals have a "strong sense of integrity, ethics and morality, and place these values above personal desires and wishes. The measure of spiritual health, then, is integrity."

DR. EDWARD BACH

Edward Bach, a British physician who lived earlier in this century and was a superb metaphysician, stated in his wonderful little booklet, *Heal Thyself*, that "the real primary diseases of man are such defects as pride, cruelty, hate, self-love, ignorance, instability and greed; and each of these, if considered, will be found to be adverse to Unity." He felt that these were the real diseases. Pride he considered to be a "lack of recognition of the smallness of personality and its utter dependence upon the Soul." As another example, he considered cruelty "a denial of unity of others and a failure to understand that any action adverse to another is in opposition to the whole." The following are Bach's thoughts on a few of these primary diseases:

> Hate is the opposite of love, the reverse of the law of creation.
>
> Self-love is a denial of unity and the duty we owe to our brother man by putting the interests of ourselves before the good of humanity and the care and protection of those immediately around us.
>
> Ignorance is the failure to learn, the refusal to see truth when the opportunity is offered.
>
> Instability, indecision and weakness of purpose result when the personality refuses to be ruled by the Higher Self, and leads us to betray others through our weakness.
>
> Greed leads to a desire for power. It is a denial of the freedom and individuality of every soul.

Bach felt that each illness, then, was "the result of the primary defect: pride leading to rigidity and stiffness of the body; pain being the result of cruelty to others; hatred leading to loneliness, violent uncontrollable temper, mental nerve storms, and condition of hysteria." Excessive narcissistic self-love led to "neuroses, neurasthenia, and similar conditions" and ignorance led "to short sightedness, impairment of vision and hearing." Instability of the mind led to the same quality in the body by creating disorders of movement and coordination. Greed finally led to the individual becoming "a slave to his own body."

The part of the body affected was no accident, according to Bach. Diseases of the heart occur when there is a lack of love toward humanity; an affected hand denotes failure or wrong-doing in action; brain disorders indicate lack of control in the personality, etc. He concluded that "there is nothing of the na-ture of accident as regards disease . . . Disease in general is due to some basic error in our constitution." By errors of constitution, Bach meant defects in attitude.

TORKOM SARAYDARIAN

Torkom Saraydarian, in his *Irritation, The Destructive Fire*, states that "there are many causes of disease, but there is a cause which is not sufficiently emphasized, explained and publicized—this cause is irritation." He lists some of the causes of irritation, which include hatred; stress of temper; a sense of being abused, deceived or exploited; thoughts of revenge; complaining; self-interest; self-sufficiency; self-satisfaction; criticism; gossip; quar-reling; ingratitude; demanding; forcing; intolerance; an inferi-ority complex; impatience and hurry; conscious distortion of facts; noise; agitation through watching criminal behavior; dis-asters or crimes; excessive sexual activity; hallucinogenic drugs; acid rock music, etc.

All of these, according to Saraydarian, create a poison that he calls "imperil . . . which slowly descends upon our nervous system as we burn our etheric and astral bodies through irri-tation; it cuts off channels of electricity which flow through the network of our nervous system." This then leads to illness throughout the body. He feels that irritation and imperil "do not attack those whose consciousness is focused within their heart and head" because loving understanding can dissolve it. Imperil creates "a blockage of life electricity on the network of the mechanism; malfunctioning of centers and glands found in the mental, astral, etheric and physical bodies; overgrowth of cells to acquire energy; starvation of cells and degeneration of the body."

On the mental plane, imperil creates "insanity, negativity, the urge for crime, depression, suicidal drives, and separatism." Saraydarian believes that imperil blocks the ability of the soul to radiate "beauty, love and light." To protect ourselves from imperil, there are many different approaches, including roses, freesias, wormwood oil or tea, barley, musk, joy, love, appreciation, recognition of divinity in others, self-sacrifice, self-forgetfulness, harmlessness, psychic energy, conversation about the Divinity, prayer, heavy labor, periodic change of residence, contentment, happiness, good nourishment, proper sleep and complete rest, orderliness, patience, humility, sleeping under the stars, spiritual living, "expressing the virtues of the soul, of divine ideas and beauty in our daily life, compassion, detachment from negativity, hostility and destructive attitudes and behavior."

FIRSTHAND RESEARCH
WITH INTUITIVE DIAGNOSIS:
Caroline Myss

In April 1985, I met Caroline Myss. I was very impressed with her well-educated and intelligent approach and asked her to assist me in clinical problems. Since that time, and prior to the beginning of the work on this book, I have spent many hours talking with Caroline, both in person and by phone. She has done readings for me on several hundred patients. Her accuracy and insight have been truly awesome. Looking back, and feeling that we had not done an adequate evaluation or report on that intuitive work in the early seventies, I asked Caroline if she would be interested in doing a book with me in which we would first demonstrate her accuracy in making diagnoses, give her readings on the root cause of these specific illnesses and then look at the root causes of a variety of illnesses in general. The result is this book, *The Creation of Health*.

RESEARCH WITH CAROLINE MYSS

When I began the research project with Caroline, I did not resort to a formal questionnaire such as that used in the earlier-mentioned research project. I was more interested in seeing just what she could do from a straightforward, clinical point of view. In most circumstances, the patient was present in my office while I talked with Caroline by phone. Initially I would just give her a patient's name and birthdate, and Caroline would then start telling me her impressions. Most of these had to do with the patient's personality conflicts. As our partnership evolved, I began to ask her to be as specific as she could about the physical abnormalities and, eventually, she began intuitively "entering" the patient's body and speaking as if she were the patient. I encouraged her to go through the patient's body in a systematic way, examining the relative health of each organ system. She was remarkably accurate.

Just how good is Caroline as an intuitive diagnostician? In this section, we shall present data which indicates that she is 93% accurate. Whatever your expectations may be, 93% is a fantastic accomplishment. In order to protect patient confidentiality, we have not given actual names, birthdates or other identifying data.

Caroline was told only the patient's name and birthdate. For convenience here, we will present a simple chart indicating patient number, Caroline's diagnosis and mine.

Patient #	Caroline's Diagnosis	C.N. Shealy's Medical Diagnosis
1.	Schizophrenia; homo-sexual	Schizophrenic (I can't confirm homosexuality but *very* disturbed sexually.)
2.	Migraine headache, myofascial pain	Migraine headache, myofascial pain

3.	Depression, sexual problems	Depression; sexual neurosis
4.	Venereal herpes	Venereal herpes
5.	Alzheimer's syndrome	Alzheimer's syndrome
6.	Rheumatoid arthritis	Rheumatoid arthritis
7.	Connective tissue weak; chronic pain	Mixed collagen (connective tissue) disease; chronic pain
8.	Stroke	Cancer of breast
9.	Severe spinal pain; stress; weight 249	Severe spinal pain due to arachnoiditis (post-surgical scar); stress; weight 250 lbs.
10.	Depression	Migraine headaches (certainly depressed also)
11.	Ruptured disc	Ruptured disc
12.	Depression; sexual abuse	Depression; sexual abuse
13.	Inflamed spine	Rheumatoid spondylitis (inflammatory spinal arthritis)
14.	TMJ syndrome, headaches	TMJ syndrome, headaches
15.	Severe low back pain; homosexual	Ruptured spinal disc, lumbar; homosexual
16.	Generalized nerve weakness; leukemia	Polyneuropathy (severe nerve damage); probable cancer—not found but strongly suspected by three physicians

17.	Back pain after accident	Post-surgical back pain (earlier accident)
18.	Stroke; abdominal pain	Stroke; abdominal pain, unknown cause
19.	Bone marrow hollow— ribs brittle	Severe osteoporosis (brittle bones!)
20.	Depression; low back pain	Depression; low back pain
21.	Pain after disc surgery	Post-surgical (disc) back pain
22.	Severe psychological fear	Worker's Comp neurosis (same thing as Caroline!)
23.	Intestinal area in trauma; severe psychological distress	Abdominal pain, severe anxiety and depression
24.	Much spinal pain; pelvis malaligned; much fear	Generalized spinal pain; severe anxiety (anxiety is due to fear)
25.	Generalized pain; severe fright	Generalized pain; severe anxiety
26.	Cancer of pancreas	Cluster headaches
27.	Worker's Comp injury; back pain	Chronic low back pain; Worker's Comp injury
28.	Much spine pain; depression	Generalized spinal pain; depression
29.	Severe fear; painful scarred spine	Severe anxiety; post-surgical back pain
30.	Very low energy; poor digestive absorption	Severe neurasthenia; spastic colon

31.	Left testicle malignant, spread to left kidney	Cancer of left testicle, metastasis to left kidney
32.	Nerve degeneration	Polyneuropathy (nerve degeneration)
33.	Chest pain, due to trauma	Post-surgical chest pain, left
34.	Spinal pain; much fear; huge corpulence	Post-surgical back pain; agitation; obesity
35.	Accident and upper back pain	Post-traumatic thoracic (upper back) pain
36.	Neck pain; much damage there	Post-surgical neck pain
37.	Much energy missing from pelvis—anemic; unresolved guilt over abortion	Vaginal bleeding, unknown cause; 2 previous abortions
38.	Cancer, spread into lymph system	Cancer of breast with metastases
39.	Sexual dysfunction; post hysterectomy	Rectal/vaginal pain; post hysterectomy
40.	Severe exhaustion	Neurasthenia (severe exhaustion)
41.	Problem with umbilical area; weak intestinal tract	Post-surgical abdominal pain (congenital atresia of bile duct—umbilical area)
42.	Malignancy of brain	Metastatic brain cancer
43.	Huge body; much weakness	Obesity; polyneuropathy

44.	Body from neck down in trauma; close to bowel cancer in etheric body	Post-traumatic back pain, 4 months later developed cancer of the colon
45.	Migraine; maladjusted homosexual; depression	Much back pain; maladjusted homosexual; depression
46.	Spine like a tube of sludge	Rheumatoid spondylitis
47.	High anxiety; much fear	Severe anxiety
48.	Back pain; anxiety	Post-surgical back pain; anxiety
49.	Wasting of brain	Alzheimer's (Note that earlier Caroline had used the term Alzheimer's)
50.	Electrical storms in brain	Epilepsy (same as an electrical storm)

I have not seen anyone more accurate than Caroline, not even a physician!

MORE PROOF: PSYCHOLOGICAL DIAGNOSES

There is no clear-cut method for diagnosing psychological hang-ups so I can't present a similar body of data related to psychological problems. I can, however, share with you some of the notes I've taken while working with Caroline. These notes represent the highlights of much longer commentaries. In the following descriptions, I have used a first name, but not the patient's actual first name, primarily to indicate that these are real people and to specify the sex of the individual. There is no detail here that could possibly reveal the identity of the particular patient. Most of these readings were done by phone conversations between Caroline and me; the patient was sitting in my office and, as before, Caroline was given the patient's full name and birthdate but no other information.

CHARLOTTE—"She has a useful vibration. Did she tell you she is sexually inadequate in relations with her husband? She feels her husband is not attracted to her. There is no energy in that area. There is stress up the spine and into the neck. She has had this problem for many years and she has no good sense of self in her sexual area. I think her husband has had affairs and she knows it. There is a sense of unfaithfulness. I also question whether she has had an affair with a younger man. There is much energy residual there."

Interestingly, this woman's husband had become impotent because of the problems between them, and everything that Caroline states is correct. They have since divorced.

JANE—"Did you check her for TMJ syndrome? Her jaw is so tight. She sleeps that way, as if in an alarm reaction. She has a rigid smile because it hurts. She has a fear of inadequacy despite many accomplishments. There is much tension in her abdomen and this is because of her feeling of inadequate power. Her female energy level is low. She is out of balance and reaching for what she needs there. She also has pain in her right hip. Treat her temporomandibular joint and teach her about issues of personal power which are contributing to her problem."

Again, it is difficult to put this sort of discussion into clinical perspective but the accuracy is absolutely uncanny.

BOB—"This is a choice. No one else can put the pieces together. He stopped taking responsibility for his life and his need is self-responsibility. He has a fairly healthy body and is allowing it to deteriorate because he doesn't want to fight for his life. There is a lot of child energy about him. Tell him to stop thinking and start doing. He needs to focus on someone else. He needs to focus outside his own dung heap of self-pity. He indulges in junk foods such as sugar and he basically has an addict personality. Monitor his diet. He needs to understand and hear emotionally. He can block anything."

Again, this is an absolute direct "hit."

LILLIAN—"Her crisis is a fear of inability to protect herself at her job, personally or in her environment. Her heart is in a state of alarm. She has never learned to communicate. Tell her that her problem is hysteria and the greatest problem that she has now is her fear."

My diagnosis was that this lady had hysteria or a conversion reaction.

PHYLLIS—"Her strongest area of dysfunction is an enormous problem in the emotional quadrant. Despite the fact that she is fifty-two years old, she feels more like a frightened, insecure child. She needs emotional therapy. She can talk a good line intellectually and she can rationally respond, but her emotions really control her. She has tried to control them and has let her left brain be the dominant factor. She may say that her heartache no longer bothers her but her psyche tells us otherwise. She had much rejection starting in her late teens or early twenties. Her back and spine are not working well. The structure is limping along. Her hands—the knuckles look swollen. There is a lot of nervous energy there. Her intestinal area is in trauma. I think she may have had some kind of bleeding from her esophagus or stomach, perhaps an ulcer. Her marriage is where her emotional problem began. She started denying her unmet needs when she was first married."

In this particular lady the biggest problem was her feeling of total dissatisfaction with her marriage relationship.

DICK—"He feels like a macho man, very strong, but he has the fear level of a sixteen-year-old revolving around issues of responsibility. His life lesson is to learn the nature of power, to transcend the physical and get beyond that. He lives totally and fully out of his second chakra and he can't handle all of that. It is throwing him into a need. His only power, up to this point, has been sex. What he is missing is the power of the heart. How well does he communicate? He has no action in his upper chakras. He must get out of his second chakra or he will become unable to enjoy even sex. He won't understand what you are talking about. He needs to get a vaster overview of life, to think about meaning and purpose. He needs to develop discipline, to expand his notion of power and responsibility and to be more humanistic. You and I cannot move him. All you are witnessing is a soul fighting its contract. The fact that he is in your office is a good kick in his astral butt. Just tell him there is more than he has been willing to consider."

Again, a remarkably accurate analysis.

CHARLES—"I sense stiffness and fright. He feels like concrete. There are vast chords of fear in him. His major problems are responsibility and power and feelings of inadequacy. I suspect he has either pain at the base of the spinal cord or sexual impotentia. There is severe dysfunction in his abdomen. It feels in trauma. There are many obstructions to energy in his colon and stomach. Has he had rectal bleeding? At the top of the stomach there is a very bad disturbance, but all of this revolves around issues of power and responsibility. He is not grounded to life. Age seventeen to nineteen was a crisis time in his life. He has the archetype of an orphan. Recommend past-life therapy to him. Nothing in his life will help him connect otherwise. He feels like a lost little boy. The core is in his family roots. He can't nurture his body without establishing roots. He can be in therapy all of his life unless he reestablishes those spiritual roots. Connection with his father is important. Ask him what happened before age seven. Nurturing was absent. I'll bet he wasn't breast fed. I'll bet he was a problem child and was threatened with being sent away. He had much fear of that."

Again, this reading was so accurate that it has helped the patient to begin moving in a proper direction.

ROBERT—"The first thing I notice is hernias. There is much blood in his second chakra. There has been trauma to his abdomen, sex-genital area. He has a very high pain quality. I'll step into his body now. 'I have a lot of melancholy feelings. My energy is pessimistic. My relations are not working. I have lost my power. It is bleeding out of me. My chest hurts. I smoke a lot. I have experienced many weight gains or losses but I am very overweight. I have spinal stress like cysts along my spine. I have suffered from many stress headaches. I tend to drink but I have cut it down in the last two years. My hair is thinning. There are large pores on my skin. I have some skin lesions. I feel very heavy around my heart. I have pain and numbness in my left arm. My liver is not functioning well. I have no hope or reason to live. My thyroid is thick and I have trouble with emotions.' He'll tell you,' Don't talk to me about this.' He has varicose veins and sciatica. He feels stabbed in the back. His biggest problem is his inability to reconcile his feelings of obligations to his children and to life. He feels that he has been negligent."

Again, this was an extremely accurate reading. This man had even had a gastric stapling to help him lose some of his gross obesity.

JOANN—"She has a powerful psyche but not under control. She has metaphysical extremes, exaggerated and depleted of energy. There is much physical pain. She must have had a great deal of trauma at about age thirty-three. Her entire physical structure feels painful. The major site of her dysfunction is in the pelvis. Her pelvis and lower spine are misaligned. There is great dysfunction of energy there. I'll bet she is unable to function sexually. Her chakras are blocked. She is frightened, insecure, has a great fear of lack of power and security. She doesn't feel safe in any way. She feels greatly overburdened. She must deal with the issues of her first chakra. Her excess weight is a form of protectionism. When she had to take on responsibility, she began to overeat to compensate. The shifting of power between her and her husband started her current problem. No one can correct her pain problem unless she deals with these issues. She must become conscious of the level of resentment and the fears which occur and still are there."

If you had known this woman, you would be as awed as I was by the accuracy of those highlights.

Actually, I have known a number of brilliant individuals including, for instance, one man who holds over eighty patents in the hydraulic field (such as hydraulic brakes and hydraulic steering for modern automobiles, trucks, airplanes and farm machinery). It is quite obvious that almost all of the information that led him to develop these highly technical, scientific, physical principles came to him intuitively. The same is true of virtually every successful physician and business person. Intuition is such a critical part of humanity that we take it for granted.

In an outstanding reference to intuition, a German physician named R. Gross reported, "There is no sharp dividing line between health and disease; they merge into each other." In relation to diagnosis, he emphasizes that ultimately all diagnosis is based upon intuition that "combines sensory perceptions with associations, mental impulses, hardly definable presentiments and feelings." Gross comments that inadequate use of intuition leads to "numerical medicine and enormous waste of effort." Finally, he mentioned that the number of "diseases" recognized in 1956 was thirty thousand, with this number expected to double within ten years. The flexibility of mind required to scan such a list is easily recognized. As he stated, although "our brains operate in accordance with the rules of logic—we arrive at several diagnoses with different grades of probability." Ultimately intuition leads us to the choice of a specific diagnosis, and "experience shows that technical progress has never improved the quality of human relationship." Thus, although computers may offer us technical assistance in evaluating the numerous possible diagnoses, intuition will remain the most valued tool of competent physicians.

As we proceed through the rest of this book, there will be an opportunity for us to present other examples of Caroline's insights into specific aspects of personality and how these relate to specific illnesses, but I can only conclude this brief analysis of Caroline's level of accuracy by stating that any physician who, at the conclusion of an initial history and physical exam, is as accurate as Caroline is with just a name and birthdate, would be one of the most revered diagnosticians of all time!

CHAPTER FOUR

Intuitive Diagnosis and the Human Energy System

(M y s s)

WHAT IS INTUITIVE DIAGNOSIS? ·

The most frequently asked questions that I hear are, "What is intuitive diagnosis?", "How do you do a 'reading'?", "What do you perceive when you do a 'reading'?" and "What does it 'feel' like?"

These are logical questions, to be sure; yet each time they are asked, I struggle for an answer and not because the answer is complicated. Rather, the assumption most people make is that using intuitive skills causes a reaction in your body that is equal to reaching for a live electrical wire while knee deep in water. People want "intuition" to be electric, dramatic, magical or mysterious. They want to believe that there are certain experiences of power well beyond the ordinary that are available to "mere mortals," or that the "power" is connected to the supernatural. Either way, I always disappoint them when I reply that intuitive skills are none of these things.

In describing what it feels like to use intuitive skills, I ask them to remember what their living room looks like. Frequently, people close their eyes for two seconds and then signal that they have a complete picture of their living room in their "mind's eye." Then I ask them, "What does it 'feel' like to remember your living room?" This is the point at which the struggle to communicate the answer to this question begins.

Intuition does not 'feel' like anything physical. It does 'feel' like a dream or a memory in the sense that intuitive sensations are very delicate and, as with a dream, the slightest external disturbance can turn the dream or the intuitive impression into a fog.

Intuition is your emotional apparatus upgraded to a perceptual skill. We sense our emotions, as a rule, in response to something. We emotionally respond to everything in our world: relationships, weather, news and job stress. Rarely, if ever, do we project our emotions ahead of us into a situation with the clear intention of receiving information about that situation. To the rational mind, the idea of projecting emotions ahead of our physical body into a situation other than the one we are physically in is preposterous.

Now, imagine this scenario. You meet someone at a dinner party and immediately both of you experience a strong attraction for each other. You agree to meet the next evening for dinner. That night and all through the following day, your mind and emotions are projecting ahead of your physical body. You are imagining what the person might wear, what you will talk about and how he or she will respond to you. Even though this is called daydreaming or fantasizing, are we really describing two different intuitive activities? Fantasies are, in fact, extensions of feelings that are generated by certain experiences, and based upon those feelings, we create our projections. Because we use the word "fantasy" or "daydream," we avoid any arguments from our rational mind.

The fact is that most people take their fantasies and daydreaming activities far more seriously than they may be comfortable admitting; after all, isn't the experience of unfulfilled expectations actually the experience of unfulfilled emotional projections? You project and hope and visualize that the situation will turn out a certain way, and when these mental/emotional images are not physically met, you are disappointed. Your very real "projections" failed to materialize.

Intuitive diagnosis is using emotional energy, only in a more highly directed manner. Rather than the random and seemingly uncontrollable manner in which emotional responses continually pour into us, intuitive diagnosis relies upon the ability to harness this emotional energy in such a way that it works as a vehicle for gathering information.

In doing a diagnostic reading, I project emotional energy toward a patient. I do this by concentrating on the patient's name and age. The emotional responses that I then receive contain data about that patient's emotional, psychological and spiritual stress. This information is my indicator as to what physical dysfunctions exist in the patient's body.

Accuracy is critical in doing intuitive diagnosis. When I first met Norm at a conference in the spring of 1985, his initial question to me was, "How accurate are you? I don't need anyone telling me a person's 'energy' is in distress. I can see that myself. I need you to be able to see what I cannot see." I told him that I did not know how accurate I was since I only had been involved with intuitive diagnostic work for three years at that point, and then only intermittently. I had begun to meet with people in private counseling sessions in 1983 and had focused primarily on helping them work through emotional stress. Though I often received intuitive information on the health of their physical bodies, I mainly limited my advice to emotional issues.

Norm wanted information on physical problems and so I agreed to try.

Two very significant factors came into play at that point in my life and in my work. The first was Norm. Inasmuch as my background lacked formal training in any medical discipline, I did not have the slightest idea of how the physiology of the human body works.

I felt tremendously anxious about proceeding with this work because I lacked any amount of self-confidence and I never wanted to work with people who were ill. I was trained as a journalist and had started to work in the field of publishing books. Until I met Norm, I considered this part of my life as a type of curiosity that I could participate in at my leisure. I hardly considered it a "profession." Moreover, because the nature of this skill is associated with "psychic" abilities, I was extremely concerned about the associations of fraud and "crackpot" that go with the territory.

Norm never tested me from the position of wanting me to prove to him that this skill existed. He already knew it was possible to develop exceptional perceptual abilities, and thus his interest in my work was from the position of whether or not I could be accurate enough for his purposes. His attitude was his first gift to me. His second was his tremendous patience in slowly but constantly working with me to develop my capacity to "see" inside the human body. Because he never made me feel as though I had failed if I could not complete a reading thoroughly enough, or even if I missed the presence of a disease, I always retained the desire to try again.

The other factor that increased my accuracy in working with Norm was due to the physical reality of our living twelve hundred miles apart. The system we use is this: Norm telephones me while the patient he wants me to do a reading on is sitting in his office. Unlike working with a person seated opposite you in an office, this system allows for a totally impersonal connection. I never physically meet his patients. The impersonal nature of this connection permits me to receive information that a more personal connection would otherwise tend to block, because it is too difficult for me to look someone in the eyes and tell them, for example, "Yes, your cancer is spreading." When I did do personal counseling sessions, strong emotional feelings would often develop between the client and me. By the end of an hour-long counseling session, I found that I became susceptible to the fears and hopes in that person and thus I could no longer offer "clear" information.

Since beginning this work in 1983, I have developed a system of interpreting the underlying significance of emotional, psychological and spiritual stresses. While I am still learning, and no doubt will always be learning, I have come to recognize certain consistent patterns in the human design that are a part of all of us.

Specifically, we all need to love and to be loved. When love is missing from our lives, our health diminishes. We all need to have something that gives our lives meaning. Without meaning, our health slowly, but most certainly, evaporates. We all hurt over the same issues, we all have fears that lessen the quality of our lives and we all have pain, regrets and grief that we are trying to heal. And we all have to work on developing our self-esteem and feeling good about who we are. We are, in spite of all of our efforts to be different, remarkably alike.

What makes us unique is a combination of physical makeup, personality traits, life experiences, talent and intelligence, cultural backgrounds and so on.

What makes us ill, however, is identical. A strong dose of negativity or fear will contaminate any human being regardless of nationality, social background, education, wealth or talent. Poison is poison, no matter who imbibes.

In teaching this material on intuitive diagnosis, I emphasize two points prior to introducing the information on the Human Energy System.

The first is that I consider myself and my work with Norm to be always "in progress." Our research continues with each patient that we see and with each workshop that we give. There is no such thing as a school of thought (including traditional medicine) that does not inherently contain exceptions and contradictions. We still remain mysteries to ourselves, and there is much we have yet to learn about "reality" and the cosmos that will, no doubt, fill in the gaps of our learning.

As such, I encourage students to study this material realizing that the findings Norm and I are presenting should be viewed as a beginning contribution rather than a final product. We have years of work ahead of us, and we have our own mysteries to follow in this work. Nothing would give me greater pleasure than to present a complete system that explains down to the last detail the relationship of our emotions to physical illness. Such is not the case.

This material represents our first steps toward finding a deeper understanding of how each individual participates in the process of creation—in particular, the creation of health or disease. We have found certain emotional and psychological patterns of stress to be consistent in people who become ill. Moreover, we are realizing that these patterns of stress are not "general." Our evidence indicates that specific diseases are intimately connected to specific types of emotional and psychological stress. Because we have only begun to research this part of the human experience, the material presented in this book should be understood as part of the foundation of this study upon which others, including Norm and me, will continue to build.

The second point I emphasize with students is the definition of the word "negativity." This is a word I use frequently in describing the quality of emotions that is associated with disease. Negativity refers to emotions that are destructive, such as hatred, rage or fear.

Negativity is not used as a description of the quality of character of any of the people in this book, and this is a point worth emphasizing again and again. Deeply ingrained in many of us is the belief that illness is a punishment. We cling to this because we would also like to believe that good people are somehow protected from bad things, such as illness. It is tremendously difficult for us to let go of this association because illness does cause suffering, pain and grief.

The reality is, however, that understanding why people become ill is not a study in crime and punishment, no matter how much we would prefer to look at it that way in order to make sense out of suffering and death. Why we become ill is much more complex than an act of punishment, and illustrating that point is part of the basis of this book.

THE HUMAN ENERGY SYSTEM

Much of my personal experience in working with intuitive diagnosis corresponds to the teachings of the Eastern spiritual traditions in terms of understanding the human body. This is not so surprising considering that the Eastern traditions emphasize the human being as a system of energy and the Christian tradition emphasizes humanity's experience in the physical world. I mention this comparison, not because I am personally associated with any Eastern spiritual tradition, but because the Eastern tradition speaks of the "energy" of the human being, and their language includes terms that are specific to what I need to describe.

Of particular value from the East is the description that we are a combination of mental, emotional, psychological and spiritual currents of energy that come together to form the physical body, and that our bodies have energy centers called "chakras." The term "chakra" is the Hindu word used to refer to each of the seven major energy centers in the human body. Each of the seven centers, located at sequential points along the spine, is responsible for maintaining the health of specific organs and bodily functions. As illustrated on the opposite page, these centers correspond to major nerve centers.

Energy is continually flowing into our bodies through the top of our heads and, as it travels down the spine, the energy "feeds" each of the chakra centers. The mechanism of physically breathing is the counterpart to this "nonphysical breath," which

The Flow of Energy Through the Body

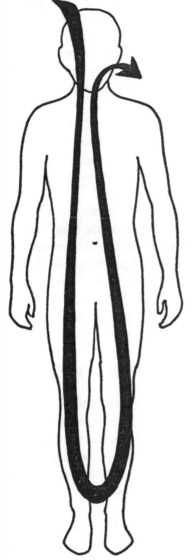

Energy comes into the body through the top of the head, circulating through the body, and is released through exhaling.

is called in the Eastern traditions "prana," meaning "life force."

The flow of these currents of energy is regulated through our bodies by our beliefs and attitudes, which create all of our fear patterns, our concepts of reality, our understanding of God and the Universe, our memories, and all of the information that we have stored in our brains through the experiences we have had and through our various channels of upbringing and education.

In doing an intuitive diagnostic workup, I begin with an analysis of the person's entire energy system. Starting at the top of the head, I sense the "quality" of energy at each of the chakra centers. By quality, I am referring to the vibration of energy that is being transmitted from each center.

As a reference point for what I am describing, think of the difference between the feelings you would sense from a person who loves you and the feelings you would sense from someone who is angry with you. No words would need to be exchanged since the quality of the vibrations being transmitted by both individuals would easily be understood at an intuitive level.

As I sense the quality of energy throughout a person's body, I look for "hot spots" or areas in which the vibration is noticeably different than it should be normally. These hot spots indicate the presence of bodily dysfunction and the exact nature of the illness.

Identifying the physical presence of an illness, however, is only the first step in this process. Equally important, or perhaps even more significant, is helping a person to understand how and why an illness has developed. This is the complex part of an intuitive reading because it involves identifying a person's emotional, psychological and spiritual stresses.

POSITIVE STRESS VERSUS NEGATIVE STRESS

"Stress" is a small word that covers a vast amount of emotional, psychological and spiritual territory. It is important to be clear about exactly what is meant by the use of the word "stress."

First, not everything that is stressful is destructive. Some forms of stress can be very positive, such as the stress that motivates people to perfect their work.

The type of stress that breaks down the body, however, is "negative stress." Yet what qualifies as "negative stress" is totally subjective and, as such, varies from person to person. Pain tolerance, people tolerance and situation tolerance is experienced in very different ways. Some people can handle a great deal of stress, while others respond immediately to stress overload.

Fear and emotional traumas are major contributors to the creation of stress. There is, however, no limitation to the number of fears or emotional traumas that a person can have.

In doing an intuitive reading, it is not necessary to identify every stressful experience a person has had, nor is it necessary to unearth every fear within a person's unconscious mind. The critical factors that I look for are those stresses that are the most *intense* in a person's life.

By intense, I am referring to patterns of stress that may be either conscious or unconscious and that exert *control* over an individual. In other words, when a fear becomes an obsession, a person is, in effect, controlled by it. When anger becomes someone's motivating force, then anger is controlling the person. The loss of emotional or psychological control creates the type of internal conflict in a person's mind and body that allows illness to develop.

The chakra energy system is a natural organizer of human stress in that each chakra center responds to specific human life issues. If a "hot spot" is noticed around the base of someone's spine, this indicates that the underlying emotional and psychological stresses are directly related to the life issues associated with the first chakra.

There is a wonderful, natural logic or body intelligence that is in evidence as one studies the flow of the chakra system. In learning about the life issues that are associated with each chakra, one can begin to understand what stresses are likely to disrupt specific areas of the body because every stress is "site" specific. The stress that accompanies the fear of failure, in other words, will not cause trauma to one's throat or one's ankle. The fear of failure directly relates to the issues of the third chakra and, therefore, the stress that accompanies this fear will directly affect the stomach, upper intestine, pancreas, liver or spleen.

We are not carelessly designed creatures. Everything about us has purpose, logic and intelligence built into it, including how and why we become ill. The emotional, psychological and spiritual stresses present in our minds travel, like oxygen, to every part of our bodies. When stress settles in a particular area of the body, it is because that part of the body corresponds to the type of stress we are experiencing.

LIFE ISSUES AND THE CHAKRAS

From my perspective, the life issues that are present in the chakra centers correspond to our natural process of maturing as human beings. That is, the first chakra relates to primary matters of life, namely, physical safety and security. The second chakra also corresponds to issues in the physical world, but from the viewpoint of more personal physical matters, such as finances. The quality of our health, therefore, is influenced by how we respond to the process of maturing that is reflected in each of these centers of energy.

It is important to realize that though each chakra center will be discussed separately, each is a vital part of a whole system of energy called the human body. The vocabulary necessary to teach this material creates the impression that each chakra operates somehow independently of the whole system, and that is inaccurate. Far better to consider that the chakra system is like a relay game with seven players constantly receiving identical information and responding to that information according to their individual skill.

The chart on the opposite page illustrates in general terms what specific issues relate to each of the seven energy centers. Beneath the chart is a more thorough explanation of the life issues as well as the major patterns of negativity and fear as-

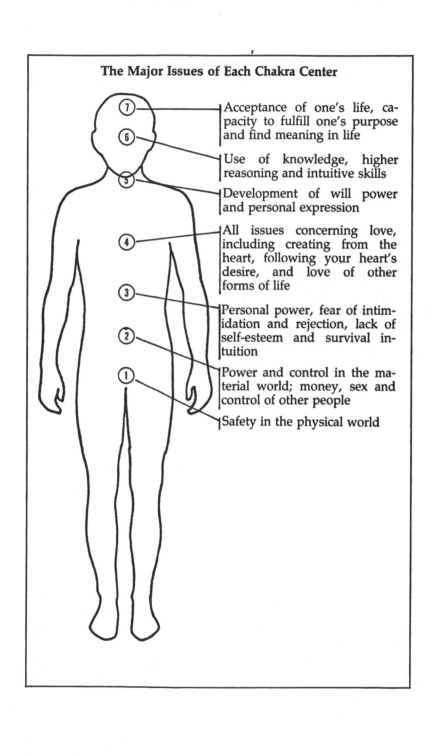

The Major Issues of Each Chakra Center

7 — Acceptance of one's life, capacity to fulfill one's purpose and find meaning in life

6 — Use of knowledge, higher reasoning and intuitive skills

5 — Development of will power and personal expression

4 — All issues concerning love, including creating from the heart, following your heart's desire, and love of other forms of life

3 — Personal power, fear of intimidation and rejection, lack of self-esteem and survival intuition

2 — Power and control in the material world; money, sex and control of other people

1 — Safety in the physical world

sociated with each energy center that are most frequently experienced. I have also included a brief listing of the diseases that
are most likely to develop in each area of the body as a result
of an abundance of negativity in these energy centers. By com-
paring the two chakra charts, you can begin to develop a sense
of the connection between specific issues of stress and how they
relate to each area of the body.

In teaching this system, I refer to each chakra as a bank
account that requires investments to be made on a regular basis.
Investments are made in the form of "wisdom chips." "Wisdom
chips" represent the acquired learning derived from one's life
experiences.

If these investments are made on a regular basis, then we
have wisdom to draw on during the moments of crisis that occur
within each of our lives. We have reference points, in other
words, within our personal realm of experience that let us know
we will make it through each crisis.

If we lack an ample supply of wisdom chips, then the
energy we withdraw comes directly from the basic energy level
we need to run our physical bodies, thereby depleting our physical energy system. This is the mechanism through which the
physical body becomes weakened.

THE FIRST CHAKRA

This energy center corresponds to issues of safety and groundedness in the physical world. Safety and groundedness refer to
how secure a person feels in the world at large. For some people,
the world is not a "safe place". They feel overwhelmed at the
prospect of providing the essentials of life for themselves, such
as a home and a means of income. The first chakra is located at
the base of the spine. Its energy primarily affects the health of
your legs and overall strength to support your physical body,
as well as the hip joints and base of your spine and overlaps
into the pelvic area of your body.

Mythical heroes such as Hercules illustrate what it means
to have full dominion over the physical world: Hercules is un-

defeatable in terms of the forces present in the external world. We associate him with remarkable physical stamina and mental cleverness at being able to maneuver the physical elements of life in such a way that they serve his needs rather than dominate him. Indeed, this quality of dominion over the physical elements of life is what makes Hercules a hero, and this aptitude is primarily first chakra energy.

Another characteristic of the first chakra relates to how well a person can "materialize" his or her dreams. That is the meaning of "groundedness"—the ability to bring an idea or desire from the mental stage into the physical world. This process of bringing our ideas into physical form is directly connected to the process of feeling safe and secure in the physical world. It is through this process that we "lay down roots" for ourselves and earn feelings of belonging, because what we bring forth onto the earth we must nurture. This requires commitment and consistency and these are characteristics that are essential to emotional and physical health.

The first investment of wisdom chips begins with infancy in having our primary physical needs for safety met as babies. Without this foundation strongly in place, the maturation process cannot proceed in a healthy and balanced way. The insecurities that result from feeling unsafe in one's physical environment become the controlling influence in the next stages of personal development, like unfinished business that will not rest until it is brought to completion.

As we grow through the normal stages of development, we continually renew our relationship with this primary issue of safety. The requirements for safety as we mature through our lives change with each stage: childhood, adolescence, adulthood and old age. Each stage holds challenges with the physical world that we are meant to complete. Becoming a competent adult is a process that is built through these challenges. The wisdom acquired in adolescence becomes the reference point for adult challenges. If there is not wisdom to draw upon—in other words, a depleted bank account—then the individual is likely

to fill in the gaps of his or her development with fear and insecurities.

The specific patterns of fear and insecurity that correspond
to the first chakra center of the human body relate to the issue
of physical safety. The most common are the following:

- The fear of not being able to provide the necessities of
  Life for oneself or one's family.
- The feeling that the external world is a threatening
  place and that you are unable to stand up for yourself
  or protect yourself. (This does not refer just to physical
  protection; it includes the fear and vulnerability that accompany human rights violations or the reality of
  being in a situation with no legal rights whatsoever.).
- The insecurity of feeling that no place is home, that
  you do not "belong" anywhere.
- The fear that comes from not being able to trust that
  you can materialize your goals.
- The feeling that you are totally on your own, unsup-
  ported by anyone and completely alone in this world.

Remember, the essential factor in the development of disease is
the *intensity* of the fear. While many people share some variation
of these fears, a person becomes physically vulnerable when any
of the fears exerts *control* over a person's emotional and psychological health.

Some of the more common dysfunctions that can be created
as a result of these fear patterns are chronic lower back pain,
sciatica, varicose veins, rectal difficulties, tumors and cancerous
outbreaks located in these areas of the body.

THE SECOND CHAKRA

This energy center, your second chakra bank account, relates to
issues of power in the external world—specifically, financial and
sexual power as well as power in relationship dynamics and
personal power in terms of business and social interactions. It

is located in the genital region of the body. The physical organs of the body that are primarily nourished by the energy of this chakra are your sexual organs, lower intestine, lower vertebrae, pelvis, appendix and bladder.

In continuing our pattern of following the developmental process, the second stage of child development is the "what's mine" stage. This is second chakra energy at work within a child's consciousness. As the child continues through the developmental stages into adulthood, the challenges of working through the "what's mine" stage become the challenges of learning to relate in a healthy and balanced manner to the material world.

The most important wisdom chips that a child needs to acquire for this chakra are those of sharing, of learning to relate with respect to other people and learning self-worth without self-worth being totally associated with material objects. When self-worth becomes attached to external objects, such as money or power, a person's self-worth is then determined solely by how much material gain is acquired. The absence of money, therefore, equals an absence of self-worth.

In adulthood, the lack of self-worth lies at the root of imbalances in all forms of relationships that exist within the material world. This includes our relationships to money, power (social, political, economic and sexual) and issues of dominance and control in personal and professional relationships. Obsessiveness in these areas is an imbalance indicating that one is compensating for the absence of self-worth.

The patterns of fear and insecurity that are associated with second chakra development are the following:

- The feeling that you have no power in terms of what happens to you sexually. This includes the experience of being used or abused sexually as well as the experience of being in particularly manipulative and controlling relationships.
- Feeling inadequate sexually, or having a dislike for sexual activity. This includes the stress that accompanies

feelings of resentment over the sexual authority of
one's partner or of the opposite sex in general as well
as feelings of dislike or guilt surrounding one's own
sexuality and sexual preferences.

- Fear of childbirth or guilt feelings about the manner in
  which you parented your child or children.
- Feeling a lack of self-worth as a result of having a minimum amount of financial power. This includes experiencing feelings of resentment over being controlled
  financially by others.
- Resentment resulting from being manipulated by other
  people. This includes the feeling of being victimized by
  one's circumstances, such as race, color or sex.
- Feeling so personally insecure that you need to manipulate other people in order to establish control levels in
  your life.
- Participating in any level of dishonesty in your financial, sexual or interpersonal relationships.
- The fear of never having enough, which includes the
  fear of poverty.

Some of the more common dysfunctions that result from these
particular stresses are, for women—all female dysfunctions such
as menstrual difficulties, infertility, vaginal infections, ovarian
cysts, endometriosis, tumors and cancer of the female organs;
for men—impotency and prostate difficulties, including cancer
(these dysfunctions are associated with loss of financial or political authority, in particular). For both male and female, common dysfunctions include pelvic and lower back pain, herpes
and all other sexual diseases, difficulties with slipped discs, all
sexual problems, and bladder and urinary difficulties.

THE THIRD CHAKRA

The third chakra is located in the stomach area of the body or
what is referred to in the Eastern traditions as the solar plexus.
The physical areas of the body that it primarily corresponds to
are the abdomen, upper intestine, gallbladder, kidneys, liver,
pancreas, adrenal glands, spleen and middle spinal area.

Following the "what's mine" stage of development, a child enters into the process of developing Self-hood. This is the learning phase that teaches the basic principles of personal empowerment and interpersonal relationship skills. It is the "survival instinct" center of the body as it corresponds to how well a person learns to trust his or her own instincts regarding how to direct their own life.

During this stage, a child will begin to explore personal choice through learning to vocalize opinions and preferences. Learning how to relate to other people begins during this phase and that includes learning how to respond to feelings of intimidation.

It is crucial that a child experience respect and validation for his or her expressions of individuality during this time, as this becomes the foundation for self-confidence, self-respect and belief in oneself. These are the "wisdom chips" that are first acquired in association with this chakra center.

The third chakra, or the solar plexus, is a particularly sensitive part of the body. In the language of energy, it is the area of the body that is the main "receiver" for the first impressions a person receives in every situation he or she enters, including the first impressions received from people. The aptly-named "gut reaction" or "gut instinct" is a highly intuitive response generated from the impressions received through the solar plexus. Its sensitive nature gleans impressions on the energy level that inevitably prove to be more accurate than physical impressions.

This is, more specifically, the activity of intuition. The solar plexus is the center of intuition that provides guidance on the daily activity of human life. The type of guidance or feedback that is characteristic of "solar plexus intuition" is the type that is so natural that most people respond to it all the time without thinking about what the source of this guidance is.

For example, in every situation involving human interaction, our "instincts" are always on the alert as to whether or not we can trust the people we are interacting with or the information we are receiving. Automatically, we scrutinize the feedback we are receiving in these social interactions and we rarely notice that mentally we are asking ourselves questions like, "Can I trust this person?" or "Is what I am being told true?"

For every one of these questions that we privately pursue within our minds, we receive answers. The answers may come in the form of a feeling or the proverbial gut reaction. The source within us that is providing this information is our own intuition. And the source from which our intuition forms its particular data is based upon the "energy data" that is penetrating our own energy systems through our solar plexus.

To some extent, solar plexus intuition is designed to assist us with survival data. Information that is basic to daily life, such as trusting people, mechanical instructions, directions, counsel about business enterprises—even gut reactions that assist in the decision-making process around hiring employees—comes through the intuition channel of the solar plexus.

It is essential to the creation of health—meaning all levels of health: emotional, psychological, physical and mental as well as healthy life skills—that a person feels adequately empowered to serve as the primary decision-maker in his or her own life. The decision-making process should rightfully be considered as a fundamental survival skill in life. The capacity to fulfill this role for oneself is rooted in the personal belief that one is capable of responding effectively with people in basic life interactions without fear of manipulation or victimization. This also includes developing an essential amount of self-confidence so that one can direct the decision-making process that is built into every person's life. The quality of intuition that operates from the third chakra is nature's way of assisting in this process of becoming personally empowered. It is the ability to trust one's own instincts.

There are certain patterns of fear and anger that can become a part of an individual's psyche and interfere with or entirely prevent this cycle of maturation from developing into its fullest capacity. While these patterns of negativity affect a person's entire life in that they cause seriously limiting behavioral problems, they are rooted in the absence of a strong foundation in personal power.

In adults, the lack of personal power breeds any number of insecurities and inner crises—from the inability to trust others, to the inability to trust oneself or to reach out for ways to respond to one's own emotional needs. The patterns of fear and anger that indicate a person is suffering from a tremendous lack of personal power are these:

- Fear of intimidation, which prevents you from establishing relationships or situations that are based upon equality.
- The fear of assuming responsibility for yourself, your needs, your commitments, your finances and your thoughts, attitudes and personal actions.
- Resentment over having to take responsibility for another who is either emotionally incapable or refuses to take responsibility for him or herself. The resentment is increased when a person also feels incapable of challenging the irresponsible partner and thus remains in an untenable situation through the negative choice not to challenge it.
- Fear that results from believing you are incapable of handling the decision-making process in your own life.
- Anger which results from having your own power of choice violated, forceably limited or invalidated by others.
- Anger which results from feeling neglected or overlooked. This often results in people who develop the pattern of constantly giving to others while denying their own needs because of a fear of not being loved.
- Fear of being criticized or the need to criticize others in order to feel empowered.
- The anger and frustration which result from the inability to break free from being controlled by the expectations of others.
- The pattern of taking anger out on "safe and helpless

victims" because of lacking enough personal courage to challenge the source of one's anger.
• The fear of failure.

It is crucial to note that the quality of health is affected not only by our fears and feelings of anger but by how we behave as a result of living with those negative patterns. Releasing anger in inappropriate ways, such as through child or spouse abuse, drugs or alcoholism, promotes the deadly cycle of guilt, self-hatred and the loss of self-respect. Health cannot be maintained when a person becomes consumed in self-hatred. Indeed, nothing positive can be created in a person's life when inwardly that individual is ashamed of the behavior in his or her life.

The most common physical dysfunctions that are created through the energy of these particular negative patterns are arthritis, ulcers and all related stomach problems; colon and intestinal problems, including cancer; pancreatitis, diabetes and cancer of the pancreas; kidney difficulties (also second chakra-related); liver problems, including hepatitis; gallbladder problems; adrenal gland dysfunctions; chronic or acute indigestion; anorexia and bulimia; nausea and flu.

THE FOURTH CHAKRA

This energy center is located around the heart. The parts of the body that receive their major energy from this chakra are the heart, lungs, shoulders, ribs, breasts, diaphragm, esophagus and the circulatory and respiratory systems.

Once a child develops a sense of personal power and self-esteem, learning to give love and attention to others as well as to receive it becomes the next stage of personal development. This stage includes the first lessons in learning about love of self as well as love of life itself.

Issues relating to learning about the nature of love are, not surprisingly, the major focus of the heart chakra.

In learning to give love, to share love and to be concerned

about the well-being of others, a child steps out of the "center of the Universe" role that can so easily develop when a child is doted on by family members. If this role is not gently removed through this natural maturation process, it could result in self-centered, thoughtless and demanding behavior as an adult.

Conversely, children who are neglected or abused develop an entirely different idea of love. Far from being in a position to love openly and trust others, abused and neglected children develop serious emotional problems and relationship difficulties. Not only does loving become associated with pain, but the human being cannot stop the instinct to reach out for love. Therefore, in spite of the pain, abused and neglected children enter a cycle of continually associating pain with every level of human interaction, oftentimes losing the capacity to distinguish love from abusive forms of behavior.

The dominant pattern in their personal lives that is created as adults is a larger version of what was experienced as a child. Ultimately, the adult in this circumstance lives a life compensating for the fact that the "wisdom chips" relating to the nature of love that should have been invested in his or her bank account as a child are missing. It becomes enormously difficult as an adult to invest in any healthy adult relationship until this bank account is appropriately replenished, and this requires healing, beginning with returning to one's childhood.

The fourth chakra is the center chakra of the body. It is the center of your body and, metaphorically speaking, love is the center of your life. A person can effectively handle any number of crises or stresses if he or she has a strong, loving support system.

Moreover, as we peel away all of the layers involved in the process of personal (and oftentimes professional) decision making, inevitably what remains at the core of why we choose what we do is that we are really choosing the path that will bring us love. Even if the words we use to describe our goal are financial security, social acceptance or political power, for example, love is still the primary motivator behind our choices. Ultimately, without love, remaining healthy, much less healing oneself, is almost impossible.

In reviewing the previous chakra centers and, specifically, their relationship to the process of personal development, what is clearly visible is that one level of development builds upon the next one. Without an adequate sense of personal power, for instance, it is not possible to learn to give love and trust others without manipulation or insecure behavior.

Emotional neglect can also lead to a person's becoming bitter, insensitive and perhaps even cruel. Abusive emotional behavior is acted out not only with other people; emotional neglect can lead to the abuse of animals, for instance, or a deep insensitivity to the needs of other forms of life including, in the broadest sense, the needs of the earth itself.

The absence of a strong foundation of love creates an inner climate in which particular patterns of fear, anger and resentment can develop in place of love. Without love, it's easy to be frightened by life.

The following list includes the more common experiences of fear, anger and their consequent behavioral patterns that can contaminate the energy of the fourth chakra.

- Fear of not being loved or the belief that you are not worthy of being loved.
- Harboring guilt as a result of participating in personal acts of rejection or emotional neglect.
- Resentment that develops from seeing others receive more love and attention than yourself.
- Fear of showing or sharing affection.
- Developing guilt feelings as a result of using anger, hostility or criticism as substitutes for love.
- Feeling emotionally paralyzed by experiencing too much loneliness.
- Experiencing emotional contamination as a result of

harboring too many negative and judgmental feelings toward other people or other forms of life.

• Experiencing emotional contamination as a result of holding on to old hurts and past resentments.

• Developing emotional fears and bitterness as a result of believing you cannot forgive or directly refusing to forgive.

• Continually creating relationships that are emotionally unfulfilling or abusive.

• Guilt from feeling you have not successfully fulfilled your emotional commitments.

• Doing something or being with someone when your "heart is not in it".

• Too much grief and sorrow, resulting in, literally, the development of a "broken heart".

These emotional traumas and sufferings create "emotional congestion" or what is frequently referred to as emotional blockages. In addition to the dysfunctional emotional behavior that results from these patterns of negativity, the physical body also responds to these stresses.

The more commonly experienced physical illnesses are heart conditions including heart attacks, enlarged heart, blocked arteries and congestive heart failure, asthma, allergies, lung problems including cancer, bronchial difficulties, pneumonia, circulation problems, and all upper back and shoulder problems.

THE FIFTH CHAKRA

The fifth chakra is located in the throat. The energy from this center flows primarily to your thyroid, trachea, esophagus, neck vertebrae, throat and mouth, including your teeth, gums and jaws.

This chakra center corresponds to the development of personal expression and, especially, the use of individual will-power. Consider once again our study of the maturation process of a child. The age of seven is considered to be the "age of

reason," the age at which a child (hopefully) has acquired sufficient knowledge of right and wrong, good and bad, appropriate
and inappropriate behavior that he or she can learn what it
means to be held accountable for personal actions, albeit in small
ways.

Consider even more deeply that in teaching accountability,
we are teaching a child about the nature of cause and effect—
that thoughts, words, mental and emotional intentions, as well
as actions, have consequences. Cause and effect is the study of
the use of willpower and its relationship to what is created in
our personal worlds. In the language of energy, the act of using
personal willpower is equal to the act of commanding energy to
take form according to the map of emotional desire and mental
intention that one is holding in one's consciousness. Thus, the
expression, "That's not what I had in mind," is given genuine
authority when you actually realize that "having something in
mind" does, in fact, precede every action of personal creation
in which you participate.

Individuality and self-expression are realized through personal actions of creativity. As a child grows into adolescence
and young adulthood, he or she is expected to assume more
responsibity for creating and achieving personal goals, beginning with school and home responsibilities. The experience and
parental/teacher guidance that are meant to accompany a child
on this first stage of learning about cause and effect are the initial
"wisdom chips" that are invested into the fifth chakra bank
account. Through this stage of development, the responsible
use of individual willpower is explored.

Apart from the obvious learnings of personal responsibility
that accompany this cycle of a child's development are deeper
and more subtle life tools that are meant to take root during this
time. The study of cause and effect also teaches a person about
the signficance of learning to "follow one's dreams" and that
you can "do anything so long as you believe in yourself." In
order to succeed at realizing your dreams, you have to hold on
to your goals, keep your intention clearly focused and make

choices that empower your ambitions. The study of cause and effect—actions and consequences—is, in fact, the study of the power inherent in each of us to create our own realities.

The essential difference often noted that separates the human being from the rest of the members of creation is the attribute of willpower—indeed, of free will. It is the one human attribute that is believed to be our universal "gift from God." The reference that free will is a gift from God suggests that what is deeply ingrained into human nature is the *need* to create, the *need* to contribute something physical to this life that is a validation of our being alive. We are born—and designed—to create. That is why we have mind, consciousness, choice and free will. This attribute of willpower and personal choice is our greatest power.

The stifling of, or interference with, the development of personal willpower during childhood creates the foundation for any number of difficult challenges that a child will need to overcome as an adult. Unfortunately, it is very easy to traumatize the development of personal willpower in children.

The experience of having no voice in the choices made for you as a child, or of having your choices ridiculed or criticized, creates fear of personal expression. This fear eventually becomes the inability to believe that you have any voice in the creation of your own reality. How could anyone who has no experience with personal cause and effect believe that this process of self-creating reality does, in fact, exist?

On an even deeper level, our very nature as human beings exudes creative energy. We create in every moment of our lives—from simple creations such as meals and the decorating of our homes to creations of art work, music and poetry. We cannot stop creating even if we try. Every time we flex a muscle—be it a physical, mental or emotional muscle—we influence creation. We are programmed to create. The experience of having our basic creative nature violated as children is equal to trying to de-program the essence of the human design.

It is not possible to de-program the creative powers of the

human being. What is possible, however, is to interfere with this process so profoundly that the instinct to create finds destructive and negative channels of expression. Creation will find an outlet—this cannot be prevented no matter how domineering or controlling the opposition is to this form of personal expression.

When violations occur in the process of development as a child, negative outlets are discovered. It is important to realize that a violation includes the absence of instruction regarding personal responsibility. Children who are given the impression that "anything goes" are as apt to find negative forms of expression as are children who are ridiculed. In our very beings, we know what we need to learn as children in order to become effective adults, and part of that inner knowledge is that we know we need to learn how to be responsible for what we create as well as to learn what it means to create responsibly. We need to know how to communicate on our own behalf. We need to know how to handle the consequences of our actions. When children are not taught this, they realize, even if only subconsciously, that they are lacking something inside of them that is essential to know in order to live as an empowered adult.

Self-expression and creativity are crucial to health—and not just physical health. The creation of a healthy life—as well as a healthy body—requires that a person maintain dominion over his or her life. This includes having the inner capacity to speak up on behalf of one's own needs.

The inability to communicate your feelings, your ideas, your sorrow, your anger or your joy is like pouring concrete around your heart and into your throat. This blockage aborts the growth process and causes destructive behavioral patterns to begin that are guaranteed to contaminate every intimate relationship.

To compensate for the fear of self-expression, individuals will expect any partner they are involved with to have the skill of mind-reading. They will require that their partners know what they are thinking or feeling without having to put it into words.

Another equally negative pattern is the practice of denying the existence of emotional feelings as a way of compensating for the fear of one's emotions.

Irrational outbursts of anger, rage or physical abuse are also connected to the inability to cope in a responsible way with fears. Dishonesty is yet another negative behavior that can develop as a result of inadequacies in the development of self-expression.

Some of the more common fears, anxieties and negative behavioral patterns that are prone to take root in a person's consciousness as a result of an inadequate foundation in the use of willpower are these:

- Fear of self-assertion—this often develops into patterns of allowing yourself to be victimized by others because of the inability to communicate on your own behalf in an empowered way.
- Fear of expressing your emotional needs, feelings or opinions. This fear almost totally blocks any level of creativity.
- Becoming dishonest or lying as a way of covering up feelings or denying responsibility for personal actions.
- Using your will to control or influence the lives of others to your own advantage.
- Regret and self-directed anger that comes from the inability to say, "I'm sorry", "I love you" or "I forgive you".
- The inability to express grief, hurt and sorrow. This includes the inability to shed tears.
- Collecting regrets as a result of not being able to speak up for yourself when opportunities have come along in your life.
- Allowing your own willpower to remain undeveloped by expecting someone else to make your decisions for you.
- Exaggerating and embellishing the truth, a misuse of fifth chakra energy. This includes the habit of gossiping.

Some of the more common physical difficulties that develop as a result of blockages caused by any of these negative patterns are the following: raspy throat and chronic sore throat problems, including throat and mouth cancers; gum difficulties, teeth problems and jaw misalignment (called TMJ); scoliosis (curved spine), stiff neck; laryngitis; tonsilitis; tension headaches that form at the base of the neck; swollen glands and thyroid conditions.

Also, in a category of its own are addictions to drugs, alcohol, cigarettes, sugar or food and any other form of addiction that indicates an inability to command your own power of will and challenge the fears or limitations present in your life.

THE SIXTH CHAKRA

The sixth chakra is located in the center of your forehead. This is also called the "third eye" or the "eye of wisdom," since it is recognized as the doorway through which higher wisdom and intuition enter a person's awareness.

The brain, eyes, ears, nose, pineal and pituitary glands are the physical regions of the body that are primarily nourished by the energy of this chakra center. This energy also assists in the physical functioning of learning and the development of intelligence and reasoning skills.

Returning to the stages of child development, we are now discussing the development of intelligence. At the very least, a child needs to acquire reading, writing and basic mathematical skills. However, that is just the beginning of understanding the content of this chakra.

A child must also learn to think and to reason. There are levels of sophistication to "thinking skills." Rudimentary thinking skills relate to being able to handle the basic challenges of life as they emerge daily, i.e., thinking about paying the bills, shopping, getting the children to school, planning what to wear, preparing dinner for your family and playing sports after work. This category is comprised of those parts of life that we do not have to think too deeply about because they form our day-today routines. They are repetitious and consistent. These are the parts of life that we rely upon to remain the same. Consequently, we do not often "think" about the more ordinary parts of our lives. In fact, we frequently prefer not to think about our lives until some form of chaos upsets the calm of our routine.

Then what? How well do we "think" when chaos strikes? What do we "think about" under crisis?

This quality of thinking requires more advanced skills. Specifically, the skills required to maneuver through the crisis situations that occur in all of our lives are those that allow us to find the meaning and purpose inherent in all of life's cycles, including disease and death.

This process is called "transcendence"—rising above the temptation of self-pity (the "why me?" syndrome) and harnessing the strength to create anew. Transcendent thinking is a learned skill requiring the development of methods of introspection, self-examination and a philosophic or spiritual outlook about the purpose of life, one that includes the idea that living and learning are synonymous. A philosophy/spirituality of this quality demands that a person continually study his or her own life from the perspective that Life is a teacher and that what is being taught to you through the avenue of your personal experiences is essential for you to know.

If that quality of thinking can take root in a person, it is then possible to introduce a more advanced thought along those same lines that suggests that no matter what happens in someone's life, it is always a necessary change for the good of that person's entire well-being. This does not mean that crisis and change are not painful nor that trauma and personal loss are experiences that are easy to heal.

What this philosophical/spiritual position does maintain, however, is that the possibility of living one's life free from trauma is extremely remote, if not impossible. That being the case, is it not the way of wisdom to consider that perhaps learning is built into all of the experiences of life—both painful and pleasurable ones—and, therefore, preparing oneself to know how to seek such learning is essential? The alternative to this way of thinking is to believe that nothing holds meaning, that all events are random and that life moves from one cruel tragedy to the next, with no discernable path of intention to its rhythms and cycles.

How does one learn the skills of introspection and self-examination? This learning should, appropriately, begin during childhood through the guidance of parents who are able to instruct their children in the techniques of thinking through their difficulties. Children, by nature, ask "why?" regardless of what they are trying to understand—be it crisis or a board game. They should be given answers appropriate to their level of understanding.

During their moments of anger, fear or rage, they should first be permitted to express these feelings and secondly, these feelings and their significance should be discussed and never disregarded. In addition to discussing feelings, whenever appropriate, children should be taught how to think and react appropriately to the events in their lives. They also should be taught to discern the significance these events might hold for them. Occasions such as birthdays are, to some extent, rites of passage. Certainly, entering the teenage years is that. These are events of transformation for children, like miniature initiation experiences.

These rites of passage hold great significance to them. They signal entry into more responsibility and greater degrees of personal authority. In other words, they have *meaning* to them and this meaning needs to be recognized and honored. This type of teaching becomes the foundation for the perception that life—both life in general and their personal lives—is composed of deeply meaningful events. In the process of learning that life is not a casual occurrence in this Universe, a child also learns that meaning and strong personal values go hand in hand.

There are two scales of value in life—visible values and invisible values. There is much about our physical lives that is of great value—our work, our health, our families, our friends, our homes and material goods, our nation and our planet. There is also much about our inner lives that has great value: our capacity to be compassionate, understanding and loving and our capacity to know how to live an honorable life, to fulfill our commitments, to use wisdom in decision making and to know how to make decisions, recognizing the effects they might have on the lives of others.

If nothing in childhood is recognized as significant or as having any transcendent value beyond physical gratification, how, as an adult, will that adult relate to life? Where will that adult find meaning? How will that adult THINK about life?

For many people, the questions of the meaning and value of life are more than philosophical. They are the essence of a spiritual world view and form the basis for a personal spiritual practice.

Spiritual thinking and spiritual perception are associated with sixth chakra power. Spiritual thinking is a higher order of reasoning that allows the search for purpose and meaning in life to find its natural avenue of expression.

An unmeasurable number of people hold dearly to the belief that life is a spiritual creation and that God is always guiding the evolution of the human experience. There are also numerous people who do not believe in a God or in an afterlife or in any form of spiritual communion. Those who believe in God do not necessarily agree upon what God is, or upon the nature of divine intelligence. Those who don't believe, simply don't believe.

Though it has been debated for hundreds of years, the existence of a God, or of any invisible divine force, cannot be proven to the satisfaction of the scientific or agnostic mind. The type of "proof" available—miracles, healings, apparitions, personal faith and other phenomena of that nature—means nothing to those who seek something more tangible or repeatable in terms of scientific methodology.

There is, however, one attribute of the human being that is seemingly acknowledged across the many lines of thinking about such matters, and that is the existence of the human "spirit"—whether accepted poetically or literally.

When the spirit of someone is not present, the creation or physical matter that belongs to that person disintegrates. We all know the expressions, "to break one's spirit" or "team spirit" or a "nation's spirit." These are references to the power and *reality* of the human spirit.

Anyone who has witnessed the gradual lessening of someone's spirit (or enthusiasm) for life, for a relationship, or for his or her work knows what it is to see the physical part of that person's life shrivel into dust. Without the participation of the human spirit, nothing can remain in healthy physical form.

This is absolutely real in the world of healing. Those who heal have Spirit. Spirit is essential to the healing process, and when any individual is unable to engage the power of his or her own spirit on the healing journey, that person is preparing to die.

The human spirit is capable of development not just surfacing in times of great crisis or when acts of patriotic heroism are required. It has specific qualities and potentials that are as real as the talent for music or science. These qualities are also part of the energy of the sixth chakra.

For those who believe in a spiritual Universe, the human spirit is recognized as the connecting link between our physical world and the nonphysical world of Divine Intelligence.

Spiritual development is the process of giving attention to the deeper capacities and qualities of human nature and working to perfect them. The discipline of nonattachment, for example, is the practice of becoming so personally empowered that you are able to interact in every situation in your life, contributing the highest degree of insight and wisdom, without needing to control the outcome of events.

The sixth chakra is particularly recognized as the entry point of intuition, wisdom and inspiration. The quality of intuition that is associated with sixth chakra energy differs from the intuition of the third chakra center. Third chakra guidance relates to assistance provided on daily, practical matters. Sixth chakra intuition is of a higher, more universal and transcendent nature, providing individuals with insights relating to the spiritual significance of their lives and of Life itself.

Intuitive skills can be developed into precise tools of perception, as in learning intuitive diagnostic skills or the ability to expand one's reasoning faculties according to Universal Laws and Principles.

As discussed earlier, the developmental process for achieving in spiritual terms requires that a person learn the language of awareness: introspection, self-examination and personal accountability. These are the tools that then serve the individual as he or she pursues a personal spiritual discipline, such as meditation or prayer.

The absence of these skills permits fear to reign supreme within a person's consciousness. Such a person lacks any effective coping mechanisms. When such is the case, the inability to reason, to challenge oneself to see the broader perspective at work in one's life, to lift one's sights beyond the limitations of one's personal grief, always will lead that individual to live according to the perceptions of negativity: judgmentalism, prejudice, fear, anger, self-pity and victimhood.

An extraordinary number of fears and negative behavioral patterns are capable of contaminating sixth chakra energy. The following items represent only a sampling:

- Fear of looking inside oneself, of self-examination and introspection.

- Fear of one's own intuitive skills, which leads to creating blockages of one's inner sensitivities.

- The misuse of intellectual power, as in participating in the creation of anything that will harm life or in deliberate acts of deception.

- Using one's reasoning skills against oneself, as in developing psychological and emotional denial mechanisms. This is the practice of denying the truth, which

leads to an inability to discern one's own reality with
any degree of clarity.

- Fear that results from believing you are intellectually
inadequate.

- Jealousy and insecurity over the creative abilities of another person.

- Fear of being open to the value of other people's ideas.

- An unwillingness or refusal to learn from your life experiences. This often leads to blaming other people
constantly for everything that goes wrong in your life
and to an endless pattern of repeating the same painful
and difficult learning situations.

- Behavior that is paranoid the anxiety which arises from
feeling that you don't know yourself.

Some of the more common dysfunctions that originate with sixth
chakra blockages are brain tumors, brain hemorrhages and blood
clots to the brain; neurological disorders; blindness; deafness;
full spinal difficulties; migraine or tension headaches; anxiety or
nervousness, including nervous breakdowns; comas; depression, schizophrenia, grand mal seizures and other forms of emo-
tional/mental disorders and learning disabilities.

THE SEVENTH CHAKRA

The seventh chakra is located at the crown of the head. The
physical parts of the body that correspond to the energy of this
center are the major body systems: nervous system, muscle system, skin and skeletal structure.

In the language of energy, the seventh chakra is the entry
point of human life force itself—an invisible current of energy
that endlessly pours into the human energy system, nourishing
every part of the body, the mind and the spirit.

Returning to our child analogy, consider that once a child
has made the passage through all of the previous stages of maturation, this child begins the process of seriously acquiring personal attitudes, values, ethics and impressions about life in

general and where in that whole pattern of life he or she fits.

Attitudes, values and ethics have power—specifically, the kind of power that makes or breaks the quality of one's life. They provide the guidepost for one's life, the standards one aspires to and holds oneself in alignment with. The qualities that universally command respect for human beings—courage, humanitarianism, selflessness—flourish inside a person who has built a strong inner foundation based upon positive attitudes and values.

Attitudes are magnets. They attract to us people, opportunities and events that are of the exact quality of our strongest or dominating attitudes. If we are pessimistic, full of complaints and negative attitudes about life, we will surely find ourselves in like-minded company—if for no other reason than that optimists annoy pessimists.

More significantly, however, our attitudes work according to the Universal Law of Attraction—like attracts like. A belief in "bad luck" creates bad luck. A belief that life is full of rich opportunities that can change the course of our lives in a flash brings exactly those types of opportunities into your life.

At a more personal level, negative beliefs about oneself, such as the belief held by many people that they are unlovable, create relationship dynamics in which being unloved or rejected is experienced. All you need to do to test this hypothesis is to write down a list of your attitudes about life and see if, in fact, they are not strong determining forces in your life.

The quality of a person's character is developed, indeed groomed, from the combination of attitudes, values and ethics to which that person adheres. "Character-power" is real and it is also a magnet, drawing to each individual challenges equal to the quality of that person's spirit.

Consider the challenges of Gandhi. He drew to himself those struggles that were a match for the power and quality of his character and his spirit. One can only speculate that accomplishments of the magnitude of Gandhi's are illustrations of the power available to the human being when one's character and one's spirit operate in unison, but I believe that this alignment was a part of Gandhi's inner power.

Most of us focus the energy of our lives on a lesser scale than Gandhi. Nevertheless, within each of our lives are challenges in which we are afforded the opportunity to act according to the dictates and strength of our spirits. Confronting an addiction to drugs or alcohol is one of the most common dilemmas of a life-challenging nature that people face. This falls into this category because addictions of this magnitude negatively affect the whole of one's life. They interfere with a person's ability to accomplish what he or she was born to do.

We create our own realities. The tools that we use to engage the process of creation are all invisible. They are our attitudes, beliefs, values, ethics and emotional energies. Negative attitudes about life diminish the life force itself. Like damming up a river, negativity on this scale is equal to disregarding continually the value and purpose of one's own life. The life force gradually, but continually, becomes weakened. The body, the mind and the spirit begin to suffer from "energy malnutrition." If this downward spiral continues unchecked, the spirit experiences energy starvation. Eventually, it becomes impossible to replenish the spirit and the body consequently dies.

The process of creation continues during downward spirals. So long as we have breath, we have the power to create. What is created is always a reflection of the energy present in a person's system. When downward cycles are created, depression results. A person's life force becomes literally depressed and void of vitality. The body begins to feel like lead and exhaustion becomes a person's constant companion. This is one example of what spiritual starvation feels like.

Because of our orientation toward physical matter, the idea of Life Force may not be easily appreciated as having validity, much less as having power to it. Yet it exists. During an intuitive health evaluation, the strength of an individual's life force is my indicator as to how committed that person is to remaining alive.

A healthy life force has vitality and very clear focus to it.

This aspect of focus is very significant because it means that the person has a level of awareness regarding where he or she invests the energy of their life. In other words, it indicates that a person is mindful of his or her personal value and, as such, invests energy, time and attention with care, thoughtfulness and wisdom.

People who practice this quality of awareness are not as controlled by the tumultuous nature of external reality. They possess self-knowledge (albeit in varying degrees), they know who they are and they know what they expect from themselves. Discernment, the capacity to think with wisdom and clarity, requires self-knowledge. You must know yourself in order to make choices that do not throw your inner self into crisis.

The following is only an introduction to the types of fears or behavioral patterns that interfere with the health of the seventh chakra. Because this chakra relates to issues enveloping the whole of one's life, the patterns of negativity are likewise of the same caliber.

- The crisis of living a meaningless life.
- Spiritual crises, such as the absence of faith.
- Crisis that accompanies the inability to trust in the natural, supportive processes of life.
- The absence of courage and faith in oneself.
- Living according to the energy of negative attitudes that prevent an individual from seeing opportunities to change.
- Fear of self development—this includes the fear of knowing oneself.
- The negative behavioral patterns that result from an inability to think and reason beyond the limitations of one's own personal needs.
- The negative behavioral patterns that result from an unwillingness to grow and change in order to accommodate the challenges of one's life.
- The inability to see the larger pattern at work within one's life.

The types of illnesses that can result from these patterns of negativity are nervous system disorders; paralysis; genetic disorders; bone problems, including bone cancer; and debilitating illnesses such as multiple sclerosis and amyotrophic lateral sclerosis (ALS).

THE CHAKRA SYSTEM AS A SYSTEM OF PERCEPTION

As you become familiar with the seven chakras from the perception of how they reflect the natural cycle of maturation, it becomes possible to work with this system as a way of studying yourself and where you are most likely to be challenged in any given situation.

The seven levels of maturation that have been discussed also reflect the seven basic questions that arise in every situation we face in our daily lives. Consider the scenario of a business meeting. As you enter the room, instinctively you scan the room to get a sense of the physical conditions present, including where you feel comfortable sitting during the meeting. This is a first chakra question—physical safety and security.

Second, you will evaluate your preparations and your relationships with those present. You will sense where the power struggles are most likely to occur and with whom. This is second chakra energy—control and power in terms of relationships and physical concerns.

Third, you will brace yourself to present your data or defend your position. You will gather your personal power and focus it so as not to lose your sense of inner control. Or, you will become aware that you are intimidated by the circumstance. In either case, this is the process of evaluating the third chakra concern of personal power.

Fourth, you will bring your emotions into the situation along with your personal need to be accepted and appreciated. This is fourth chakra influence.

You will want to affect the situation, to make your presence known and to exert some level of your own willpower into the meeting. You will want to contribute your energy and this is fifth chakra energy.

How well you think is always evaluated in a meeting and this is sixth chakra energy.

As you leave the meeting, automatically you will evaluate how your performance or any of the decisions made will affect your professional and personal life. This is the energy of the seventh chakra.

The cycle of the seven chakras repeats itself constantly in our lives, in every one of the situations and relationships in our lives. Wherever you sense a difficulty, review the chakra system in terms of its sequence of issues and locate where you feel blocked. Then work on the block to empower yourself effectively. This is one extremely powerful form of preventive medicine.

OTHER CONSIDERATIONS:
GENETICS VERSUS KARMA

Where does the influence of genetics fit into this system of health analysis? The genetic factors present in the human body are recognized to be very real, like the given material one then develops.

Admittedly, all of the visualizations one can do will not increase one's height nor change a person's blood type. The tenets of holistic health do not purport to be able to alter a person's genetic structure, but rather to find methods through which a person can achieve the maximum condition of health given the physical reality of his or her body.

However, it also must be noted that because all of the holistic technologies are only in their developmental stages, and because we have yet to tap the full potential of our mind in terms of its ability to influence the body, the answer to the question of genetics remains open-ended. At present, we are unable effectively to challenge genetic limitations. Who knows what we will be capable of fifty years from now.

The question of genetics is intimately connected to the

question of karma (the Universal Law of Cause and Effect); do we choose our physical makeup based upon karmic ingredients, or are we born once and subject to the random genetic patterning of our parents?

This is, of course, another unanswerable question. I can only offer an opinion based upon my experience. For me, the factor of karma is a reality.

While past-life information is not always a part of an intuitive diagnosis, whenever there is a significant connection between a person's present physical condition and a previous lifetime event, that connecting link is present in a person's energy system. It seems as though the individual's unconscious mind is working to unearth the memory, to bring it into the light of day. And because we are not consciously open to this type of information, it emerges through dreams or through unusual fears or patterns of behavior that we develop in our present lifetime.

For a very long time, I could not accept this reality. I thought it useless to the healing process to inform someone that the reason they were suffering in this lifetime was because of some deed they did four hundred years ago to someone, and that it is just unfortunate that they could not remember either.

What I have learned, however, is that in almost every instance where past-life information surfaces, the individual is able to connect the data to something that is present in this lifetime. In one reading, for instance, a woman contacted me because of throat problems that had been with her through most of her adult life. No physiological cause could be found for her condition.

During her reading, I saw that she had been a nun in a monastery approximately three centuries ago. During her life as a nun, she had been put under silence for an incredible number of years as a punishment. Apparently, she had never commited a wrongdoing and because she was unable to clear this, the sense of injustice and the desire to scream out against this injustice followed her to her grave. In this lifetime, not only was this woman born into a Catholic family, but she had been plagued since the time this disorder surfaced with nightmares of being punished while in a monastery. Until this reading, the dreams had made no sense to her. Shortly after the reading, her condition improved.

I am hardly in a position to make definitive statements about the larger cycle of life and about the cosmic process of death and rebirth. I can only comment within the scope of my experiences.

As such, I have come to believe that nothing, absolutely nothing, about our lives occurs outside our personal power of choice. The problem is that we have underestimated this power, believing that the power of choice belongs only to our conscious minds. We have no reference point for realizing the vast amount of choice that occurs through the power of our fears, attitudes and unconscious minds.

Moreover, we base our reasoning regarding choice upon whether or not we are happy, healthy and financially successful. In other words, as has often been pointed out to me, if we do indeed choose our lives, then why aren't we all "blessed" with a Swiss bank account, fame and health? Why would anyone choose to be born into poverty? Or into an abusive home? Or into a country experiencing war?

These are logical questions, to be sure, but they also reflect very human concerns, human values of success, human fears and insecurities. Moreover, if these concerns truly reflected the purpose of the creation of life, why haven't more people achieved these goals? Why are challenges far more abundant than money and happiness?

The possibility does exist that in the nonphysical state as spirits, our perceptions and our values are free of these earth-laden concerns and that the scale upon which we "choose" the particulars of a lifetime reflect the desire to expand our aware-ness according to Universal values of immortality and conscious-ness. In other words, we choose a lifetime that serves our learning and not our "earning power." As such, we would then

choose even our genetic makeup as a factor that serves our
learning.

Assume for a moment that this degree of choice might, in
fact, be the case. Add to this possibility that in the nonphysical
state, a single lifetime is like a drop in the bucket of eternity.
We, of course, value our lives from the perspective that this is
all we've got. But what if that were not true at all? What if, while
in the nonphysical state, we were given the opportunity to evaluate the sum of all of our learnings in all of our lifetimes in order
that we could fill in our gaps?

What if, for instance, a soul had such a life review and that
during that process of evaluation, the soul realized that it had
never learned about the nature of compassion but had preferred
to ignore the sufferings of other people. The soul might indeed
choose to learn compassion and create a lifetime to accommodate
that choice.

What types of circumstances teach compassion? One learns
compassion because one personally experiences the struggles
and pain of the human condition. Compassion is not learned
when one is focused on learning how to build empires. Compassion can be learned either through having to serve those in
need or through being a person requiring the compassion of
others. And so it is that a lifetime designed to teach compassion
is created. It may be that just such a choice created a Mother
Theresa.

From my perspective, I accept the continuing cycle of life
as a reality. Not only has this reality been repeatedly verified
through my work, but I have found that it provides the foundation for believing that this Universe is a fair, just and compassionate system. Whatever it is that we are and the
circumstances that we find ourselves in, we have earned. The
option that we are born only once to circumstances beyond our
control, meaning that we thrive or starve without reason, is
unacceptable to me.

Karma is the basis for the teaching that "what goes around
comes around" and that we had better "do unto others as we

would have them do unto us," because we will, indeed, always find ourselves on the receiving end of what we give to others.

ENVIRONMENT

The influence of our environmental conditions also plays a vital role in the creation of a person's health. As our environment continues to weaken as a result of pollution, the hole in the ozone, acid rain and nuclear fallout, pesticides and herbicides, we cannot help but become more susceptible to the massive amounts of poison infiltrating our systems each moment.

Certainly everyone cannot move into the country to live, and even the country is not all that healthy any longer. The reality many people are facing, however, is that the conditions of city living limit even the healthiest of health regimens. For example, people who run each day in New York City are breathing in car exhaust fumes and polluted air. This is equivalent to smoking.

In doing health evaluations for people, the environmental effects are showing up more and more frequently. Anxiety from sound pollution and irritations from polluted air are becoming commonplace.

We have yet to realize what the effect of the disruption in our ozone will create. Certainly, it is not difficult to imagine that there will be a rise in skin cancer, as the direct rays of the sun are disturbing to the human body. Moreover, the reality of nuclear waste material, nuclear fallout from tests in our atmosphere and nuclear wind, created as waste from power plants, is real.

We also have not begun to realize the full impact of the use of chemicals in our food and water supply. Since we have no extensive studies available that reflect the effects of the ingestion of chemicals on our mood sensitivities or our intellectual capabilities, we cannot make substantive statements about the impact of chemicals. We can only assume, as more and more reports surface about the high levels of pesticides that exist in our food supply, that this is a substantial negative health factor.

THE IMPACT OF VIOLENCE

We are a violent species—not by nature, but by choice. We have become so addicted to violence that we are no longer able even to realize our addiction, much less appreciate the impact violence has upon the human spirit and the physical body.

We entertain ourselves with violence, and we communicate to each other in violent words and, very often, violent acts. We permit violence to animals and to the environment. Worst of all, we consider these endless acts of violence as an acceptable part of human nature, as if we cannot be held responsible for them.

Television brings the violence of war into our homes in the evening news reports, but can we actually emotionally distinguish this very real violence from the entertainment that follows the news programs?

We live in a culture laden with victims of child and spouse abuse, interracial abuse and abuse of the poor. The homeless on our streets are victims of economic violence. Our schools are filled with violence and the streets with gang warfare.

This is only a comment on the abundance of visible violence. We are also invisibly violent. Thoughts of anger, violence and judgment wage wars inside of us, destroying our spirits and our bodies.

While we may believe that we are designed to handle violence and that it is a given part of the human experience, that is not so. We have simply become so acclimated to this distortion of our own basic natures that we no longer realize we have become poisoned.

My personal belief is that we are a species filled with violent illnesses because we ourselves are filled with violent emotions. Violent energy within a person destroys both internally and externally. The violent energy that exists within a person's energy system is a major contributor to the creation of disease in that person's body, though it remains a medically unmeasurable factor.

SUMMARY

The study of the human energy system and of the power of our own natures is the study of the dynamics of creation itself and of the vital part we play as participants in the process of the continuation and maintenance of life.

Human history is an illustration of our cycles of learning about ourselves, of shedding the limitations of one system of thought in order to reach for greater heights of our own self-awareness. Just as the advent of scientific thought disempowered the superstitious mind, so also will this emerging consciousness of co-creation challenge the belief that any one of us is born a victim.

Knowledge of the human energy system will eventually merge with traditional medicine. This is already happening in small ways, but as more becomes known about the "physics of the mind," this knowledge will have to be incorporated into our understanding of how disease and health are created.

CHAPTER FIVE

The Journey of Healing

(Myss)

REDEFINING THE HEALING PROCESS

What does it mean to heal? You might think the answer is obvious, but it is not.

Within the traditional medical model, healing means, quite simply, treating a disease until the disease is cured. Cured means successfully treated with drugs and/or surgery until the symptoms disappear.

The holistic model of health has introduced the study of the relationship among the mind, the body and the spirit. Recognizing the influence of emotional, psychological and spiritual factors is redefining the nature of the healing process. Studies in this area strongly indicate that the healing process must be expanded to include giving much-needed attention to the inner life of the human being.

This shift in perspective is also broadening our understanding of what qualifies as legitimate illness. For example, alcoholism is now recognized as an illness, whereas previously it was thought to be a "habit" or a lack of willpower. Likewise, depression and other sufferings of the mind and the spirit are gaining ground in terms of being accepted as forms of treatable illness.

Simultaneously, the holistic movement has approached the dying process with compassion and openness, thereby including the last stages of life as a vital part of an individual's healing journey. Within the traditional medical world, the dying process is viewed as the failure to heal, thereby implying that nothing of genuine value can occur within the human being once death is imminent. Yet what has become apparent to the many therapists who work with dying people is that the last stages of life provide opportunities for completion of a person's unfinished business. The experience of shedding troubled emotions and completing long-awaited conversations with family and friends brings to an appropriate conclusion all of the energies a person has set in motion during the course of a lifetime. This is a deeply healing process that allows the necessary moment of letting go to occur without residual guilt or angry emotions being retained by family members or friends. Though grief is present, it is not grief mixed with the crippling feelings that come from not having the final opportunity to say what is in your heart.

The impact of the holistic point of view, which includes the dying process as a healing journey, is redefining what it means to heal, and it illustrates time and again that treatment of the physical body alone is insufficient. Equally significant, the study of why and how we become ill is re-sensitizing us to our own emotional nature. The study of why we break down is also the study of what we need to remain healthy. Many schools of psychotherapy, while they may differ in their particular approaches, nevertheless share one strong premise: that the human being is a deeply sensitive system of emotional, psychological and spiritual needs.

A chemical cure does not exist for emotional injuries. Nor can surgery remove painful memories of being abused as a child. The "stuff" that disease is made of requires much more complex treatment than can be given through surgery or drugs alone. It requires, for example, the process of transforming inner grief into lessons that empower rather than destroy the individual.

There are several considerations to the healing journey that have been introduced through holistic thinking. Each one contributes valuable insights into what it means to heal and how an individual engages the full use of his or her inner resources to assist in that profound journey.

We are presenting the holistic concepts alongside the perceptions held by the traditional medical model in order to illustrate the natural transformation of thought that is taking place through the advent of the holistic paradigm.

CURE VERSUS TRANSFORMATION

Consider that the word "cure" implies that something external can be taken as treatment for something that is happening internally to the human body. In terms of infections and various viruses, this is accurate. But what happens to this system of treatment when emotional and psychological stress is introduced into the picture? Admittedly, there are drugs used for the treatment of depression, anxiety and stress, but do these drugs cure these illnesses or do they simply help the person to function until the symptoms abate? Drugs are effective in treating reactions to stress, but not the core of the stress itself.

The holistic model of treatment has brought to light the need to help a person heal the stresses of his or her life as an integral part of healing the body. In order to do this, a person must be willing and able to look at all of the pieces of his or her life, including emotional injuries (both given and received), unfulfilled emotional needs, disappointments in relationships, broken promises, unfulfilled ambitions, disappointments in oneself, and other patterns of unfinished business that form a person's inner grief.

In accepting the necessity of doing this quality of inner work, you are acknowledging the need to change or transform the areas of your life that are not conducive to regaining your health. As you do this, you alter the relationship you have with your disease. Rather than considering "disease" as a condition that has spontaneously manifested in the midst of your life, you are able to think of it as a "messenger." The transformational process, then, becomes the experience of understanding the particular messages that the experience of illness brings into your life and the challenge to act on those messages in ways that are productive to your health. Inevitably, the messages will direct you toward reevaluating who you think you are and what you realize you can live with versus a much more authentic appraisal of your real needs and considerations.

To put this description in the language of transformation, disease is unconscious change (or choice by default) manifesting in a person's body because the individual either 1) lacks the courage to look clearly at what is not working in his or her life, 2) does not believe that stress affects the body or 3) lacks the skills of introspection and self-examination that allow the analysis, and thus the dissolution, of stress to take place through positive channels.

Transformation is the process of becoming conscious of the many levels on which we make our choices and learning to recognize what it is we create as a result of our choices. Choosing, therefore, becomes a conscious act rather than the unconscious activity of reacting to our fears and stresses. It is this step-by-step, self-study process that allows a person to realize that the choice to remain filled with anger, for example, is *exactly* the type of invisible, subtle choice that produces illness.

What is it that occurs within the process of transformation

that makes it so healing? Self-analysis is certainly a part of the answer, but it is the goal of analysis that is healing and that goal is *completion* and *validation*.

Completion is the opportunity to understand and bring to a close—literally and figuratively—the open wounds of your life. Completion is the counterpart to creation: We want to see the energy we set in motion in our lives come full circle. We want to see our children grow up, we want to understand why some of our relationships failed, we want to see our businesses flourish, we want to see our creativity come into physical manifestation. And we want to see the seeds of our lives produce a harvest, even if we reap that harvest long after we first planted the seeds.

Wherever there is incompletion in our lives, there are strings attached, though these attachments may be unconscious. We remain tied through the invisible strings of our creative energy to all that we have set into motion, like hundreds of umbilical cords attached to our energy systems.

This is, perhaps, the dynamic that is responsible for causing us to recreate certain situations in our lives until we learn the lesson and can finally break the pattern by applying conscious choice. Consciously, or unconsciously, we are bound to what we create. Even if what we create is painful, the desire to see our creations through to completion is stronger than our capacity to walk away from them.

Once we become aware that we are repeating the same struggles, we can position ourselves to appreciate that *different choices produce different results*. Those who marry alcoholics will, more likely than not, continue to be involved with alcoholics until they look inside themselves to see what it is about their needs and beliefs that draws that type of imbalanced relationship into their lives. Perhaps it is a need to rescue someone, or perhaps it is the only way they have experienced being needed or loved. In either case, once awareness is brought to bear upon the pattern, the pattern can be released and a more fulfilling relationship can then be created.

Validation is the deeply healing process of sharing your pain with another, not so that the other person can make it go away, but because no one can bear the inner weight of suffering alone. Somehow, if only one other person is aware of the grief we carry, the burden becomes easier to bear because the suffering no longer seems meaningless and unacknowledged.

Suffering is an integral part of the human condition. The need to share one's suffering with another, to have a witness, so to speak, is deeply connected to the transformational journey and makes a necessary distinction between ego pain and the deeper sufferings of the soul.

EGO PAIN VERSUS SOUL PAIN

Ego pain and soul pain both produce the experience of suffering. There is, however, a significant and noteworthy difference between these two dimensions of suffering. Ego pain is the result of fighting against changes that need to take place, not only in oneself but within one's physical environment as well. Soul pain comes from the process of undergoing the necessary changes that occur within one's life and require acceptance or release.

The challenge that each of us is confronted with during our periods of suffering is whether to allow pain to remain at the ego level or whether we can transform our ego pain into a process that strengthens our soul. While both ego and soul pain may seem to be somewhat indistinguishable in terms of how you feel, there is a qualitative difference in terms of how able you are to appreciate the purpose or necessary reason for the experience.

There is a quality of pain, for instance, that is very much associated with injuries to the ego. The needs of the ego are simply stated: attention, praise, admiration, acceptance, control, power, sex and money. The only variable is the degree to which a person needs this type of feedback and the extent to which a person will go to get this level of reinforcement.

Whenever this type of feedback is denied, or whenever one is on the receiving end of negative feedback, the ego hurts.

The ego will go to great lengths to get its needs met, while at the same time denying any actual ego involvement. The need to impress others, the need for "center stage," the need to feel good about one's masculinity or femininity are all ego-based.

Certainly when we hunger for this feedback and it is not forthcoming, we hurt. And this hurt can lead to any level of negativity, either self-inflicted or directed toward others. Emotional rejection can lead to an emotional "getting even." Or it can lead to self-rejection and feelings of unworthiness. Ego pain can also lead to an embittered and self-pitying personality.

A person who is in the midst of an ego crisis is also in the midst of an opportunity to transform that ego pain into a process that leads to the deepening of personal awareness and insight. This is done by becoming open to the learning that is present in the situation. Just this one shift in perspective can begin the healing process and give the pain a direction in which to move rather than remain internalized for months, or even years. Choosing to view an ego crisis as a learning experience is choosing to involve one's soul in the healing process, thereby giving the crisis a purpose and meaning, one that cannot be realized if the pain remains at the ego level.

Soul pain is the processing of that which we cannot change, avoid or otherwise remove from our lives. While much about ego pain is optional (i.e., there are many ego choices we make that we *know* are not wise, but nonetheless we choose them), soul suffering is not optional. It has a purpose and a depth to it that is not present in ego pain.

Suffering that involves the soul teaches us about ourselves—our dark sides, our inner strengths and our capacity to rise beyond our previous limitations. This level of suffering is a "shedding" process, a letting go of various parts of ourselves that interfere with the development of our inner selves.

The role that this level of suffering plays within the human experience relates directly to the higher, or spiritual, purpose of life itself. Consider these questions: Why does life continually present us with challenges? Are we meant to move toward the state of enlightenment? Why are "learning" and "suffering" such integral parts of the human experience? Indeed, what is the purpose of the experience of life?

These questions have been answered metaphysically, existentially and spiritually for centuries. Regardless of how an individual forms his or her personal conclusions about the purpose of life, the natural intelligence of Life itself flows in a cycle that continually produces challenging experiences that cause us to question our understanding of "reality" and what part we, as individuals, serve within this vast expanse of life.

The conclusions each person draws in response to his or her critical crossroads are completely subjective. My experience has been that those individuals who reach for spiritual insight during these periods emerge more deeply conscious of the possibility that Life is a spiritual journey and that the contributions we make toward our own growth and that of others is of tremendous importance.

Perhaps the paradox that is an integral aspect of suffering can be compared to the insights we are learning through studying ourselves in relation to disease. Specifically, it may be that much of our suffering occurs as a natural result of forgetting that our lives are governed by a spiritual purpose and that when we are out of alignment with that purpose, we enter into a crisis as a way of reevaluating our life's priorities. Similarly, we are discovering that many of the illnesses we create can be avoided through realizing the impact emotional stress has upon our physical bodies.

If there is a reason and purpose to the continual process of conclusions and new beginnings in life, chances are the purpose has more to do with our immortality than it does with our mortality. And to the extent that we lose sight of the demands of our spiritual path, we enter into a fog of great unreasoning and meaningless pain.

Suffering causes our attention to turn inward. Perhaps one of the greatest false goals of life is our belief that we can somehow maneuver our lives in such a way as to avoid difficulties. That is impossible, and living as though it were possible is a belief that certainly leads to the frustration of desiring the impossible. It seems that a more realistic goal is to learn to accept the cycle of Life on its terms, striving to learn from the wisdom built into the natural momentum of conclusions and new beginnings. Rather than expecting life to be something it is not (an unchanging dynamic), it would seem that our tendency to suffer would be greatly diminished if we were able to recognize the spiritual wisdom inherent in the natural, continually *changing* processes of our lives.

PERSONAL SELF VERSUS IMPERSONAL SELF

The personal self is our ego lens to the world. It is the part of us that would like to believe that we are the center of our own universe and, at times, everybody else's. Our personal self is the receptacle of our fears, our needs and our insecurities.

It is also our enthusiastic self, our love of life, our sense of spontaneity. It is the part of us that reaches for relationships, friendships and community involvement. Our personal self is the means through which we experience loving and being loved.

As a rule, we tend to live our lives through the personal lens. Our personal self forms attachments to people, places and things. It rebels against change and prefers to establish a sense of control over all the parts of our lives.

The personal self is an extension of our individual identity and personality. It is that part of ourselves that needs recognition for simply being alive.

The personal self is the part of ourselves that is challenged under crisis because it is the part of ourselves that is capable of acting from fear as well as being consumed by it. While our personal self is an asset in creating the day-to-day experiences of our lives, it is a liability under crisis.

The lens of our impersonal self, however, sees a much broader vista. It is the part of us which is connected to all of humanity and to all of life. It is that part of us which recognizes our place in the whole of life and, as such, can grasp a higher reason and purpose to each of the successive challenges of our lives.

The first wave of crisis for most individuals causes a reaction at the personal level. The diagnosis of a disease, for instance, immediately brings a person's attention to the personal level of one's life: How serious is it? Who and what will be affected? How will I handle this? Who will be there to help me? What about finances and my job? And finally, why me? For what reason is this *happening to me*?

Everyone needs to move through this stage of personal reevaluation. To remain there, consumed with self-pity, fear and anger, is lethal.

The challenge every human being confronts in crisis situations is the challenge of transcendence—of engaging the power of the impersonal self to shake free of the feelings that bad things happen only to you. It is very difficult to break free from the gravity field of self-pity and, for that reason, it is also tempting to remain enmeshed in feelings that, while very real, are exceedingly nonproductive.

Our "impersonal self," on the other hand, is capable of understanding that life is a process into which fall all of our personal experiences. Life is more than the measure of events. It is a process through which we come to know the purposes underlying our experiences. For all of us, life is a teacher, and the lessons it teaches us are remarkably similar.

The means through which we are taught may differ: disease, poverty, wealth, fame, success, failure, marriage, single life. In the long run, none of the particulars matter, since they are props that serve the learning process of that part of us that is larger than our immediate, physical selves.

It is the transcendent or impersonal self that holds the power to heal. I have learned through all of my many experiences with people who are facing serious illnesses that those who are able to separate themselves emotionally from the disease itself gain a tremendous degree of empowerment within the healing process.

For example, it is a natural figure of speech to say, "my backache, my cancer or my breast tumor." The use of the word "my" allows the illness to merge with the other personal aspects of the personality. "My" means attachment, regardless of the argument that a disease is a separate, unwanted presence in the body.

This figure of speech is counterproductive to the healing process. Not only does it suggest that the disease belongs to a person, it also implies permanence, as though the illness has become a part of one's entire being. Making anything personal adds to the difficulty of releasing it.

The healing process is enhanced when a person is able to become impersonal about the presence of an illness. Impersonal does not mean unemotional. Rather, it means aligning our emotions so that they are supportive and not overwhelmed with fear.

Impersonal means that we consider an illness in the same category as we might consider a teacher. The illness has developed because the student needs to learn something or to stop everything else in his or her life long enough to complete an overload of unfinished business. This perception is empowering because it challenges helplessness and offers a person a way of working with the disease rather than collapsing under the weight of being held hostage by it.

How does one accomplish an impersonal attitude? Certainly it is not an easy adjustment to make, emotionally or psychologically because the fears one feels in times of crisis are real, and they do not disintegrate in the blink of an eye. Yet, even though this transition to a higher level of reasoning is not easy, it is *natural*.

The human spirit naturally flows in the direction of that which enhances life. Optimism and humor surface even in the midst of tremendously difficult situations, and that is the energy of the human spirit on a rescue mission.

As one focuses attention on finding a productive and life-enhancing course to follow, it becomes a reality.

RELIGION VERSUS SPIRITUALITY

Faith is essential to the healing process. Without exception, the people I have known who have healed their illnesses credit their faith in God as the core of their strength and ability to heal themselves.

Because faith is such a powerful force, it is important to realize that what we have faith in is of great significance. Not everything a person has faith in necessarily qualifies for positive internal reinforcement. Because of the power of faith, it is critical for people to realize that they also have the power to choose carefully the beliefs they desire to empower. All beliefs, regardless of their source—be it cultural, social or religious—are worthy of being challenged *if they no longer adequately serve us in terms of helping us to cope with the challenges of our lives.*

During the past twenty-five years, a new quality of spiritual awakening has taken root worldwide. The spirituality that has emerged is very closely linked to the holistic health movement because the fundamental principles are identical. Both the teachings of spirituality and the teachings of holistic health direct a person to develop faith in oneself.

Both spirituality and holistic health encourage people to develop faith in their own capacity to create their own reality. From the point of view of spirituality, this marks a shift from traditional religious thinking in that religion encourages faith that is outwardly directed toward a specifically defined God. Spirituality encourages faith that is directed toward the God within so that individuals can explore the creative capacity of their own spirits.

The premise that we create our own reality is, in essence, a spiritual one. This teaching is, to some extent, contrary to religious positions that embrace God as an external being, because spirituality emphasizes a "God-within" reality. As a result, spirituality has redefined the practical application of faith as evidenced by the belief that we can heal ourselves through the power inherent in our own being.

As people recognize that they create their own realities,

the question that inevitably arises is, "Through what source? What is the *source* of this power of creation that runs through my being?"

The answer to this question is not found externally, but internally. The study of our own nature is the study of divinity itself in action, incarnated into each person. One may ask, "How does divinity work through me?" The answer is simple: Look at what you create. That which you create is alive; the life force in all of your acts of creation is expressed through the dynamic of cause and effect. Cause and effect is an *alive* activity. It is your energy in motion and your willpower commanding energy to create matter. What you create is a reflection of your own divinity.

Spirituality is the practice of honoring your relationship to the God-force as a *partnership*—transcending the traditional parent-child relationship that is inherent in most Western religious teachings. This involves reaching for a mature spirituality based upon principles of co-creation and personal responsibility.

The teaching that God exists outside of ourselves has proved repeatedly within my work to be a handicap to people on the healing journey and, in particular, to people who are working with holistic therapies. The reason is that most traditional religious beliefs adhere to the teaching that God, as an external force, determines whether or not a person heals, as well as whether or not a person becomes ill. In some regards, this belief is identical to the position held by traditional physicians that all sources of disease, as well as their cure, exist externally.

As a result of this belief, one automatically directs the power of his or her faith to an external understanding of God. The reason why this hampers the healing process is that it encourages the belief that disease is the result of the will of God rather than the result of the creative power of negativity.

It is remarkably difficult to tap into our own innate powers to heal when we believe simultaneously that God's will is responsible for the development of an illness and, therefore, responsible for its cure. In this situation, where do we place our faith? In ourselves or in the mercy of a God who created this suffering?

The blending of spirituality with the tenets of holistic health provides individuals with a means of understanding how they contribute to the creation of their illness, not as a result of the will of God, but rather as a result of allowing fears and other negative emotions to take charge of their lives. The relationship we develop with the Universe becomes a means of transcending this human value system of reward versus punishment and growing into a relationship based upon the principles of co-creation. The journey of healing, as well as the journey of life, is thereby freed of the burden of feeling victimized by our fate, circumstances or God. Individuals are then able to have faith and hope not only in God, but in themselves as well.

THE WILL TO LIVE VERSUS
THE WILL TO HEAL

In most cases, the first response to the diagnosis of a serious illness is, "I want to live." For most of us, it is incomprehensible that anyone would choose otherwise. And yet, many people have little realization that a vast ocean of inner power separates the will to live from the will to heal. The will to live is a reaction to illness that is generated from the personality. It is largely a fear response that is capable of producing an artificial calm and temporary feelings of courage. The statement, "I want to live" is simply another way of saying, "I don't want to die," but there is very little authentic power present in the will to live.

Wanting to heal requires more than the desire not to die. The will to heal is a far deeper commitment to the healing process. It shows the capacity to enter into the journey of complete transformation of oneself, without compromise or limitations.

A person in the midst of the crisis of an illness discovers that the disease experience automatically ignites the process of reevaluating all of the parts of one's life. This "life review" occurs naturally, like a built-in mechanism that nature provides to assist the body/mind/spirit toward returning to inner harmony.

The areas of one's life that are contributing to the creation of disease pour into one's mind during a life review, as if to say, "Look at this memory, look at this resentment, look at this emotional hurt; this is your opportunity to do something about these feelings." Though this process can be overwhelmingly frightening and painful, it is nonetheless the organic cleansing of one's inner self that must occur in order to heal.

The will to heal is the capacity to face this life review with courage and the resolve to make choices that can lead to the creation of health. For many people, this is the part of the healing process that they cannot fulfill. Confronting one's life openly and honestly inevitably means change. Oftentimes, the prospect of facing the changes necessary for healing is too much for a person to handle, and thus, denial—a characteristic of the will to live—takes over.

Admittedly, if the task of responding honestly to the inner difficulties of our lives were easy, we would all be much healthier. But we are creatures who continually struggle with openness and honesty, and thus, we communicate our inner stresses and unresolved personal issues through the avenue of unconscious communication—namely, disease.

In many cases, the information that is received in an intuitive reading indicates the specific inner stresses that a person is experiencing which have contributed to the creation of a disease. Yet, in the majority of these situations, people choose to continue their stressful patterns despite the outcome of inevitable suffering or even death.

In one instance, a woman suffering from chronic pain, continual anxiety and severe bronchial congestion refused to quit smoking. Her response was that she had tried repeatedly to quit smoking and knew that she simply could not manage without cigarettes. I emphasized to her that she was choosing to remain in pain and ignore the natural warning signs that her body was transmitting to her, which indicated the loss of health to her bronchial area. Nevertheless, she remained a smoker.

Another woman who suffered from arthritis, migraines,

diabetes and obesity, flatly refused to alter her diet in any way. While she bemoaned her drastic weight situation, she said that she never was a person with any willpower, and "that's just the way I am." I pointed out to this woman that she was choosing to live a *lifetime* of constant pain and a doubtless premature death rather than undergo three months of uncomfortable but empowering and health-inducing discipline. Her response was, "That's right."

A man, faced with cancer of the colon, had a lifetime pattern of resentment built around his professional career. From his perspective, he had always been the person overlooked for promotions or any type of increased responsibility and authority at work. His emotional response to this pattern had been to become bitter, withdrawn and very, very angry. As he lay in his hospital bed, he would relive his countless experiences of professional rejection, playing the conversations over and over in his mind of "What I should have said," and "How I should have quit my job long ago or refused to do what I was told." His anger grew more potent as the days went by. His wife and I pointed out to him that while he could not undo the past, this was his opportunity to release these feelings that had tormented him for years and that his life was more valuable than a job promotion. Though he could intellectually grasp the understanding that his anger was harming his body and that he could not heal filled with this deep reservoir of negativity, he felt so justified in being angry that, ultimately, his anger won and he died. All the while, however, he continued to state that he wanted to live. True, he did want to live, but he did not want to heal.

The will to heal is the ability to approach one's life prepared to change and/or let go of all that is not contributing to one's inner well-being. This journey of transformation cannot be done in a compromising manner. It is not enough, for instance, to release negativity only part way, or only partially to forgive someone. And it is not enough to admit that one *knows* what he or she needs to do, but not act on those changes. Disease thrives on procrastination and excuses. The mental response to healing—knowing what one should do but taking no action—is the activity of the will to live; in other words, it is talking one's way through healing rather than actually *doing* anything.

Fortunately—or unfortunately—energy cannot be fooled. It is not possible to lie to oneself in terms of the behavior of energy. Energy is honest—it responds to exactly what is in someone's heart and mind. Even if the heart and mind are in conflict, as is the case with many people, a person's energy will act in accordance with the conflict and the healing process will reflect that inner turmoil.

Healing requires transformation. And for that reason, it should be recognized that healing is a matter of courage. It requires a tremendous amount of inner strength to choose to change familiar patterns of thinking and living, particularly when one is physically weakened. Yet, it must be realized on the part of those facing illness that the will to live—referring to the desire not to die—does not, and cannot, result in health. Healing is a path of action.

TIME VERSUS THE PRESENT MOMENT

Time plays a critical role in the healing process, perhaps far more than most people realize. We are normally very unconscious about the factor of time. Certainly, we are accustomed to thinking in terms of time: It takes time to heal, it takes time for a drug to work, it takes time for people to change.

The healing technologies of the holistic field, however, are challenging our relationship to time. The technique of visualization, for instance, is producing strong evidence that the body responds to the messages of the mind exactly as they are transmitted. Visualizations done in present tense, that is, in the now, are far more effective than are visualizations that build "time" into the healing process. As people visualize their bodies as fully healthy, they are encouraged to image their bodies as healthy *now*—not tomorrow, not in the future and not soon. But *now*.

The implications of this factor of time, as experienced with the technique of visualization, suggest the possibility that healing, as well as the creation of a disease, can occur instantly. This evidence also suggests that the process of creating one's reality is a moment by moment experience that can shift, either positively or negatively, in the proverbial blink of an eye.

While we are literally programmed to look forward in our lives, to plan for tomorrow and to set goals far in advance of where we are at the present moment, the fact is that this practice is detrimental to healing. It may be that focusing a vast amount of attention on our "tomorrows" is also detrimental to the rest of our lives, aside from our health. The reason is that this tendency draws our attention away from what we must deal with in the immediate moment. Rather than responding in a productive manner to our present concerns, whether they be healing our bodies or creating career opportunities, we generate anxiety by projecting our present difficulties into our tomorrows. What we need to realize is that in doing this, we are using our stress to create what we will experience "tomorrow." In other words, projecting ahead instead of living in the present moment keeps our stress, or illness, alive because we "program" it into tomorrow rather than use our energy to heal today.

As we learn more about how we create our realities through the energy of our thoughts and feelings, we can somewhat logically conclude that whatever it is we will face tomorrow is somehow being created today—now—in this present moment. It requires a tremendous amount of discipline to create consciously, that is, to pay attention to what we are feeling, to what we are thinking and to what we are doing, with the understanding that it is these "energies" that influence and give form to our physical realities.

It is particularly crucial to create with consciousness when health is the goal, especially in light of the possibility that creation is an instantaneous process. Perhaps the essence of "miracle cures" resides in the ability to focus our attention so clearly and thoroughly in the present moment that the condition of disease is immediately transformed.

ILLNESS AS TEACHER

In certain instances, an illness or a handicap exists in a person's life not as a result of negativity but as a necessary vehicle that the soul requires in order to accomplish his or her life's task. Helen Keller is perhaps the most dramatic example of this type of situation. Her "handicaps" proved to be her greatest gifts, ones from which all of humanity has benefited.

There are many such instances in which people courageously respond to the apparent limitations of their physical bodies by developing the extraordinary capacities of their spirits. They exist as inspirations for each of us who requires proof that the true strength and power of the human being resides within the human spirit.

THE CHALLENGE OF RESPONSIBILITY

Health is our most precious commodity. No matter how much material success a person has, or regardless of the highs that are a part of an exciting career, if a person's physical body is racked with pain or disease, the pleasures of the physical world are meaningless.

Yet, what has become the greatest mystery to me in my work with people who are confronting illness is how frequently individuals will choose to continue unhealthy habits of mind, body or spirit *knowing* that these habits are contributing to illness. To put this another way, I have come to realize that the promise of health does not necessarily motivate a person either to heal or to change habits that almost certainly guarantee the creation of an illness.

Curiously, not even intense states of pain nor the threat of death are able to motivate some people to change their lifestyles. Repeatedly, I have had experiences with individuals who know what they should do, but choose to continue what they are doing rather than change. They prefer to rely upon drugs, surgery or mental games rather than create more productive lifestyle patterns.

After years of being perplexed by this phenomenon and

frustrated with people who *could be healthy but choose otherwise*, I have concluded that the promise of becoming a healthy person, (and all that that means—vital, energetic, pain-free) is not the ultimate motivator for change that many might think it is. Health is the result of a commitment to live a more conscious life—to become more responsible for one's emotional health and well-being—and that is the overwhelming challenge to many people.

Certainly, this commentary does not apply to everyone. There are numerous people who are extremely conscious about their health habits. And there are numerous people who participate very consciously in their healing process. However, my experience has been that the majority of individuals with whom I have worked find the challenge of transforming their stressful patterns to be an overwhelming ordeal. For many, this represents too much change, too suddenly. Consequently, the older, more familiar patterns of thinking and behaving remain dominant.

A physician who is very much a part of the holistic model of health care remarked to me that he has no argument whatsoever with approaching healing through holistic concepts. His difficulty is getting his patients to recognize the value in seeing the connection between their emotional stresses and the health of their physical bodies. He concluded that, in the majority of cases, his patients remained closed to holistic thinking because it seemed like "too much work" and they preferred, instead, to rely on the doctor to heal their illness.

There is a profound lesson about human nature contained in this dynamic and that is the lesson of compassion. Built into each of our lives are countless challenges that highlight what we fear and what we find difficult to confront. Regardless of what these challenges are, the underlying purpose inherent in every one of these situations is the opportunity to respond in ways that increase our awareness of our own inner strength and power.

Given this perspective, it is possible to consider that all of us continually exist within the process of healing. Indeed, the journey of life could be thought of as a journey of healing, accomplished step by step through the acquisition of self-knowledge and personal awareness.

At times, the healing taking place in someone is obvious because it has produced a physical dysfunction that needs attention. But in many individuals, the healing process they are involved in is occurring outside the experience of a physical illness.

The personal crises that fill our lives are all opportunities to release patterns of fear and negativity that stand in the way of our becoming whole and empowered. The condition of physical illness is just one of several responses we can create as a result of how we cope with these challenges.

We are accustomed to believing that genuine healing has occured ONLY WHEN the physical body has returned to either a pain-free or disease-free condition. Just as we undervalue the role that our emotional and psychological factors play in the development of an illness, we also undervalue the healing of our inner selves as not being authentic. If we do not see "proof" of healing on the physical level, we tend to disregard the possibility that any degree of healing has occurred. Yet, healing, most often, is a gradual process of returning to balance in which the inner steps necessary for a person's recovery to full health are taken bit by bit.

In truth, each of our lives contains fears, confusion and pain. In this, we are all identical. It is not necessary to become physically ill to realize we are often controlled by insecurities. The experiences in our lives—our relationships, our careers, our lifestyles—all contain elements of what frightens us. Knowing this provides us with a scope of genuine compassion so that when we are with someone who is ill, including ourselves, we are able to realize that they (or we) are in the process of healing much more than just the physical body. Whether illness strikes in our bodies or in our individual life environments, it brings to each of us the same challenge—to heal that which we fear about ourselves and about life. And regardless of where and how we encounter our illnesses, the path of genuine healing will always direct us toward expanding our capacity to take more responsibility for our inner selves and the power of creation that exists within us.

UNDERSTANDING
THE ORIGIN
OF DISEASE

CHAPTER SIX

The Popular Way to Die: The Big Three—Heart Disease, Cancer and Stroke

(S h e a l y a n d M y s s)

HEART ATTACK

(S h e a l y)

Heart attack, the common name for this most prevalent disease, suggests a more metaphysical cause than science has accorded. Why do we call it an "attack"? I suspect that this word goes back many centuries since sometimes individuals who are having a coronary occlusion, or heart attack, grasp the chest, and it must have appeared to someone many years ago that the individual was trying to pull off an attacker. The word "attack" is still used in medicine, although coronary occlusion and myocardial infarction are the more scientific terms.

The number one cause of death in the United States and most of the Western world, heart attacks are most often thought to be the result of hardening of the arteries or atherosclerosis. In general, atherosclerosis is thought to be caused from deposits of cholesterol in the walls of the blood vessels. When the heart is affected, a blood vessel becomes occluded and a "heart attack" or myocardial infarction occurs. High levels of blood cholesterol and low levels of HDL (high density lipoprotein) are major predisposing factors. The precipitating factor is probably a surge of adrenalin.

Statistically, cigarette smoking is the greatest single associated factor in setting the stage for a heart attack. Smoking causes an 84% increase in adrenalin. Smokers are four to five times as likely to suffer a heart attack. Smoking is not specific for heart disease; it is a catalyst for most diseases, including cancer of the lungs, bladder and cervix, emphysema, flu, bronchitis, pneumonia and even wrinkles. Most of the inflammatory diseases or "itis" illnesses are increased in smokers. The generalized nature of these illnesses results from inhibition of prostaglandin E1, a natural, powerful anti-inflammatory agent damaged by nicotine. As indicated above, nicotine is also a powerful stimulant of adrenalin production.

Coffee intake, when it exceeds five cups per day, is similarly risky. And there is some evidence that excessive coffee consumption is associated with an increased incidence of cancer of the pancreas as well as heart attacks. Caffeine, the chemical pick-me-up of coffee, is a strong stimulant of adrenalin production.

To some extent, the degree of obesity is correlated with the likelihood of coronary artery disease. A weight of more than 10% above ideal shortens life expectancy. Obesity is also associated with an increased incidence of high blood pressure, diabetes and stroke. And obesity increases adrenalin production.

Atherosclerosis is also highly associated with nutrition. Both a high fat diet, especially animal fats, and a high sugar diet are associated with increased heart disease. Low levels of fiber, sugar and fat are also associated with increased cancer of the colon and breast, diabetes, gall stones, appendicitis, high blood pressure, varicose veins, hemorrhoids, diverticulosis and adrenalin production.

Type-A personality and depression are also psychological contributors to heart disease. Time-conscious, excessively driven Type-A individuals share with depression and "hot reactors" an excessive amount of adrenalin. In the final analysis, heart disease seems to be one of the prime stress diseases. But note that the *stress* reaction, basically an increase in adrenalin, is created by physical, chemical and emotional pressures. And even physical inactivity was reported by Hans Selye to produce a stress reaction. An inactive lifestyle is also associated with coronary heart disease.

In addition to heart attacks, there are dozens of other diseases of the heart, ranging from congenital malformation to bacterial and viral infections, defects in the valves of the heart, congestive heart failure, or dropsy, and irregularities of rate and rhythm. Various and sundry etiologies are suspected for the plethora of heart diseases. Admittedly, however, the spiritual or metaphysical crises are not generally included in the differential diagnosis of heart disease or any other disease!

Indeed, it is the "why" that intrigues me as a scientist. Why me? Why that patient? Why not another patient who seems to be even more obese, who smokes even more and who has a stronger family history of illness? James Lynch's wonderful book, *The Broken Heart*, comes closer, in my opinion, to the real cause of most coronary artery occlusion than either Type-A behavior or low HDL cholesterol.

Some individuals appear to be much more what Dr. Robert Elliott has called "hot reactors." They respond to relatively minor stresses with a great physiological response: increased pulse rate, increased blood pressure, increased output of adrenalin or epinephrine or norepinephrine. I suspect from clinical observations that these individuals also tend to be more psychothymic in their personality. That is, they have more mood swings from high to low. Thus, they are affected more by depression, and it is my strong suspicion that the depth of depression is the time when a heart attack manifests itself.

My father was an example of this. He was divorced suddenly by my mother after over twenty-four years of marriage. He went into a deep depression. He had always smoked two and one-half packs of cigarettes per day, and his cigarette smoking increased to about three packs per day after the divorce. Fifteen months later he was remarried. On his honeymoon, he suffered his first of three heart attacks. He had married on the rebound, and it was not a happy marriage. Eventually, it led to his second divorce.

My father was never willing to give up cigarette smoking and, in fact, said to me on more than one occasion, "I'd rather be dead than quit smoking." He remained severely depressed and died of his third heart attack. One *could* blame it upon his family history; five out of six brothers died of heart attacks between the ages of fifty and fifty-four. Or one could blame it on these other factors: He drank three to five cups of coffee a day; he smoked three packs of cigarettes a day; he ate a high fat diet; and he was very active in business but did not do any specific physical exercise. On the other hand, I believe that it was primarily the depression resulting from the divorce of my mother that precipitated the specific heart attack.

Ultimately, as I see it, when we choose our parents (and I believe that we choose our parents on a spiritual level before we are born), we set up a genetic code. If you have chosen a family history that has a particularly weak cardiovascular system, especially as related to the heart, then you need particularly to pay attention to nutrition, physical exercise and mental attitude.

The "No Fat Added Diet" is my recommendation for a nutritional program, and this will be discussed in detail in a later chapter. Physical exercise also will be discussed, but exercise needs to be emphasized here for those who have a genetic predisposition to cardiovascular disease above almost any other illness, with the possible exception of depression.

THE ENERGY FACTORS RELATING TO HEART DISEASE

(Myss)

The energy perspective of illness differs from the physical interpretation of disease in that an energy evaluation is naturally inclusive of the whole process of life and not limited to understanding the activity of one particular organ or system. As such, it is necessary to discuss the creation of illness or health within a framework that accommodates the issues and cycles of life. The fundamental principles of the holistic paradigm of health suggest that health and disease are the natural extensions of how well we live and cope with the demands of our entire lives.

From that perspective, then, let us discuss the energy factors related to heart disease.

We are, by nature, a tribal species. We need each other and we need to be needed by each other. We need to give love as well as receive love. We thrive when we are loved and we are diminished in strength and vitality without love.

Yet in spite of the simplicity of our needs, we remain deeply confused about the nature of love. It seems that we have separated our natural capacity to love and be loving from the activity of living. Most, if not all, of us exist somewhere between the simplicity of our needs and the complexity of our fears and insecurities that share the space of our hearts.

It is no surprise, then, that heart disease is the leading cause of death in this country, as well as in several other nations. We are more accustomed to disguising, denying and protecting our emotions than we are to understanding and fulfilling them. The demands of our societies, and therefore our lives, are such

that we lead with either our fears and insecurities or our intel-
lects—or both.

We are afraid of our emotions, as several psychologists in
recent years have noted. But why? What is the power inherent
in our emotional natures that is so frightening? One answer is
that opening up emotionally makes us vulnerable and we do
not like to be vulnerable. That is perhaps an accurate answer,
but not a sufficient one.

Emotions have the power to cause us to be honest in ways
that do not necessarily serve the demands of our lives nor our
way of living. Emotions tell the truth. If we open ourselves to
feel what others are feeling, we then must either act on that
input or consciously act against it, thereby denying our own
emotional experience. This is valid both in terms of how we
interact within our personal lives and how we interact in the
larger, impersonal area of our institutions. Consider that we go
to great lengths to keep emotional input out of business, politics,
government and other major decision-making institutions. We
are, as a whole, not prepared to respond to the emotional input
of other people and of the other kingdoms of life.

Consequently, we live more according to the demands of
self-protection than the requirements of our emotional nature.
We require openness, honesty, love and trust. We live according
to the limitations of fear. To put this another way, we spend
more energy acting *against* ourselves than in harmony with the
essential loving design of our species.

From my perspective, this is the reason that heart disease
is the leading cause of death. Because we so fear living according
to what our emotional natures require, we have become desen-
sitized to the reality that we *are* emotional beings and not just
intellectual decision-making systems of flesh and bones.

The statistics on heart disease serve as evidence that our
natures are not going to change to accommodate the demands
of our society and our fearful way of living. It would appear
that if we truly intend to understand the root cause of heart

disease, we need to begin with evaluating what is preventing the natural flow of love through each person's life.

A discussion of four major heart illnesses is included in order to illustrate more specifically the emotional stresses that contribute to the creation of these diseases.

ENERGY ANALYSIS OF HEART ATTACK

(Myss)

A heart attack is literally an attack of the heart chakra brought about through the inability of the individual to acknowledge, and therefore process, the emotional stresses of his or her life. The key to focus on is "process"—the ability to handle emotional reactions. People who prefer not to think about the meaning or significance of the events and relationships of their lives (usually because it upsets them or they feel unable to control matters) are more prone to create heart attacks than are people who know how to cope with internal stress. In the language of energy, a heart attack is an explosion of energy attempting to break through or break down an emotional barrier that a person has created.

What creates this type of block? In general, the energy behind a heart attack is mainly caused by warehousing fears and anger related to a sense of failure, the inability to meet the increasing emotional demands of personal relationships, and the inability to process emotional disappointments in relationships. Also strongly associated with heart attack personalities is the need to maintain control. Logically, the fear of losing control, or of having control and responsibilities taken away, is extremely common in people prone to heart attacks.

As these emotions build in a person's body, the stress levels brought about by intense fears and feelings of anger create "walls" around the heart. The individual, usually unconsciously, begins to warehouse his or her fears and anger and focus attention even more intently upon the external circumstances of his or her life.

People inclined toward creating heart attacks have in common a tendency to believe that they can handle anything that occurs in their lives (self-control) and therefore are not open to discussing their stresses prior to the experience of a heart attack. It is also very difficult for these individuals to admit having feelings that relate to fear of failure. There is embarrassment and shame associated with these feelings and, therefore, discussing them is doubly difficult, if not impossible.

The tendency toward harsh judgments is also a characteristic that contributes to the stress of the heart area. Judgmentalism is frequently combined with anger, fear and prejudice. The attitude that a group of people, or an individual, or some other form of life has less value that oneself is an attitude that results in negative thought and action.

An individual with the characteristics described is usually not prone to self-examination of these attitudes. Rather, what is more common is a strong emotional denial mechanism that prevents the person from registering the natural body signals that are transmitted when the body has reached a level of stress intake that places health at risk. These signals are always emotional in nature—namely, an increase of anxiety and restlessness, the inability to sleep and depression.

This general dysfunction relates to an inability to release emotional injuries and past hurts. Forgiveness also is difficult, and the more prevalent tendency in people susceptible to heart attacks is to hold on to resentments rather than to work consciously toward releasing these experiences.

CONGESTIVE HEART FAILURE

It is essential to derive a sense of satisfaction from what we do and from the relationships in our personal lives. When this inner sense is absent, we often say, "My heart's just not in this any more." That expression, used so casually, communicates not only a feeling we all can relate to very easily, but also a very real physical stress. It implies that what a person is doing in terms of occupation, or the quality of that individual's relationship(s), is sadly lacking in emotional health. The need to fulfill one's heart's desire is not satisfied. And the result of this is "emotional congestion," usually accompanied by depression, melancholy and strong feelings of being detached from one's life. This creates congestive heart failure.

BLOCKED ARTERIES

Blocked arteries, as a rule, are created through the warehousing of guilt feelings and fears related to disappointing the expectations of others. Guilt weighs heavily on a person's consciousness and, like cement being poured slowly into someone's body, it eventually hardens.

MITRAL VALVE PROLAPSE

This condition is common in women and is rapidly on the increase. This dysfunction is created through an inability to recognize and therefore respond to one's personal needs. We, as human beings, are meant to explore and develop our emotions. In the process of doing this, we develop ourselves to our fullest potential. We challenge our fears, we move forward with creative expression and we grow.

Just as heart attacks relate more to the emotional fears and patterns of anger that are prevalent in men, mitral valve prolapse also is rooted in emotional denial but lacks the intense levels of anger that are required to generate a heart attack. This is a condition of emotional confusion and frustration, of not knowing how to direct one's emotions, and of continually not having one's own emotional needs met with satisfaction.

A WORD ABOUT BROKEN HEARTS

Broken hearts are real. Every human being has his or her limits when it comes to absorbing grief, hurt, rejection and despair.

While children are remarkably resilient, their hearts can be shattered easily. Without the developed ability to understand why they are neglected, abused or criticized, children absorb negativity in their hearts.

Adults have their limitations as well. There does come a point at which a person is incapable of "getting up again," of trying one more time to recover from the loss or absence of love in one's life. This is the crisis of a broken heart, and it can create a heart attack—it can stop the heart completely.

CASE REPORTS

RICHARD

(S h e a l y)

Diagnoses: Myocardial infarction; hypertension; obesity; ruptured intervertebral disc.

This fifty-six-year-old businessman considered himself in good health except for chronic high blood pressure. When first seen, he had a blood pressure reading of 170/100, and at 5'11" in height, he weighed 263. Despite adequate treatment and autogenic training, biofeedback and recommendations for appropriate nutrition to achieve his desirable weight, the patient did not follow the program outlined. There was a significant conflict in his marriage brought about through his wife's attitudes, which he described as rigid and restrictive. He was not willing, however, to get into a discussion of his marital problems.

Eight months later, Richard suffered a heart attack. He recovered from that and has since lost sixty pounds. He has no residual cardiac symptoms. He still has not dealt with the marital discord, and it is of some interest that, more recently, he has suffered a prolonged bout of low back pain and sciatica. Also, about a year after recovery from the heart attack, Richard developed an acute ruptured disc, which responded to conservative therapy.

ENERGY ANALYSIS

(Myss)

Richard is an individual whose emotional development has not expanded to include the capacity to cope with the needs of another person, specifically, his wife. His temperament is such that he finds thinking about personal problems and deeper reasons for stress a source of irritation and frustration. As a result of Richard's emotional makeup, he is prone to episodes of rage and anger. He emotionally withdraws from his wife when he is angry and is inclined to blame others for not changing to accommodate his needs.

Underneath these unproductive behavioral patterns are fears of criticism and failure that are strongly embedded in Richard's consciousness. He associates introspection and the willingness to discuss problems with "giving in" and admitting he is wrong. Therefore, he was closed to any suggestions of discussion since this frightened him at a very deep level. There was very little room for compromise in Richard's attitudes and in the manner in which he expressed wanting to live his life. As his marriage progressed and his wife continued to change and develop herself, he found her changes threatening to their familiar pattern of marriage. From the perspective of energy blockages, these stresses were the contributing factors to his heart condition.

Following his heart attack, which was a traumatic form of emotional release, Richard continued with his attitudes of anger and resentment over his inability to control his wife's life. As described in Chapter Four, issues of control over the activity of another person reside in the second chakra area. The second chakra corresponds to the sexual organs of the body as well as to the hips and lower back. Richard transferred his stress to his hip joint, producing sciatica. Sciatica, an inflamed nerve ending, is created from anger or frustration over a situation that one cannot "stand" any longer but one feels unable to change it.

Eventually, the anger he was warehousing in this area of his body spread to his spine and he created a ruptured disc.

FREDA

(S h e a l y)

Diagnosis: Mitral valve prolapse.

This thirty-five-year-old teacher consulted with us in December 1986, complaining of fatigue and insomnia. She has a lifelong history of exercise intolerance and had recently been under marked increased stress in her job. She is in her second marriage and says that she has a very satisfactory relationship.

At my suggestion, a consultation was obtained with Caroline. According to Caroline's information, Freda's dysfunction was related to emotional trauma that was unresolved and therefore plagued her unconscious.

At first, the patient felt that she had not had any major love trauma. However, during the consultation, she mentioned to me that she had had a previous marriage that had been unhappy. Her husband had been verbally abusive. When she finally got up the courage to tell him that she was leaving him, he actually physically abused her. Even after the divorce, she continued to live in fear of him.

Interestingly, one year later, he died in an accident. She admitted that she felt both a sense of sadness and a sense of relief, since she no longer needed to be afraid of him. Also of interest, Caroline noted that Freda exhibited repressed sexual energy. I asked her how often she was having sexual relations with her husband, and it turned out that she and her husband have had sexual relations an average of once a month during the past year. She felt that it was because of her fatigue and insomnia but did not feel that it had created a strain on her marriage.

ENERGY ANALYSIS

(Myss)

Freda's energy was depleted of vitality at the time of her reading. The pattern of avoiding her deeper feelings and emotional needs, which she had developed during her first marriage, was contributing to her exhaustion and increased irritability. Because she was now involved in a harmonious and loving relationship, Freda preferred to close the door on her previous marriage, thereby leaving her unfinished business to settle into her unconscious mind.

During the years of her first marriage, her relationship with her husband became more and more distant. When she would try to speak to him about what she was feeling, he became critical of her or changed the subject. This man was a person who found emotional discussions very threatening. As a result of this severe lack of communication and emotional support, the marriage disintegrated. Each resented the other. Freda responded by becoming more withdrawn and cold, and he responded with critical attacks and hostility.

My sense of Freda's condition is that she had to reduce her own awareness of what she was feeling and of how deeply she was hurting in order to cope with the lack of emotional support in her marriage. She began to deny her own feelings by telling herself that "Things could be worse," or "I'll be all right; I've always been able to handle things," or "Maybe I expect too much."

Eventually, the emotional blockades Freda had created led to her condition of mitral valve prolapse. Her relationship with her first husband had left her feeling emotionally rejected. When she married a second time, Freda feared intimacy as much as she was drawn to it. She still had unfinished business with her first marriage that related to healing herself and releasing the residual fear and anger. Even though she continued in her pattern of telling herself that "It wasn't so bad," this emotional confusion was, in my opinion, the root cause of her fatigue and exhaustion.

FRANK

(S h e a l y)

Diagnosis: Coronary artery disease with angina pectoris.

This forty-one-year-old ex-priest had left the priesthood one and one-half years earlier and had married an ex-nun. He gradually developed severe angina pectoris, which prevented him from walking more than a few hundred feet without developing chest pain.

He had been seen by a cardiologist and had a stress test that indicated severe coronary artery disease. He was strongly urged to have a coronary angiography and a cardiac bypass. The patient did not wish to undergo the surgical procedure and felt that his problem was due to cumulative stress.

He was approximately twenty-five pounds overweight and had been through tremendous social changes in the previous two years. He was treated with a low fat diet, autogenic training, biofeedback and counseling. Within two weeks, he was able to walk two miles. Since that time, he has had only one or two episodes of angina pectoris and has continued to do well.

Frank is currently pursuing a Ph.D. in Counseling Psychology.

ENERGY ANALYSIS

(M y s s)

Major life changes are traumatic, regardless of how prepared one believes he or she is to cope with them. Under the best of circumstances, it is not easy to let go of familiar roles and obligations. One's mental, emotional, psychological and spiritual patterns can continue to function according to the old form even though the old form is no longer appropriate to who you are and what you want. Time and patience are required in large measure during the transition periods, along with the capacity to anticipate episodes of emotional confusion, uncertainty, disappointment and guilt.

Frank's decision to leave the priesthood and to marry represents the crisis of a major life change. It marked the ending of an entire way of being in the world and a releasing of ordained responsibilities.

Even though Frank felt that his decision to leave the priesthood was appropriate for him, he found himself confronting the challenge of starting over again in the outside world. The persona of being a priest, and all that that role communicates in terms of identity and what one represents to the outside world, no longer existed.

Frank had to face the challenge of finding himself all over again and of shedding his former identity and role that had become so familiar to him. This meant shifting values and goals and creating a totally different plan for his future. Moreover, leaving the priesthood is similar to a divorce in that it represents the termination of a bond made from a deeply felt heart commitment.

The stress of this transition brought about Frank's heart condition, as he himself was aware. The fact that he realized the connection between his inner stress and his physical condition gave him an edge on healing his condition, as he could immediately benefit from a stress-reduction program.

STROKE

(Shealy)

A stroke is diagnosed where there is sudden focal loss of brain function. Most often it includes weakness or paralysis of an arm and/or leg and frequently is associated with difficulty speaking. Loss of vision, numbness, epilepsy, tremor and unconsciousness are all potential results of a stroke. Although strokes are often the result of atherosclerotic blockage of a blood vessel to or in the brain, similar symptoms may result from hemorrhage. And hemorrhage may occur from spontaneous rupture of a blood vessel, high blood pressure, an aneurysm (congenital defect in blood vessel), a blow to the head or even any one of a dozen or more illnesses indicating damage to the blood clotting mechanism. Also, some metabolic chemical problems may mimic a stroke.

Just as heart attack is the result of lifestyle, stroke also is significantly related to similar habits. High blood pressure is a major precursor. High blood pressure occurs primarily from obesity, excessive consumption of salt or inadequate intake of calcium and magnesium. Psychological hyperreactivity with excess norepinephrine (adrenalin) is a key factor in high blood pressure. The average American eats 10 to 20 grams of salt per day. The ideal is 2 grams.

Diabetes is another major contributor to atherosclerosis and stroke. Most diabetes is preventable or reversible with a high complex carbohydrate (starch), high fiber, low fat diet combined with adequate exercise and good mental retraining.

As in all major illnesses, smoking has a tremendous negative influence and almost doubles the chance of having a stroke. Finally, excess alcohol intake is statistically associated with a higher incidence of stroke.

Differentially, then, physicians must look for a potential *treatable* cause of the sudden neurologic catastrophe. This particular diagnosis is often called a "cerebrovascular accident" or CVA, a remarkable misnomer. Except for some trauma, it can rarely be considered an "accident." It is of considerable interest that the strict medical terminology is cerebral vascular accident.

Given these considerations, one cannot help but wonder why a person with a blood pressure of 230/140 does not have a stroke, whereas another person with a blood pressure of 160/95 has a stroke. Surely it cannot be only a genetic predisposition.

It appears to me that the total psychological and social stress of the individual is a more likely precipitating factor. Perhaps the level of adrenalin at a given moment provides the trigger. Unexpressed and unresolved anger and resentment are key co-creators of high blood pressure. "Terminal" frustration also may be the trigger for a stroke.

ENERGY ANALYSIS OF STROKE

(Myss)

As Norm described, a stroke causes a sudden loss of brain function. The question I focus on when doing a health evaluation is, "What would cause an individual to shut off the activity of the brain?"

As in most illnesses, a warehouse of negative energy is amassed prior to the dysfunction physically manifesting. The specific patterns of stressful behavior I have noted that contribute to the creation of a stroke relate to having a dominant and oftentimes obsessive need to control one's physical environment. This pattern develops in a person who finds it difficult, if not impossible, to trust the intention or activities of others. The marked lack of trust is a very significant factor in the creation of a stroke.

Because lack of trust is a major issue, certain fears become a compulsion. Specifically, the individual continually fears for his or her own financial and material security and well-being. Sometimes this is a conscious fear and sometimes it is unconscious. This fear has strong associations with feelings of vulnerability and the belief that the external world is unsafe. Consequently, it becomes crucial to be the person in charge of all decisions and all activity in one's work and living environment.

These patterns of fear and compulsive feelings of distrust cause a specific physical reaction in the body. As the energy of these negative stresses accumulates, it triggers charged emotional responses in the form of frustration, rage, anger and, of course, fear. The individual is challenged to remain "in control" while these high-voltage currents of electrical energy are racing through the body, like the explosive energy of a geyser waiting to burst through the earth. This energy can be temporarily released in small dosages through several conventional channels, such as emotional outbursts, reestablishing control in the business or home environment, alcohol or other means that bring temporary relief.

The reality is that what this type of temperament requires is behavioral modification that allows the individual to cope with daily stress effectively rather than internalizing it and allowing emotional explosions (or implosions) to act as release mechanisms.

When a stroke does occur, it is an indication that the individual can no longer process the effects brought about by the particularly threatening or overwhelming stimuli from the outside world. The energy causes an eruption to occur and the brain shuts down. It is important to note that while the emotional stresses that create a stroke in people are remarkably similar, this similarity does not transfer to personality types. In other words, if one were to apply the description of stroke characteristics to human personalities, one would assume that only Type-A extroverts are stroke candidates. That is inaccurate. Internal stress of this nature is just as likely to be found in a mild-tempered individual as it is in a person with an explosive personality. It is easy to make false assumptions about these gentler individuals simply because they tend to internalize rather than externalize their stresses.

CASE REPORTS

ROGER

(Shealy)

This fifty-two-year-old attorney was examined for left-sided facial pain. He had a history of a stroke in 1981, at which time he developed paralysis of the left arm and leg. The leg and arm recovered, but he continued to experience pain on the left side of his face, which is generally called thalamic pain syndrome. Although he had no high blood pressure, he had had diabetes for five years at the time of his stroke. The patient responded well to d-phenylalanine with virtually total control of his pain.

ENERGY ANALYSIS

(M y s s)

Roger's energy indicated that he was experiencing an accumulation of stress brought about through wanting to take on more professional responsibilities. He faced the challenge of having to release authority to other individuals in the law firm in order to meet his own expanding obligations. This was a particularly difficult challenge for Roger since he had always taken full responsibility for his clients.

It is important to note the significance of diabetes. Though we will be discussing this disease in depth in a later chapter, it must be pointed out that diabetes is a disorder that is connected to issues of responsibility. There are several variations of the types of responsibility issues that contribute to diabetes, and in Roger's case they had to do with the belief that releasing responsibility to other people implied that one was failing to fulfill professional commitments.

According to the findings of his energy evaluation, the combination of his issues regarding the sharing of authority with his need to be personally in charge and responsible for all professional activities brought about the crisis of a stroke.

ALICE

(S h e a l y)

This seventy-four-year-old lady was experiencing problems of severe left and central abdominal pain, which had been present for eight years. Because of her pain, she had an exploratory operation and a partial removal of her colon two years earlier, even though no specific abnormality was noted. The operation had been done with the intention of bringing her pain, of unknown cause, under control.

The patient was first seen by us in September 1984, and her pain was reduced 50-60% with acupuncture, autogenic training and biofeedback. In August 1985, she had a stroke with loss of vision, decreased hearing, slurring of speech and paralysis of the right arm and leg. She regained most of the use of her arm and leg. Following that stroke, her pain became much worse and she has been less well controlled with continuing acupuncture.

ENERGY ANALYSIS

(Myss)

The energy reading on Alice indicated that once she became seventy years old, her concern over her capacity to take care of herself increased dramatically. In particular, Alice feared becoming financially and physically dependent. Because this fear became such a powerful force in her consciousness, Alice started to lose confidence in herself to the extent that usual activities of her life began to become potential health threats to her. Ultimately, she lost all sense of physical safety and her tremendous sense of vulnerability took over, resulting in a stroke.

LARRY

(Shealy)

This seventy-year-old man developed severe pain in the left buttocks and hip area one year following a stroke that had left him paralyzed in the left arm and left leg. He had regained 50% of function in those extremities. His pain continued despite extensive and intensive physical therapy, acupuncture and local nerve blocks, as well as transcutaneous electrical nerve stimulation. The patient tended to be rather irritable and refused to quit smoking.

ENERGY ANALYSIS

(M y s s)

Larry's energy revealed that he had always been determined to have his own way in his life, regardless of how reasonable or unreasonable his choices were. He found cooperation impossible and, in almost every situation, he perceived all external dynamics as "power plays." As a result, Larry could not trust anyone or anything in the outside world. He was suspicious of everyone's motivations and found it difficult to listen to the suggestions of others, even medical professionals, who offered him assistance. Because of his temperament and general outlook on life, Larry was easily threatened by change and certainly by the loss of control over his life and environment. His stroke was brought about through these stresses combined with his highly angry temperament.

KATIE

(S h e a l y)

This thirty-six-year-old lady has a Ph.D. in learning disabilities and teaches this subject. Six years ago, about one week following a mild case of flu, she developed sudden paralysis of the left side of her body along with confusion that cleared over a several-month period. She was left with mild clumsiness of the left side and an intense feeling of internal discomfort, especially in the left side of her face.

ENERGY ANALYSIS

(M y s s)

Katie's reading indicated that she was a compulsive over-achiever with a strong need to gain a position of authority in her field. Her professional ambitions consumed her thinking processes, most often to the exclusion of her emotional needs. Katie believed that her intellectual accomplishments satisfied and *controlled* her emotional needs. As a result, she was not inclined to give her internal emotional concerns the attention required to enable her to work through her fears related to her need to accomplish.

Under stress, Katie tended to focus her attention on what was happening in her professional environment rather than developing techniques adequately to challenge her insecurities. Eventually, the stress overloaded her system and her brain shut down. It was, unfortunately, a very dramatic means through which to signal Katie that her emotional nature needed as much attention as her intellectual development.

CANCER: THE EPIDEMIC OF GUILT AND FEAR

(S h e a l y)

Cancer is the third most common cause of death and, prior to AIDS, the most feared disease in the Western world. Scientifically, it is generally conceded that most, or all, human beings produce cancer cells daily. A *relatively* healthy immune system destroys these cells most of the time. Ultimately, cancer represents a defect in the body's complex of Killer Cells, T-Cells, B-Cells and antibodies.

But what triggers this defect? Strong correlations have been demonstrated with chemical toxins, genetics, excess radiation, nutrition, viral infections and depression. Cigarette smoking is a common "culprit" in cancer of the lungs, bladder and cervix. High fat, low fiber diet is associated with cancer of the breast, uterus and colon. Excess sunlight exposure is responsible for an increased incidence of skin cancer. Inadequate beta carotene (vitamin A) and low levels of vitamin E and vitamin C are found in most cancer patients.

To most scientists and clinicians, however, the overwhelming evidence that depression clobbers the immune system is apparently threatening because it raises the probability that cancer, the most dreaded and "physical" disease, is just as "psychosomatic" as a peptic ulcer. Recent studies in psychoneuroimmunology may make earlier extensive psychological research more respectable. Of some interest, also, is the observation that individuals with allergies are *less* likely to develop cancer. Their immune systems are "overactive."

It is now widely reported that cancer often is diagnosed one to two years following a devastating emotional crisis. Indeed, 75% of the cancer patients I've treated have reported that they actually wanted to die for the six to twenty-four-plus months previous to the diagnosis. Such an overt admission of a "death-wish," the ultimate emotional trauma, usually has been considered the fabric of a psychoanalyst's couch and certainly an attitude lacking any impact upon the physical body.

Such traumas most frequently reported in individuals prior to a cancer diagnosis include: divorce; death of a spouse, child, parent or close friend; sudden job loss (which includes loss of security, authority and social prestige); absence or loss of meaning in one's life; any major social disruption or trauma; loss of home; rape; severe financial loss or gain; disruption of roots (moving); and emotional rejection.

Most of us feel secure emotionally when there is relatively little change. We crave stability. In a society in which, in one generation, we have lost the extended family and the nuclear family, almost any additional change becomes more threatening to our sense of security or to the *illusion* we maintain of having control over our lives. These events cause us to realize the limitations we have over control of external events, circumstances and people. Many of the changes described above can provoke feelings of guilt, failure and/or just plain fear of the unknown.

ENERGY ANALYSIS OF CANCER

(Myss)

Through my work, I have come to believe that cancer is created through excessive fears, guilt feelings, the inability to cope with change, self-hate or denial, and unfinished business. All five of these "root causes" have one crucial element in common in the manner in which they affect people. They each cause a major disruption to occur in an individual's emotional, psychological and spiritual development. In other words, when the natural cycle of growth is interfered with, unnatural growth occurs in the form of cancer cells.

In my opinion, cancer, more than any other illness, teaches us that we are alive in order to learn and that it is essential for us to challenge those obstacles that prevent us from exploring our own development. When cancer forms, it is an indication that something taking place inside of us has sufficient force to prevent us either from successfully entering into the next phase of our lives or from furthering our emotional, psychological and spiritual growth. Health cannot tolerate prolonged obstacles to one's growth.

Nor can we hope to fulfill ourselves if we essentially do not like ourselves. Rather than giving ourselves necessary care and attention, we will treat ourselves (consciously or unconsciously) as unwanted and unloved people. We will create relationships and experiences that do to us exactly what we are doing to ourselves. And chances are, we will blame "life" for our unfortunate conditions rather than look to ourselves as the source of our difficulties.

In my workshops, I often teach participants to imagine that their bodies are like an enormous piece of cheesecloth. Ideally, all of the feelings and experiences we have in each moment of our lives should pass through us like wind through a cheesecloth. We retain the learning inherent in each moment, but we release the package (the event, relationship or situation) in which the learning came. I repeat that this is the *ideal*. Cancer is a leading cause of death because living up to this ideal is incredibly difficult. We are far more inclined to hang on to the package and ignore or avoid the learning.

Fears, guilt feelings, the inability to cope with change, self-hate and unfinished business retard growth because we remain stuck in experiences that handicap our capacity to move forward with our lives in creative and productive ways. Rather than moving through the cheesecloth, these negative patterns lodge in the open spaces, forming blockages. These blockages prevent the wind currents (other experiences and lessons) from entering a person's life. Eventually, the blockages so interfere with the natural process of growth that the system (the body) breaks down, indicating that attention is needed in order to return the system to health.

Consider, as an example, the experience of suddenly losing one's job. This is, of course, a tremendous emotional, psychological and physical trauma. It is also, as the Chinese adage teaches, an opportunity for change. The essential factor in this crisis, as in all crises, resides with how well a person *responds* to this situation.

An optimistic response creates opportunities. That does not mean a person denies the emotional impact of the experience nor overlooks the effect that the loss of a job has on one's financial situation. These are real concerns, obviously. Yet endings are also beginnings. Every plant produces seeds before it dies, providing naturally for the next generation. We also make provisions for *our* next step, whether or not we consciously recognize this. Because we are all part of the intelligence of nature, we, like all members of nature's kingdom, experience change *according to what our growth requires.*

The inability to accept the natural cycle of change interferes with growth and that interferes with health. It is impossible to stop the process of movement and growth. A negative response to change will produce negative growth. A seedling eventually requires transplanting to a larger pot. If this need for change is not acknowledged, though the plant may fight desperately for its life, it will die, never having reached its full maturity. We are no different.

Fear, guilt, unfinished business, self-hate and the inability to move forward in one's life are the equivalent of remaining cramped in a pot that cannot support the next phase of growth.

The following case studies provide a deeper understanding of how cancer is created and also healed.

CASE REPORTS

RUTH

(S h e a l y)

Diagnosis: Cancer of the breast with "spontaneous" recovery.

This forty-six-year-old woman was first seen in November 1985 for a recurrent mass in her right breast. She originally had a benign cyst removed in 1978. In 1981, the lump returned. Eventually in April 1983, the tumor broke through the skin with hemorrhaging. At that time, cancer of the breast was diagnosed and she again had a simple partial mastectomy with removal of the mass.

Six months later, the tumor returned and, at the time she was seen, she had a huge tumor that had already burst through the skin. There was pus and blood oozing from the mass. By clinical observation, this should have been an extremely malignant cancer. She was advised to have a complete mastectomy. The patient decided to do a great deal of praying and visualization and waited another month from the time she was seen. When she underwent surgery a month later, the mass was totally removed but pathology showed it to be totally benign—a great surprise to the surgeons.

ENERGY ANALYSIS

(M y s s)

The breasts, of course, are the nurturing, life-giving glands of the female body. As described in Chapter Four, the area of the breast corresponds to the energy of the heart chakra. This means that the issues of *love* and *nurturing* directly influence the health of a woman's breasts.

There are multiple variations to the love and nurturing scenario that can affect breast tissue. For some women, cancer develops in response to an inability to nurture, which results in guilt feelings and self-hate. Others experience fear and identity crises as a result of not accepting the natural closure of the cycle of motherhood when children leave the home. Who will need them, and what do they do when their roles as "mothers" are no longer primary?

Ruth was a woman who found it impossible to love or nurture herself. She gave continually to others while denying that she ever required love or attention herself. Underneath her persona of the emotionally self-sufficient woman were feelings of resentment over never receiving love and nurturing from others.

Yet Ruth could not see what she was creating. The negative feelings she warehoused resulted in an energy block that, naturally, located in her breast. Her choice to postpone surgery and to pray and visualize represented her first major act of *self-love* and *nurturing*. She finally focused her capacity to love others onto herself, recognizing that she deserved as much love as she gave to others.

In my opinion, the influence of her change in consciousness and her awakening to what it means to love oneself immediately brought life and health back into her body. Rather than remaining in her pattern of self-denial, which was a tremendous obstacle to her growth and development, Ruth released her resentment and negativity, thereby healing the cancer.

HARRY

(S h e a l y)

Diagnosis: Cancer of the testicle with metastasis.

This thirty-two-year-old man was first seen for management of severe left lumbar back pain. He was addicted to narcotics for this pain. He had a previous history of having had cancer of the testicle which had spread to the spine and later to the left kidney. He was a heavy smoker who was unwilling to cooperate in any kind of treatment program other than the use of drugs or surgery. Incidentally, his vitamin B_6 level was 1.5 mcg/liter. The normal range is 3.8 to 18 mcg/liter.

ENERGY ANALYSIS

(Myss)

Harry exemplifies the psyche of a person frozen in fear about life. His cancer originated in his testicle, which is the second chakra region. As stated in Chapter Four, this area of the body corresponds to issues of control, finances, sexuality and external power.

From the time Harry was a young man, he developed the pattern of quitting and thus resenting others who tried. He learned to manipulate and become uncooperative as a means of processing his fear and anger. Harry continually gave in to excuses and the "easy way out."

As a result of these negative patterns, Harry brought his own growth to a halt. He felt insecure about his capacity to take care of himself, earn a living, develop his own skills and interact with others as an equal. Even faced with the challenge of cancer, Harry would not consider that he needed to change his attitudes and outlook about life substantially. Not surprisingly, Harry opted for drugs and surgery as a treatment, but he was by no means "cured."

HORTENSE

(Shealy)

Diagnosis: Cancer of the breast with metastasis to the liver and later to the brain.

This forty-eight-year-old physical therapist was seen for assistance in managing metastatic cancer of the breast to the liver. The patient had been on chemotherapy and radiation treatments and decided to use visualization and nutritional support to gain control over her cancer. She was placed in a two-week intensive autogenic training/biofeedback program. On the last day of the training, she felt as if a spiral of energy left the area of her liver.

One week later, there was no evidence of cancer in the

liver. One year later, the patient developed mild cranial nerve symptoms of loss of taste on one side of the tongue and numbness on the left cheek. A CAT scan of the brain was negative but the clinical impression was probable metastatic cancer to the brain.

At that time, consultation was obtained with Caroline and this was shared with the patient. Her symptoms gradually came under control and she has remained free of the brain symptoms for years.

ENERGY ANALYSIS

(Myss)

According to Hortense's energy reading, she was a person who simply had become exhausted from the emptiness in her own life. She was alone and very lonely. She did not have anyone to love, and the satisfaction that she drew from her job had long since diminished. Life had become an effort and, prior to the diagnosis of cancer, Hortense could not imagine that anything would change the empty path her life was on. Resigned to her "fate," she became depressed, and the emptiness that she felt from a life of being alone, unloved and uncared for, took over. Breast cancer developed as the natural response to her particular crisis.

The metastasis to the liver is also significant to note. The liver is an organ that is nurtured by the third chakra, which is the center of one's personal power. Hortense was exhausted from the continual effort to keep herself going and involved with life on her own. As she looked toward her future, all she could imagine was several more years of having to cope with life and all of its challenges alone. The liver, which cleanses the blood of toxins, also represents the "cleansing of toxins" that are emotional. Hortense could no longer cope with keeping her emotions positive, or cleansed, by herself.

Until the cancer developed, Hortense had not considered that she could change much of the empty space in her life by changing her attitude and making different choices regarding her personal and professional activities. The experience of cancer helped her to realize that she not only *wanted* to live, but that she had the power to change the way she was living.

This insight, coupled with a renewed sense of meaning and new beginnings, allowed Hortense to release her cancer and to start living her life by being open to a positive future.

MARK

(S h e a l y)

Diagnosis: Post-traumatic pain syndrome; severe depression; cancer of the colon; high blood pressure; diabetes.

This sixty-one-year-old man was experiencing severe pain in the lumbar spine, left buttocks and hips, as well as depression. He had been involved in an accident in which he had run into another car that was stopped in front of him just as he came over a hill on an interstate highway. The man in the other car was apparently dead from a heart attack, and the coroner ruled that this had not been Mark's fault. Mark, however, developed a severe depression and would not forgive himself for hitting the other car, even though everyone assured him that there was nothing that could have been done to avoid the accident.

The patient was 5'10" tall and weighed 225 pounds. He had a diagnosis of diabetes that came on following his accident. He had a long-standing problem of high blood pressure for which he had been on antihypertensive drugs. When first seen, he was taking Elavil, an anti-depressant drug, and Tranxene, a tranquilizer (which also causes depression). He stated that he had pain, which was 80% as bad as pain could be, and was restricting his activities 90%. He was quite tender throughout the neck as well as the lower lumbar spine and left sacroiliac joint. The patient was treated with intense biofeedback, autogenic training, acupuncture, nerve blocks, transcutaneous electrical nerve stimulation and a lot of counseling. Any time he was in therapy for a week or two, his depression would lift and his pain would be modified. Upon returning home, he again would go into a deep depression.

The first reading done by Caroline was in July 1985. At that time, she predicted that if he did not improve his attitude, he had a high chance of developing cancer of the bowel. In November 1985, he was operated on for cancer of the colon. When we had first seen him in July, he had had no symptoms suggesting any problems in the colon.

In February 1986, Mark was again in a deep depression. At that time, he was told about the earlier reading by Caroline and given the intense recommendation that he immediately develop a more positive outlook on life and challenge his ongoing depression.

Also, during that reading, Caroline predicted that Mark would die in August if he did not alter his emotional patterns. It was recommended that he retire from his job as a manager of a trucking company and devote his life to his wife and his farm. He continued to have a moderate degree of depression and pain but was somewhat better after a time. His greatest residual problems remained his left sacroiliac and left hip pain and depression. He died of metastatic cancer two and one-half years after his original accident on August 31, 1987.

ENERGY ANALYSIS

(Myss)

Mark's depression was the first and most obvious energy block in his system. Depression always reduces both the flow of energy through the body and the quality of the energy that actually enters the body.

Mark had literally given up the desire to live, even before the car accident involving the man who was found dead of a heart attack at the wheel of his car. This incident merely provided Mark with a legitimate and obvious crisis upon which to focus, since the deeper issue was much more difficult to handle.

Mark's energy revealed that he saw himself as someone

who was no longer useful. He could not cope with the aging process and the loss of his virility and physical strength. He had a very gentle nature, yet underneath that he prided himself on physical strength and capability.

I saw the probability that cancer would develop in his second chakra region because his energy was particularly blocked in that area. This indicated to me that his sense of external power and authority was being threatened, and that he lacked the ability to enter into the next phase of his life. He feared dependency, and growing older represented to him the ultimate condition of uselessness.

The accident that so consumed his attention represented deeper issues still in that Mark could not forgive himself for not becoming all he had wanted to become in his life. His inability to forgive himself existed long before this particular incident. Yet in encountering this situation, he had created an experience through which to deal with his negative attitude toward himself. Mark was, unfortunately, unable to challenge the grip his depression had over his consciousness, in spite of the loving support of his family.

ALICE

(S h e a l y)

Diagnosis: Widespread metastatic breast cancer.

One of my most challenging patients, Alice, offers some interesting considerations. She came for treatment in April 1974, apparently dying of widespread metastatic breast cancer. Vomiting, unable to be out of bed most of the time, she was depressed and uninterested in being "brainwashed." But on the seventeenth day of training in self-regulation, following a twenty-minute insight exercise on forgiveness, Alice had a miraculous sudden relief of pain. Three months later, there was no clinical nor x-ray evidence of cancer.

A year later, looking very healthy, Alice told me, "Norm,

during that exercise, I suddenly realized how much I hated my family, and I decided that I wasn't about to let the bastards kill me." She went on to say that when she got well, "My husband committed suicide." Actually, the story is even more unusual. Three years earlier, her husband had almost died of kidney failure. She had nursed him back to health after a kidney transplant from her favorite son. During that doubly stressful event, her breast cancer flared up.

When she developed cancer, her husband rejected her and treated her as though she had leprosy. He considered cancer contagious, a curse and inevitably fatal. Even though he had had no problem with kidney rejection in three years, he became increasingly agitated as she became well. He then developed rapid kidney rejection and "committed suicide" (Alice's comment) by dying of kidney failure.

A year later, her dog died. She became quite depressed and her pain returned. Extensive testing revealed no evidence of recurrent cancer. She then stated, "I now realize that I cannot afford the luxury of depression!" In another session, she also recalled that she had, at age sixteen, set her life script to die at age fifty-eight of cancer. Her favorite grandmother had died of cancer at age fifty-eight when Alice was sixteen.

Despite her cure from cancer, Alice suffered a great deal from multiple complications of extensive x-ray and chemotherapy. She died eight and one-half years after her cancer cure, of *kidney failure* caused by the chemotherapy. Her autopsy revealed *no* cancer in her body. She died just shy of fifty-eight years of life, and of kidney failure, the same illness that had claimed her husband. And despite much insight gained by this lovely, sweet lady, she still died at her pre-set script time of fifty-eight years of age.

Although Alice turned her cancer around in one of the most miraculous cures that I have seen, she apparently did not reset her "life script." We know that individuals who stop smoking before they develop serious major illness reverse the increased risk of cancer within ten years. Theoretically, one should be able to reverse one's life script as well, given the capacity to challenge and transform one's core beliefs.

CONCLUSION

(S h e a l y)

Throughout the latter half of this century, cancer has been the most dreaded disease. At least 75% of the patients with whom I have personally worked have wanted to die before they developed cancer. Usually this is the result of depression because of a problem with a love relationship.

But what about the 25% of people who seem to have a remarkably positive attitude and so much for which to live? Although they weren't "wanting to die," they almost invariably had major psycho-social stresses. My own belief system is that cancer, as with all other illnesses, is always a multifaceted disease. That is, there tends to be, at least in some families, a predisposition toward cancer. This means that there may be a genetic weakness in the immune system.

There is no question that chemical pollution of various sorts predisposes people to cancer, as do cigarette smoking and excessive exposure to radiation, as well as chemotherapy for other forms of cancer.

I believe that someday we will have "proven" that there is usually, if not always, a virus involved in precipitating the onset of cancer. And finally, the personality, the belief system of the individual, along with the total reaction to life stresses will be recognized as the precipitating final straw.

CHAPTER SEVEN

Acute Diseases and Injuries: Infections and Accidents

(Shealy and Myss)

INFECTIONS AND ACCIDENTS

(Shealy)

H istorically, infections and accidents have been the major causes of both illness and death until approximately the middle of the twentieth century. The almost 50% increase in "average" longevity of Americans is attributed primarily to the decreased incidence of death in infants from infectious diseases. Although death from infectious diseases is still a very significant phenomenon, the major and more serious infections today, and those that incapacitate people, more commonly lie on the thin line between acute and chronic disease.

In this chapter, we will concentrate on some of the more worrisome infectious diseases and accidents. Although they may seem quite different, both accidents and infections represent illnesses that come on suddenly and produce acute symptoms, ranging from minor disorders to life-threatening conditions. Accidents, often created by drunk adults and teenagers, are the major cause of death in children under fifteen years of age. Adults set themselves up for accidents by being careless, usually when they are preoccupied with other concerns. In a subsequent chapter, we will focus on chronic disorders.

In general, most physicians classify as acute diseases those that have been present for less than one month. Semi-acute are those that are from one month to six months in duration and by six months, the illness has become chronic. With meningitis, except in extremely rare fungal and certain viral infections, the individual is likely to die within hours or a few days if not treated properly with antibiotics.

With the most common viral infection, a "cold," most people recover fully within a maximum of two weeks. Similarly, measles, mumps and even whooping cough are only relatively acute and generally short-term illnesses from which most individuals recover within a very brief period of time.

There are literally hundreds of infectious illnesses, ranging from localized infections, such as pimples, to generalized and fatal ones like AIDS. Clinically, medicine rarely looks for a *cause* other than to identify the specific bug (bacteria, virus, fungus, etc.). But it is generally recognized that there are some genetic predispositions toward viruses (such as congenital immune deficiency syndrome) and that smokers and diabetics have many more infectious illnesses. Social scientists have concluded that malnutrition (continual low protein and low calorie intake) is a major predisposing cause of infections.

Of course, much infection can be prevented by proper sanitation, good handling of sewage, pasteurization of milk and chlorination of water. But science has ignored the most critical question of all: Why, even in an epidemic, do some people *not* become infected? The work of Hans Selye in stress physiology gave us the beginning answers to these questions. He demonstrated that stress produces an alarm reaction and, although it is important to have such a reaction if you have a tiger coming at you, as you will learn in this chapter, most of the causes of an alarm reaction are much more subtle and the stressor is not dealt with appropriately. Indeed, in today's society, chemical stress weakens the immune system, inactivity weakens the immune system and, finally, our negative emotions weaken the immune system tremendously. The new field of psychoneuroimmunology now suggests that emotions may be the final straw that causes the immune system to decompensate.

When I was a resident in general surgery, rotating through a hospital for treating only patients with tuberculosis, I was impressed with the social problems of almost all of the patients who were confined there. They were lonely, distressed individuals. Frequently, they were alcoholics.

We now know that alcohol itself is a major stressor and weakens the immune system. Most alcoholics also smoke, which has another powerful adverse effect upon the immune system, and, of course, most alcoholics are extremely depressed. Again, this sets them up, from a psychoneuroimmunological point of view, to become candidates for infectious diseases.

ENERGY ANALYSIS OF ACUTE DISEASES, INFECTIONS AND THE IMMUNE SYSTEM

(Myss)

Our physical immune system is extremely sensitized to respond to the "signals" it receives from our emotions. Just like a moat surrounding and protecting a castle, our immune systems respond to and protect us from invasion, both in the sense of "germ invasion" and "emotional invasion."

Specifically, our immune systems respond to our sense of safety. Just as the physical immune system is triggered into action when a threatening element is introduced into the system, so also does the "emotional immune system" respond with high activity when we feel intimidated, insecure and threatened, or when we need to perform in assertive or aggressive ways.

We "defend ourselves" with our attitudes. How secure we are about meeting new people, how we feel about ourselves, whether or not we are loving or hostile, trusting or withdrawn— all of these attitudes that we hold inside of ourselves form the energy of our "emotional immune system."

We gravitate to and melt into the energy fields of people who are open and loving. We feel compelled to stand next to them, sit next to them, talk to them and look into their eyes. Their energy is soothing and we feel "safe."

We talk openly about ourselves, and the sensation that comes from being with someone without the need to protect oneself is not only delicious, it is health-inducing.

When we feel threatened, however, or when we are under performance stress, we generate attitudes of a very different quality. Our attitudes and actions then reflect the need to protect ourselves and our vulnerabilities. We all fear being victimized. As such, our energy fields project a quality of energy that keeps people at a distance—we are protecting our "safety" and "defending" our energy fields from "invasion/infection."

Under normal circumstances, we are able to generate our "defensive" energy effectively. By normal circumstances, I am referring to a tolerable amount of day-to-day living stress, which is then combined with a fair amount of emotional support. In other words, the insecurity-producing activities are counterbalanced with a security-inducing support system.

When conditions are such in a person's life that effective emotional support is absent, then the chances are greatly increased that the person will exhaust his or her emotional (and thus, physical) immune system far more rapidly than would a person with support. Without a support system, the capacity to feel "safe"—meaning cared for—is practically nonexistent.

The result is that without a support system, the individual does not have the opportunity to recharge the energy of his or her immune system with feelings of safety and support. Rather, his or her "defense" system is running on high energy almost continually, and thus, burn-out occurs. Emotionally, the individual becomes exhausted with the burden of *self*-support and/ or constant "high performance."

Emotional burn-out that occurs through feelings of lack of safety, in turn, causes burn-out in the physical immune system. Unable to maintain a "defensive-proof" energy field, a person becomes susceptible to "invasion or infection," as a virus can now penetrate one's energy field.

In my work, I have noted that a pattern exists between the underlying reasons why a person suffers emotional-immune burn-out and the corresponding virus that one "attracts." Emotional-immune burn-out that is the result of a collective series of daily, rather ordinary, emotional stresses is likely to attract a cold virus. The HIV virus that creates AIDS, on the other hand, is attracted to an individual whose level of inner stress and emotional burn-out is far more intense.

In general, I believe that the human immune system as a whole is weakening due to both an increase in physical toxins in the environment and food systems, and a dramatic rise in emotional toxins generated from the highly insecure nature of our living situations. The necessary transformation of our social system has reordered the family unit and the stability of intimate relationships, producing a massive increase in the number of single-parent households, broken homes and divorces. This rise in the "instability factor" is producing an epidemic of anxiety and social/personal insecurities. We need stability and we now all live in a world in which stability no longer seems to exist.

I add only the brief comment that beyond the instability factors that are active at the personal level of life, our planetary environment also is generating unlimited and unprecedented causes of anxiety regarding our safety and our future. The possibility of nuclear war or complete depletion of our energy system (to name but two crises) contributes a constant level of stress into our collective consciousness, and this contribution should be recognized as emotional toxic waste products—as real and as damaging as chemical waste products. I believe that this contamination of our collective unconscious influences our overall health as a group and that as a result of this group stress, our immune systems in general are weakened.

The following examples of viruses and infections represent those that are most common and/or threatening. In each case, we have highlighted the specific emotional stresses that weaken the immune system and thus attract a specific virus.

INFECTIOUS DISEASES

AIDS

(S h e a l y)

AIDS—a simple word whose modern meaning confounds medical science and strikes fear in the heart of most Americans. It is estimated that at least 100 million people will die from AIDS, worldwide, within a generation. AIDS has rapidly replaced cancer as the most dreaded disease known. It is considered to be an epidemic in Ethiopia and is rapidly becoming one in the United States.

FACTORS THAT AFFECT NATURAL IMMUNITY

At birth, most infants are immune to many potentially serious infections, such as poliomyelitis and diptheria, because of a passive immunity acquired from the mother's blood. This advantage is lost by three to six months of age. Additional passive immunity is passed to the baby who nurses; colostrum, the mother's antibody-rich first milk, is almost essential to survival.

Immunity to many infections can also be acquired by immunization, the administration of a vaccine usually consisting of a killed or weakened culture of bacteria or viruses of a very specific type. Polio, measles, diptheria, whooping cough and small pox are examples of diseases in which vaccination can assist in achieving immunity.

Successful recovery from infections also conveys varying degrees of immunity. Lasting immunity is seen especially after chicken pox and most childhood infections such as measles. Each organism has its own specific way of spreading. For example, colds and flus are transmitted through the respiratory tract; cholera and typhoid are generally transmitted by contaminated water and other fluids; hepatitis is transmitted by contaminated food; AIDS, hepatitis, malaria and encephalitis are among the many diseases that can be transmitted through blood, such as by a contaminated hypodermic needle. AIDS, venereal herpes, gonorrhea, syphilis and Chlamydia are among the numerous diseases that can be transmitted by sexual contact. With most infectious agents, the incubation period is a few days to a few weeks. With AIDS, the incubation period may be at least as long as ten years or more.

NUTRITION

Adequate calories and sufficient protein are essential for the basic integrity of the immune system. Without those building blocks, individuals, especially infants, are much more susceptible to infectious agents.

ENVIRONMENTAL FACTORS

Many environmental factors affect our health, including seasonal changes, natural light, pollution and antibiotic therapy.

Although antibiotics are wonderful drugs for treatment of meningitis, ear infections, syphilis and gonorrhea, the organisms that cause these diseases can change during reproduction so that they become resistant to antibiotics. Antibiotics also have numerous side-effects and complications, and may predispose individuals to overgrowth of candida, a common yeast infection.

PHYSIOLOGY OF THE IMMUNE SYSTEM

Our bodies are composed of trillions of cells, each measuring only a few microns in diameter. Cells contain a fatty cell membrane, or outer wall, and a central nucleus that contains the genes linked together to form chromosomes. Human cells each have forty-six chromosomes and each chromosome contains approximately 50,000 genes. The genes determine the way in which the cell's cytoplasm operates.

Most viruses, including the AIDS or HTLV (more recently, the HIV) virus, invade the cell nucleus and alter chemical messages sent from the nucleus to the cytoplasm. The immune system, mostly part of our blood cell mechanism, strives to keep the body healthy. The highly specialized cells of the immune system may attack and destroy invading bacteria, viruses and the body's own cells when they go astray and become "cancer."

When a foreign material enters the body, the T-cell lymphocytes are aroused. They detect the abnormal protein and secrete chemical alerters, lymphokines, which arouse other lymphocytes, the B-cells, to manufacture antibodies, specific proteins or globulins which adhere to the specific invading antigen and coat it. Such coated antigens attract phagocytes, also called polymorphonuclear cells, the clean-up crew of white blood cells. Phagocytes devour the coated antigens.

The body is elegantly protected by the natural killer cells which destroy cancer cells. Macrophages also devour and digest cancer cells. Almost 25% of the body's 100 trillion cells are involved in the immune system. The HIV virus, AIDS, invades the cell nucleus of the T4 cells (helper or inducer cells) and shuts off the alarm system not only to the AIDS virus, but to many other antigens as well. Thus, the AIDS virus assumes control of the most important part of our immune defense system. A number of other viruses also damage the T4 cells, but in none except AIDS is the destruction so complete.

Despite widely reported fragility of the AIDS virus, it has been found to survive up to fifteen days at room temperature and to live for at least ten days in a "dried" stage. We know that AIDS can be transmitted through blood and semen. AIDS, therefore, is more common among homosexuals than hetero-sexuals because of oral ingestion of semen and anal intercourse, which often leads to bleeding as well as introduction of semen.

Homosexuals also have a higher incidence of giardiasis, an intestinal parasite that weakens the immune system. Further-more, homosexuals may have successive relationships that may involve more than one hundred partners per year.

Hemophiliacs and IV drug users are also particularly sus-ceptible to AIDS—hemophiliacs through frequent blood trans-fusions and drug addicts because they often share needles.

Given all available evidence, *prevention of AIDS* is the path of choice. The following are prevention-oriented, holistically sound recommendations for those who are not already carriers of the HIV virus:

- Choose monogamy with a partner who has long been sexually conservative.

- Avoid all street drugs.

- Avoid anal intercourse as it weakens the immune system.

- Avoid smoking or the use of any tobacco products.

- Obtain adequate regular sleep, an average of seven to eight hours per night.

- Eat a healthy diet; avoid fats and sugar; emphasize whole grains, vegetables and fruits.

- Exercise regularly, including exposure to natural sun-light as often as possible.

- Follow a stress-reduction program of thirty to forty minutes each day of positive imaging, affirmations and self-regulation techniques, such as biofeedback.

- Minimize caffeine and alcoholic beverages.

ENERGY ANALYSIS OF AIDS

(M y s s)

The AIDS virus is the most complicated of all viruses to discuss because of the emotional and social associations with this illness. Contributing to the complications of the disease are the larger planetary factors that I believe are central to the reason why the HIV virus is now a part of our lives. As described above, the human immune system is responsive to emotional issues concerning a person's sense of safety and his or her capacity to challenge and overcome feelings of vulnerability. Every person, to some extent, experiences concerns over safety and personal well-being. No one wants to be "victimized" by other people or by circumstances that seemingly are theatening in some way.

The common psychological/emotional profile shared by individuals who become infected with the HIV virus is the most intense degree of "victim consciousness" that I have witnessed in people. In using the example of a social caste system, the groups of people who first became infected are those with the least amount of dignity, self-esteem and inner power within our global community. These groups—IV drug users, prostitutes, homosexuals, Haitians, poverty-stricken Africans—exist at the lowest level of human socio-political and economic power. They form the last rung on the human caste system ladder.

For the average individual coping with personal fears of being "victimized," whether that be economically, legally or through any other possible channel, options for responding in a self-protective way are available. For example, lawyers protect people from becoming victims of poorly negotiated contracts. Human rights, at least within the United States, offers a level of social protection for the average citizen.

The quality of victim consciousness associated with HIV-infected people exists at a level of helplessness and hopelessness that is so powerful that it eclipses what little hope the person holds for ever changing the condition of being victimized.

Consider what it means to be homosexual. Regardless of whether the heterosexual community believes homosexuality to be a matter of personal choice or a propensity one is born with, the fact is that a homosexual individual cannot forceably shift sexual preference, regardless of how much social or moral pressure is applied. While many homosexual people marry and have families, this choice to "blend in" to what is socially acceptable merely disguises their suffering. It does not heal their anguish and fear of being socially and morally rejected.

For those who choose to live a homosexual lifestyle, "hiding" their private lives becomes second nature. They fear telling their family and friends. For many, disclosing this personal truth may result in the loss of a career or community standing. The exceptions exist mainly among those who become successful economically, as economic power affords a mantle of protection. Nevertheless, the fact remains that being homosexual is a threat to social and religious mores and thus, even for the financially successful homosexual individual, acceptance remains largely a matter of economic and not personal leverage.

For people who face this degree of victim consciousness, the overwhelming and debilitating factor that needs to be emphasized is that there is little they can do to change what it is about them personally or socially that makes them unacceptable or disempowered human beings. In other words, the opportunity for these people to challenge their social, economic and moral status in order to lift them beyond a powerless condition is virtually nonexistent.

Poverty-stricken Africans are bound to a seemingly endless cycle of birth-starvation-disease-death. Prostitutes and IV drug users are caught in life patterns that are emotionally and psychologically desperate and often violent. They are considered social and moral outcasts. Beyond judging their choices to live as they do, appreciate the emptiness of living a life of being used and useless. Imagine how deep must be their sense of being victimized by life that they fully live out their "victim consciousness" either through selling their bodies or deadening their feeling sensation through drugs—often both.

What about those people who contract the virus through blood transfusions or at birth from infected mothers? Does the concept of "victim consciousness" apply to these individuals?

While it may not be as obvious, nevertheless, hemophiliacs and infants born to carrier-mothers exist in an "atmosphere" of victimization. Hemophiliacs, by virture of their illness, must take precautions to protect themselves from injury and the risk of internal bleeding. This ongoing need creates a sense of vulnerability and fear of encounter with the physical world. Though this sensitivity and vulnerability is often subtle, it does place the hemophiliac in a range of consciousness that is continually filled with the need to protect oneself.

Infants and children, likewise, are vulnerable beings. They are as responsive to the emotional, psychological, physical and spiritual stresses of their worlds as are adults. Certainly, they are limited by their capacity to articulate their impressions, but these impressions nonetheless affect their physical bodies.

Infants born to women who are carriers of the virus inherit, to some extent, the "vibrational genetic code" of the mother. If the mother is a drug user and abusive to her own body, the infant will be influenced not only by her physical genetic code and body chemistry, but also by her emotional chemistry. Children are as susceptible to contamination as adults.

These people, who have become the first victims of a virus that thrives upon victims symbolically (and perhaps literally), represent a voice speaking on behalf of all life that is victimized and exists in a powerless condition upon the earth.

Epidemics, including AIDS, arise as a collective response to the stresses present in the larger atmosphere of our lives together as members of the same society and global community. Exceeding our personal life stresses, we share the influence of impersonal stresses that are the "sum of our parts" blended together. Pollution is a collective stress, as are all ecological problems. We are all affected by contaminated air.

Similarly, we all participate in the creation of our social, economic and political quality of life, both within our local and national communities as well as the larger social atmosphere of the planet. We share not only the creation of our "human atmospheric conditions," we also share in the EFFECTS of its quality. Epidemics arise in response to emotional, psychological, social, political and economic stresses shared by a group. Thus, the same stresses that produce a case of AIDS in an individual are responsible for the spread of the virus throughout the human community, including the global human community.

The AIDS virus responds to "victim consciousness." It is our theory that the AIDS virus has spontaneously emerged into our global atmosphere in response to the massive victimization of all forms of life, including the planet itself. We have always been a war-making planet. There are three factors that have been added in the past thirty years that have considerably increased the stress factor of life: nuclear power, the worldwide effect of international media and the increasing shortage in the worldwide supply of food and energy. All three relate to an increase in global pressure regarding the victimization of life.

Whereas we have always had war somewhere on the planet, the nuclear age and its corresponding technology have created the very real possibility of worldwide destruction, including the destruction of the planet itself. It is not an exaggeration to state that the planet and all of its inhabitants are being held hostage by the threat of nuclear destruction. Adults and children worldwide are now mindful that their future is no longer assured.

Simultaneously, we have the global crises of contamination of our food and water supply as well as the impending shortage of food, water and energy. These crises greatly impact the stress levels of every person's life, regardless of how conscious one is of these worldwide pressures.

Any one of these crises has enough power to threaten the quality of life on this planet. All of them combined make our future highly questionable. In fact, the reality is that all of the kingdoms of life are now subject to the victimization of their right to live. The contribution of the worldwide media network is that it is heightening our awareness of humanity's suffering and plights, and, thus, we can no longer live in ignorance of the critical nature of our situation. The media is bringing the depth of human struggles into our homes and, whether or not we realize it, the media is serving as a catalyst for causing people to think in terms of their responsibility to the quality of life on this planet.

It is our opinion that the AIDS epidemic has arisen in response to the massive victimization of life and the very real threat of the demise of life. It is global in proportion because the crises present on our planet are global.

We believe that the manifestations of the disease are also present at the global, or macrocosmic, level. AIDS results primarily in the development of two diseases: pneumocystis and Kaposi sarcoma. Pneumocystis is a terminal lung infection. By analogy, consider the massive and rapid destruction of the rain forests of South America (which produce 40% of the world's supply of oxygen) and all of the other forest areas worldwide that are being destroyed by acid rain. These forests are the "lungs of the earth" and they are rapidly becoming incapable of producing life-giving oxygen.

Kaposi sarcoma are cancerous lesions located beneath the surface of the human body. Once again, by analogy, look at the lesions that are created within the earth by nuclear explosions carried on underground. In essence, we are participating in a nuclear war waged against the planet itself. These nuclear explosions are releasing an unlimited supply of destructive nuclear energy into the earth's underground—including the earth's underground reservoir of water and healthy soil.

The result of these two devastating ongoing situations is that the entire biological and ecological system of life is now undergoing the most extensive and serious victimization of itself that has ever been orchestrated by humanity. In essence, the planet itself has manifested AIDS as a way of signaling that its interdependent systems of life cannot withstand the effects of victimization any longer.*

If all disease is created as both a learning opportunity and a manifestation of underlying emotional, psychological and spiritual stresses, then from AIDS we must learn that the victimization of life can no longer continue on this planet if we are to survive as a species. This is a learning that everyone on this planet must respond to and, for that reason, the message inherent in this epidemic has spread into almost every nation on this globe. I do not believe that a "cure" or vaccine will be found for this illness until the critical message of this virus is understood by humanity.

The following case study illustrates the nature of victim consciousness even more clearly.

ANDY

Diagnoses: AIDS-Pneumocystis, polyneuropathy, cancer of the prostate.

In May 1988, I participated in a panel presentation on the subject of AIDS. I shared with the audience my theory as to why AIDS is a part of our lives and I emphasized the need to understand its relationship to victim consciousness. Following my presentation, a gentleman in the audience asked to tell his story.

He was forty-four years old, born in New England, and was raised as a member of the Mormon faith. From his earliest memories, Andy recalled always trying to prove his manhood which, for him, was particularly difficult since he was extremely petite. He joined the service and was shipped to Viet Nam. There, he was exposed to Agent Orange.

*This material is presented in the book, *AIDS: Passageway to Transformation* by C. Norman Shealy, M.D., Ph.D. and Caroline M. Myss, M.A., published by Stillpoint International. The book includes case studies as well as a program for the treatment of the disease.

When he returned from his tour of duty, he settled back into his home area. Andy was plagued with guilt over his awareness that he was homosexual, and his fear of being discovered caused him to marry. Needless to say, his marriage was a disaster and ended in divorce. After his divorce, Andy left New England for San Francisco.

He became totally immersed in the gay culture in that city and, for the first time in his life, Andy began to open up in terms of his feelings and his own identity. He became involved in numerous sexual encounters and, in 1985, he was diagnosed as carrying the HIV virus. Earlier, he had received a diagnosis of cancer of the prostate which Andy believed was brought on by exposure to Agent Orange. He further developed polyneuropathy, a neurological condition in which the muscle system deteriorates, and he was losing the strength in his legs.

By 1987, Andy decided to return home to his parents. He wanted to tell them about himself as well as the fact that he had AIDS. He was only home a few days and had yet to speak with his parents when his father handed him a newspaper article. It was the story of a young Mormon man who had returned to his home town seeking help as he had developed AIDS. The Mormon church excommunicated the man.

Andy realized that his father was using the newspaper article to communicate the same message to him and, shortly thereafter, Andy left his parents' home for Boston. He never told them what he had come home to say.

Andy said that all of his life, he had felt like a victim— first, of his religion, then, of his sexuality, and then of Agent Orange. He felt that he was always trying to prove that he was a person of worth.

Andy is now working to help other AIDS patients and is proud of his personal efforts to resurrect his own dignity in these last months of his life.

Andy's life history is very typical of the struggles and pain of victim consciousness. Like numerous other individuals with AIDS, Andy has taken this awesome challenge and is using it to heal himself emotionally, psychologically and spiritually as well as to make a positive contribution to the lives of others.

HERPES GENITALIS

(S h e a l y)

Most people think of herpes as venereal herpes. However, even today, venereal herpes is not as common as is a fever blister, which is a first cousin of the herpes genitalis virus. In fact, some people believe that the herpes virus, which afflicts the genital organs, is just the fever blister version of the herpes virus that is "transplanted" to the genitalia during oral genital activities.

It is generally recognized that herpes genitalis is a venereal disease, and it is widely known that the manifestation of the herpes virus in the genital region is strongly related to stress.

A herpes outbreak is likely to occur during menstruation, at which time the immune system is slightly weakened. Indeed, even in men we know that herpes exacerbations are highly related to the total stress in that individual's life, so that extraordinary stress, such as exams or job problems, may lead to an outbreak. Thus, herpes is both a chronic recurrent illness and an acute one with exacerbations that often last a few days to a week or so. Just as in fever blisters, the venereal herpes virus "lives" in the body and seems to "come out" only under certain types of significant stress.

Oral herpes rarely produces a serious infection, although it can. It is generally believed that the herpes virus lives in the skin around the mouth and nares (entrance to the nose) and manifests itself only when an individual's general immunity is weakened, such as during a "fever."

ENERGY ANALYSIS OF
HERPES GENITALIS

(M y s s)

The condition of genital herpes develops most commonly in individuals who participate in sexual activity that they themselves consider to be either meaningless or, just the opposite, a desperate substitute for love. Note that the sexual activity itself is not the negative, as is so often thought. Rather, the energy blockage in the genital area is created in response to the fact that very little, if any, true emotional satisfaction is forthcoming from one's emotional/sexual activities. In other words, the individual participates in actions that do not reflect what a person really needs. Sex with a partner one is not emotionally drawn to does not satisfy the need to be loved. What is required is that the individual assess his or her needs and then make choices in terms of partners and relationships that meet those needs.

SANDY

(S h e a l y)

Diagnosis: Venereal herpes.

This thirty-five-year-old x-ray technician came to the clinic in June 1985 with venereal herpes that she had contracted one month earlier. Sandy had a long-standing history of unsatisfied sexual relations that had left her constantly unhappy and unloved. She repeatedly enters such relationships seeking a "feeling" of love and is then always disappointed. Her outbreaks of herpes are clearly related to increased stress in Sandy's life.

ENERGY ANALYSIS

(M y s s)

Aside from the obvious stresses that Norm has described, Sandy's case is valuable because it illustrates what I consider to be the activity of our "higher self." We have a "higher self" that interacts on our own behalf whenever and wherever we lack the wisdom to do so with our ordinary consciousness. To me, an illness such as herpes is a perfect example of this type of "higher-self intervention" illustrating that herpes, in this example, is an obstacle that is meant to cause us *to stop long enough to reevaluate what we are creating for ourselves* as well as the consequences of our choices. Sandy's higher self, in other words, intuitively understood that she was unable to challenge her compulsion unless she was given even more "motivation" than her loneliness.

Sandy was almost "electrocuted" by her emotional needs in that they kept her behaving in ways that produced anxiety. Even though she admitted that she recognized her compulsion to settle for sex instead of love, it was obvious by the absence of conviction from her voice that she had no intention of challenging this behavior in herself. Rather, she felt sorry for herself because she had contracted herpes. And she felt ashamed of having herpes because she considered it to be an indication that she lived promiscuously.

I pointed out to her that it was possible that her higher self created this illness as a more serious "motivator" to cause her to reevaluate how she was coping with her emotional needs, because it was obvious that her feelings of loneliness were not enough of a motivation. Were she able to respond to this dysfunction as an opportunity to break a pattern that controls her, Sandy would then become able to create different and more satisfying choices. This, in turn, would generate very real feelings of love and she would heal emotionally as well as physically.

Unfortunately, despite numerous suggestions on our part and tenative seeking on her part, Sandy has continued to flounder in this pit of low self-esteem.

SHINGLES OR HERPES ZOSTER

(S h e a l y)

Shingles or herpes zoster is a relative of chicken pox. In general, chicken pox affects children, and most individuals who have had chicken pox as children do not develop shingles as adults.

Shingles tends to affect individuals when their immune system is already weakened. It occurs primarily in older people and in those who have cancer. The herpes zoster or shingles virus affects the ganglion, or collection of nerve cells supplying a given nerve root. Thus, the outbreak of the rash, which is a vesicular rash somewhat like poison ivy, follows the nerve root path. Most commonly, it occurs in the chest but it can occur in a branch of the sciatic nerve or even into the face. When it affects the face and enters the eye, it can cause blindness.

About 10% of individuals who have shingles wind up with chronic intractable or post-herpetic pain which is a peculiar, internal burning pain problem that can be totally incapacitating for many years.

Fortunately, the pain is often easily controlled with transcutaneous electrical nerve stimulation. It can also be controlled with tryptophan (the precursor of serotonin) and Elavil (the antidepressant drug referred to earlier) or Dilantin (an antiepileptic drug).

ENERGY ANALYSIS

(M y s s)

Shingles is a disorder that is created through experiencing chronic anxiety and irritation due to feeling overwhelmed by the circumstances or demands of one's environment. In particular, the anxiety is generated because the activity in one's environment continually makes the person feel physically, financially or materially insecure and vulnerable.

It is important to note that shingles is more commonly associated with chronic anxiety than sudden anxiety. Even though shingles may develop following a certain stressful incident or trauma, the anxiety that comes to the surface during an outbreak has far deeper roots in that individual than is actually generated from that particular trauma. Years of warehousing little episodes of anxiety over one's financial situation or physical security gradually burn out the nerve endings, resulting in an outbreak of shingles.

ROSE

(S h e a l y)

Diagnosis: Post-herpetic or post-shingles pain syndrome.

This seventy-one-year-old lady was experiencing pain in the chest following shingles, which had occurred one year earlier. Treatment for the shingles and further post-herpetic pain had included a variety of antidepressant drugs which had led to three falls, with fractures of the hip and arm and continuing post-herpetic pain.

Rose entered into an intense program of autogenic training and biofeedback, and showed at least a 75% decrease in her pain at the end of a two-week session.

ENERGY ANALYSIS

(M y s s)

Rose worried continually over her physical and financial situation. As she aged, her worry-syndrome became anxiety. She saw herself losing more and more control over her physical circumstances and she feared dependency.

I strongly believe that the reason Rose responded so effectively to autogenic training and biofeedback was due to the fact that in learning to regulate her own bodily responses, Rose experienced a renewal of her self-confidence. The better she felt about herself, the less inclined she was to let her fear about becoming physically vulnerable and dependent control her.

INFLUENZA

(S h e a l y)

Among the best known viruses is, of course, the common "flu." Generally during the winter months, there is some degree of those small to large epidemics of flu almost every year. The influenza virus and its problems, which generally include an upper respiratory infection, a fever and an overall myalgia or ache, often associated with severe headache, are extremely well-known. The major epidemic in the first quarter of the century, which led to death in many individuals, also was the precursor of many cases of Parkinsonism, which did not manifest until twenty to forty years after that episode of flu had taken place. There are vaccines that will protect people from a given strain of flu, but the flu virus has a remarkable ability to mutate and change, so the immunization acquired from flu vaccine is good only for six months or less.

ENERGY ANALYSIS

(M y s s)

Certain illnesses occur as a part of Nature's cleansing program. Just as rain storms clean the air over our cities, epidemics like influenza cleanse the energy of the collective unconscious. The general stress and toxins that build up naturally and gradually in our "atmosphere"—toxins that we invisibly breathe in and consume—are discharged through the various influenza viruses.

This type of illness is not so much associated with a specific emotional issue as it is with cleansing the emotional stress that is just part of life.

COMMON COLD

(S h e a l y)

A very ubiquitous virus, the common cold virus has many different varieties of virus which cause the same symptoms, mainly involving the nose, sinuses, throat and occasionally bronchi. Secondary infections occur not infrequently in the weakened tissues. It has been known for many years that a cold only affects someone whose immune system is already weakened and that, furthermore, the cold virus is not something that is "caught."

Some researchers believe, in fact, that certain varieties of the cold virus live in the body and manifest themselves during a state of diminished immunity.

There are a number of studies, for instance, indicating that individuals who are healthy and strong and are exposed to extremes of cold without clothes on do not necessarily develop a cold, clearly indicating the strength of their immune systems.

I believe that the evidence is also adequate that individuals who take quite large doses of vitamin C do not catch colds nearly as often and recover from them much quicker. I recommend 2 grams a day plus 100 mg of B_6 or B complex.

ENERGY ANALYSIS

(M y s s)

A person becomes susceptible to the cold virus as a result of emotional exhaustion brought on by the ordinary business of living. The important factor in understanding the cold virus is that it is primarily an emotional dysfunction.

MONONUCLEOSIS AND CHRONIC EPSTEIN-BARR INFECTION

(S h e a l y)

The mononucleosis virus is a cousin of the herpes virus. It primarily affects young people, is thought to be transmitted largely through kissing, can cause very minor to extremely serious illnesses and often affects the liver and spleen. Individuals can become remarkably ill and die from severe cases of mononucleosis.

Chronic Epstein-Barr virus has been recognized only in the last few years. In this particular syndrome, patients have recurrent episodes of a wide variety of symptoms, including allergies, and more than anything else, severe fatigue. Chronic Epstein-Barr infection then becomes much like herpes to which this virus is related. That is, it appears that it can cause both acute illnesses and chronic recurrent illnesses with acute exacerbation.

ENERGY ANALYSIS

(Myss)

Mononucleosis and chronic Epstein-Barr infections are increasing in dramatic numbers, mostly in women. That is not surprising, considering the underlying psychological and emotional stresses we are experiencing in our society.

People who become susceptible to these viruses frequently feel that their emotional needs have been repeatedly violated. More than dealing with the insecurity of finances or physical well-being, these individuals are involved in unproductive relationship patterns in which their needs are not met. It is important to note that a central part of the emotional and psychological pattern of these people is that they "chronically" feel incapable of challenging the source (or the individuals) through which their anxiety is generated, primarily because of the fear of rejection. Like a seemingly endless cycle, this fear causes a continual pattern of emotional violation because a person is unable to speak up on behalf of his or her own needs, thus producing insecurity and an inability to challenge the pattern because of the fear of rejection. And so the vicious cycle of this situation repeats and repeats until the person finally gets, quite literally, "sick and tired" of the whole situation.

Frequently in men who develop the illness, the source of their insecurity is related to their work environment and their inability to challenge the professional situations that cause chronic feelings of insecurity and anxiety.

Mononucleosis and Epstein-Barr occur in people who are "sick and tired" of their nonproductive emotional patterns that result in "chronic emotional insecurity."

SARAH

(Shealy)

Diagnosis: Chronic Epstein-Barr.

This is a thirty-five-year-old woman who lives a highly stressed life. She has generalized fatigue, smokes heavily, is very nervous and anxious, and has severe and incapacitating headaches. Although this may seem to fit many women, the outstanding feature here was such intense fatigue that she often had to leave work early or could barely finish the workday and then she would collapse on her couch in the evening. This degree of fatigue was considerably greater than she had experienced before.

ENERGY ANALYSIS

(Myss)

Sarah is a person who developed mononucleosis as a result of becoming emotionally exhausted trying to create her own little world in which she would be safe. Sarah lived on a very thin emotional edge, trying to prove she was a worthy and lovable human being. Her relationship history includes multiple episodes of rejection that resulted in her believing that she needed to "try harder" in order to be loved and accepted. Her stressed life reflected her two divergent motivations; the first was to create a safe world for herself so that she would not need anyone else, and the second was to prove she was worthy enough so that someone would want her.

SYPHILIS

(Shealy)

Syphilis used to be the best known venereal disease. It is caused by venereal contact and it is an extremely chronic disease. Often, in the initial stages, syphilis passes as a very small sore on the genitalia. This is followed by a long, dormant stage in which the individual may not be ill at all. Syphilis ultimately enters a tertiary stage and then may affect all the organs of the body, especially the aorta—the biggest blood vessel in the body—the heart and the central nervous system, as well as the spinal cord. Once it enters the tertiary stage, it is not curable. Prior to that point, syphilis is responsive, the majority of the time, to adequate treatment.

It is widely believed that many individuals who have AIDS also have syphilis, but because of their weakened immune system, even the blood test for it may be inadequate in order to make the diagnosis. Many AIDS patients also have venereal herpes, Chlamydia, hepatitis and candidiasis.

ENERGY ANALYSIS

(Myss)

Syphilis is a disorder that results from negativity directed toward oneself. Specifically, the person who becomes susceptible to this virus very likely will be someone with a history of making unwise and impulsive personal choices regarding his or her emotional needs. Because of the intense feelings of self-directed negativity, the individual will tend not to bring self-respect or self-love into his or her emotional activities. In fact, the negativity toward oneself is often associated with feelings that one is "dirty." My sense is that this negative association is the result of erotic sexual fantasizing that one participates in that reflects one's own lack of self-worth and intensifies the belief that sex is "dirty."

CANDIDIASIS

(Shealy)

Candidiasis, or chronic yeast infection, is a disease that seems to occur in people who have had antibiotic therapy and whose immune system is weakened. Thrush is one form of candidiasis that occurs in the mouth and pharynx area. Candida may also infect any part of the body, including the bloodstream, but it is more common in the vagina, bladder and intestinal tract. It is generally treated with a specific antibiotic, Nystatin.

Dr. Orian Truss has written elaborately on this subject and believes that candidiasis is a commonly missed diagnosis that is responsible for many unusual and difficult to diagnose syndromes such as multiple allergies and generalized fatigue. Truss recommends treating such patients with a low carbohydrate diet, since yeast feeds upon carbohydrates, and Nystatin taken for up to a year in rather large doses. The general medical community has not accepted candidiasis of this low-grade chronic type as a legitimate illness, although many alternative health practitioners believe it is a common disease.

ENERGY ANALYSIS

(Myss)

This disorder occurs mainly in people who have been psychologically, emotionally and physically over-active and are in serious need of stablizing their lives. As in the mononucleosis virus, women are particularly susceptible, but for different reasons. Whereas the mononucleosis virus relates to issues of emotional safety, candidiasis corresponds to issues regarding the creation of a stabilized living situation, specifically what is known as the "nesting bug." The stress emerging from the unfulfilled desire to lay down roots and establish a home and family is directly connected to this virus.

Chronic candidiasis is a rather recently recognized disorder, and my opinion is that candidiasis, along with other contemporary epidemics such as mononucleosis, reflects very accurately our contemporary human stresses, lifestyles and concerns.

FRAN

(S h e a l y)

Diagnosis: Candida infection of the vagina.

This forty-one-year-old psychologist had surgery in 1985 for large fibroids of the uterus. This was an uneventful procedure, but in the post-operative stage, she developed a candida infection of the vagina that has not responded to the usual Nystatin treatment. This has been a recurrent problem for about one year. The patient is a very successful individual and has a large practice. She does feel unfulfilled and wishes that she had been able to have a child. She is not married and has thought about adopting.

ENERGY ANALYSIS

(M y s s)

Fran's situation is very common. Her inner struggle reflects what many women must confront and that is the dilemma of choosing between having a family or a career. In order to excel professionally, Fran focused all of her attention on her education and then on developing a practice. Her personal life and emotional needs were shelved during her start-up years, but as time went by, it appeared that opportunities for fulfillment of any of her personal needs for a husband and a family were rapidly slipping away. Fran would experience serious depression and grief over never having had a child. My feeling is that her personal sorrow and disappointment over not having had a family, coupled with her fear that she had run out of time, was the source of the stress that created not only her candidiasis, but her fibroids of the uterus as well.

CARLOTA

(S h e a l y)

Diagnosis: Candidiasis and infection.

This thirty-two-year-old young lady consulted me with a history of repeated tonsillar, pharyngeal infection (treated with antibiotics), fever and exhausting fatigue. She also had a problem of vaginal candidiasis. She had been treated at least fifteen times with antibiotics in a period of several years. She presently is in the midst of an extremely unsatisfactory marriage with a remarkably ego-centered husband who constantly tells her she is unattractive and that he does not love her.

ENERGY ANALYSIS

(M y s s)

The source of stress for Carlota was obviously her very painful marriage. Her long-running encounter with candidiasis was, in my opinion, a disorder created as a result of never establishing a stable home. Her husband would frequently threaten to leave her and he would occasionally arrange to meet other women. Because Carlota's self-esteem had been so damaged through his continually telling her that she was unattractive, she lacked the capacity to challenge him to any real extent since she feared he would leave her. Moreover, she believed her husband when he told her that she would never find anyone else to marry her. Carlota has not yet been able to find a way of breaking through this challenge.

BACTERIAL INFECTIONS

(S h e a l y)

There are numerous bacteria ranging from typhoid fever to Salmonella (which is generally contracted through contaminated food), to Staphylococcus infections which are known most often in boils or acne pimples. Staphylococcus is also an opportunistic infection and is the most common infection after surgery. As in all infections, it affects people primarily when they are in a generalized weakened state.

Other well-known bacterial infections are streptococci (strep throat), which can lead to scarlet fever, rheumatic fever and rheumatoid arthritis; pneumococcus, a common cause of pneumonia; Hemophilus Pertussis or whooping cough; hemophilus influenza, which are frequent infectious agents in children; Neisseria gonorrhoeae, which causes well-known gonorrhea or "clap," another venereal infection; Klebsiella pneumoniae; E. coli; Shigella; Pseudomonas aeruginosa; Brucella; Clostridium tetani (tetanus); Clostridium botulinum (food poisoning); Mycobacterium tuberculosis (TB); and Mycobacterium leprae (leprosy).

In addition, there is a group of organisms called Rickettsia which includes typhus, one of the more common causes of plague and Rocky Mountain spotted fever.

We have not gone into great detail about many of these infectious agents because most of them are not very common and I believe that the principle involved in infectious diseases is demonstrated through the cases we have presented.

It is interesting to note that on his death bed, Pasteur is quoted as saying, "It is not the germ, it is the culture medium upon which it falls." In other words, it appears that these organisms primarily affect individuals whose immune system is already weakened through an emotional or nutritional factor.

ACCIDENTS

(Shealy)

Accidents remain in the top five causes of illness and death. Generally, they are considered the result of human error or "natural" catastrophes. But in general, science ignores many intriguing associations.

For instance, at least 80% of accidents occur from "carelessness" when individuals are angry. And there seem to be strong correlations between biorhythms—the "natural" rhythms of mood, physical strength, tension, creativity—and the occurrences of accidents. This research indicates that accidents tend to occur more frequently during an individual's negative or low-energy biorhythmic cycles.

Some accidents are the result of lack of sleep, of drugs, poor nutrition and low blood sugar. Each of these stressors leads to decreased coordination, poor concentration and ultimate inability to focus adequately to pay proper attention to the activity at hand.

One of the leading causes of serious accidents is alcohol consumption. And, among children under the age of fifteen, accidents created *by* alcoholics are the leading cause of death.

As one might expect, cigarette smokers have an increased incidence of accidents. Among the many adverse effects of cigarette smoking is decreased memory and a lessened ability to concentrate on fine details. Every time a person lights up a cigarette, the norepinephrine or "adrenalin" is increased by 1.8 times baseline and this causes a marked stress or alarm reaction.

There is also evidence of an adverse effect of positive air ions upon human performance, in addition to some cases of both automobile and airplane crashes that apparently resulted from operator confusion created by the lack of negative ions in the air. Negative ions are generally felt to be more beneficial and to enhance one's feeling of well-being and calmness. Negative ions are more prominent at high altitudes, in the mountains for instance, and after a rainfall.

In a category unto themselves are Worker's Compensation accidents and automobile accidents. Although many physicians have an intuitive feeling that a high number of automobile accident victims and Worker's Compensation victims try to take advantage of the economic consequences of the accident, my own experience with these patients is that it is easier to say that my back hurts than that "my marriage is falling apart" or that "I am not successful at my job." I think that the patient is oftentimes not aware of the difference in terms of the source of pain.

If an individual is having a great deal of marital or work stress
and an accident occurs, for whatever precipitating reasons, then
it seems to the patient that the accident is the cause of all of the
feelings of anger. Obviously, the usual method of scientific attention to measurable cause and effect prevents consideration
of the broader spiritual and metaphysical implications.

JONAH

(S h e a l y)

In December 1987, a friend of mine was involved in a private
plane accident. He was a passenger in the plane along with
another man who was the pilot. The fuel gauge was defective
and the plane ran out of gas and crashed. Jonah, who was thirty-
seven years old, suffered a blow-out fracture of the first lumbar
vertebra with total loss of sensation and function in the bladder,
bowel and sexual area, but with no other major nerve injury.

Jonah initially chose not to have surgery and wanted to
return to our Springfield clinic for his medical care. He asked
me to coordinate surgery if it was to be done. I called Caroline
and asked her to do a reading. The following is a summary of
what she said.

> This accident is more of an initiation experience than it is
> an accident. He did the appropriate thing in choosing
> not to have surgery. It may take him eighteen months,
> but he will take on the journey of learning how to heal
> himself.
> My sense is that this is a sacred experience for
> Jonah. This accident was invoked as a challenge for him
> to see if he could develop himself into a healer. He could
> ultimately have the ability of Olga Worrall [a highly re-
> garded healer] and become a strong channel for healing
> energies.
> He will have to challenge his ego. This is a test to
> draw on will, inner discipline, faith and inner resources.
> If he permits his ego to take over, he will fail. This is
> meant to be a transformational experience. In one to two

months, his ego may try to exert itself over the inner spirit to regain control. Once he overcomes that, he will go on toward true healing.

In cases like this one, the accident serves as a major testing ground for initiating a person into a higher order of consciousness. This is the case with Jonah.

I then saw what Caroline was saying. The accident was a type of spiritual "outward bound" program, forcing a person to live what he or she teaches.

I later asked Jonah, before giving him any of this information from Caroline, what he had been feeling and thinking prior to the accident. He said,

> The other man and I were doing a heavy-duty death urge. We have never been able to receive love. I have been scared of being alive because I know that I have to learn to be loved. But at the time of this crash, I had a calm feeling, as if something was preparing me. The man with me also had something of a death wish. We had been discussing our feelings regarding our inability to receive love, and we also had these feelings of self-punishment needing to be expressed.
>
> When we went down, the pilot tried to bear the brunt through his legs (and he sustained severely fractured ankles on both sides). After just thinking that nobody loves me, the first thought that I had immediately after the accident was that I've got to let people love me.

After I read Jonah the material from Caroline, he said, "It is all fitting all the pieces of the puzzle together." Inwardly, for Jonah, this was a deeply transformational experience. His attitude has been remarkably positive. After I had seen the x-rays, I advised him to consider surgery to decompress the spinal cord and to have a fusion so that he could be up and about in a cast.

The surgeons gave him little hope of recovery of neurological function. Only five months later, however, Jonah has at least 85% of neurologic function, with normal erections and bladder function.

ACCIDENTS

ENERGY ANALYSIS

(M y s s)

Not every accident is as potentially rich an experience as is Jonah's. Nevertheless, I personally maintain that accidents—that is, random events in which one or thousands are victimized—are also events that are co-created. The emotional responses to the fact that many die does not, in my opinion, change the fundamental principles governing how we create our realities. The emotional responses to tragedy and death are just that—emotional responses. They are not evidence that we do not create our own realities.

Discussions about whether or not we create accidents are similar to discussions about whether or not we actually create cancer. In small dosages—such as we create colds, and our anger can cause us to cut ourselves on a kitchen knife—the idea of co-creation of reality holds up.

However, change the outcome from colds to cancer and from knives to airplane crashes, and the entire principle of co-creation gets discarded. The reason why this argument disintegrates when the stakes are so high rests with the misunderstanding people hold concerning "choice."

Certainly, no one rises on a Monday morning and says, "What a lovely day to create cancer," or "I think I'll take my plane out for a fatal crash today." That is, of course, preposterous. But more importantly, it is also *not* an accurate portrayal of the level at which choices of this magnitude are negotiated.

Choices of this importance are made at the spiritual level and, most often, the conscious mind remains unaware of this process. Bear in mind that inasmuch as death is inevitable, why is it so inconceivable that we would participate in the choice as to when to leave the physical form? The only consideration that makes that idea difficult to believe is that we lack any hard-core evidence of what lies beyond this life. If we knew what awaited us, we would have no difficulty believing that we choose when to return to the nonphysical dimension.

I separate accidents into three categories. The first is the rare incidences such as Jonah's in which the "accident" was in fact a means to a greater end.

The second category is those experiences that are created through the unconscious discharging of negative energy, in particular, anger and tension. Dropping things, breaking objects, car collisions, hitting one's knee on a desk corner are all examples of this category of accident. Realize that a person does not consciously choose to break an object; rather, the factor of "choice" refers to the quality of a person's attitudes, which is always determined by the individual. An angry attitude increases the chances for accidents. Nervousness increases the chances for accidents. In allowing these types of emotions to control you, you are choosing also to experience the consequences of that energy. In this case, the consequences are an increased potential for creating accidents.

The third category of accidents is those we consider to be tragedies in which death or serious injury occurs either to one person or to multiple individuals. As stated earlier, it is a challenge to consider that we create our own realities when the outcome is, from our human perspective, death or injury.

Yet, it is not possible for me to discount the principles of co-creation simply because my "reasonable" mind cannot produce an explanation valid enough to cope with the tragic outcome. The human spirit is capable of making choices that the human mind would never consider. For me, the concept of "accident" reflects yet another area of what we need to learn about ourselves. I do not believe that there are any such things as "accidents." Rather, there are only experiences and situations that remain unexplainable because of our lack of awareness about the dynamics and principles of co-creation.

CHAPTER EIGHT

Chronic Diseases—The Long Way Home

(Shealy and Myss)

CHRONIC STRESS

(Shealy)

Most of the diseases that fill our hospitals and lead to the greatest frustration on the part of patients and physicians are the chronic diseases, often called degenerative although they include a wide variety of etiologic agents.

If we consider it possible that Freud's description of a universal "death wish" and Eric Berne's theory of Life Script are representative of a large segment of human consciousness, it is amazing that more people aren't suicidal. Most persons depressed enough to "wish" they were dead do not dwell on that wish twenty-four hours a day. Nevertheless, there are varying degrees of depression and despair, enough in many individuals to create a constant state of unresolved and consuming emotional, psychological, physical and chemical stress. Chronic negative patterns create chronic disease.

To some extent, we each have a "cup" of stress reserves; our amounts differ in strength and size. Additionally, we have various inherent weak spots as demonstrated by the simple diagram on the following page.

As long as our total stress remains below the weak spot, we are relatively "well." When chemical, physical and emotional stress approaches the weak spot, we develop symptoms of dysfunction. As we exceed our "tolerance," we become ill. Thus, chronic illness represents the state of balance between being free of symptoms and illness. As the total of chemical, physical and emotional stress increases, we become increasingly ill. When our limit is reached, our reserves are used and we die. Reducing stress can restore health *if* we reduce the total stress below the free of symptoms line.

Conscious attention to controlling stress at all levels is crucial for restoration of health. Failure to acknowledge problems at any or all eight levels of function (see Chapter One) sets the stage for chronic disease.

ENERGY ANALYSIS OF CHRONIC DISEASE

(M y s s)

Chronic diseases develop as a result of chronically or continually dysfunctional emotional, psychological and/or spiritual patterns that remain ongoing sources of stress in a person's life. These patterns are frequently unconscious, meaning that they blend into what we consider to be our personalities or basic natures. They are the "that's just the way I am" part of ourselves that

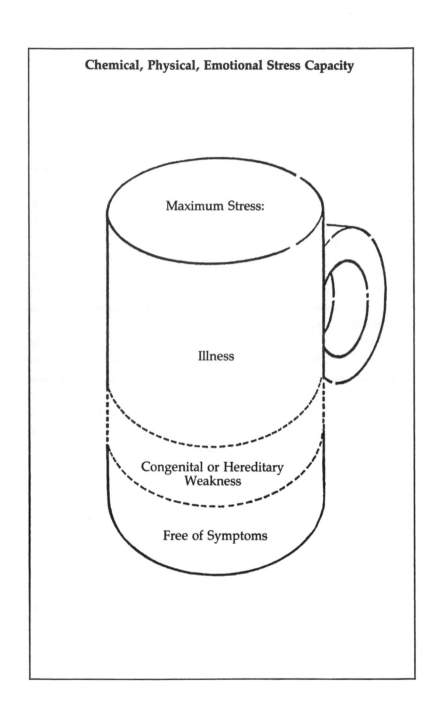

Chemical, Physical, Emotional Stress Capacity

Maximum Stress:

Illness

Congenital or Hereditary
Weakness

Free of Symptoms

we usually don't think about, much less recognize as dysfunctional.

We are often blind to our own chronic patterns. Therefore, we cannot usually unearth them without the occurence of a crisis or a disease. The use of the term "chronic" implies that these patterns tend to be negative or nonproductive—unconscious ways of responding to people or situations that ignite in us our insecurities and anxieties.

Because of the unconscious roots of chronic, stressful patterns, we find ourselves continually irritated, angry or anxious without necessarily knowing what the cause of the tension is. We make the assumption that the source of our stress is "out there" in the form of a person, place or thing. In other words, we project our inner anxiety onto everything and anything *but* ourselves. This is how cycles of chronic, dysfunctional patterns not only get created, but continue to operate in our lives.

The illnesses that chronic patterns create develop gradually and are, not surprisingly, degenerative or chronic in nature. Just as our dysfunctional patterns slowly but surely wear us down, so do these illnesses. Healing chronic ailments requires that the chronic patterns of inner stress be effectively challenged so that their capacity to exert a controlling influence in a person's life can be released.

EPILEPSY

(S h e a l y)

Epilepsy is generally understood to be a "seizure." In earlier days, it was considered a seizure or take-over by demons. Approximately one person in every one hundred people has epilepsy and, in families of epileptics, the incidence is 3%.

At least 97% of the time, epilepsy is idiopathic, meaning "we don't know" the cause. Epilepsy may include generalized or focal, uncontrollable muscle movements, or it may be only sensory (tingling or odd sensations) or behavioral in its manifestations. Behavioral seizures are called "temporal lobe" seizures and may include a variety of actions ranging from violence to catatonia, and the patient is generally amnesic after the episode passes.

Between seizures, epileptics have, a majority of the time, normal EEG's. "Causes" of seizures include trauma to the head or brain, strokes, infections and a wide variety of metabolic/ chemical abnormalities. The latter range from diabetes (high blood sugar) to hypoglycemia, inadequate calcium, kidney failure (high urea), liver failure (high ammonia), to various drugs and toxins. Alcoholics, when drunk or in withdrawal (DT's), drug addicts (even to Valium) and smokers all have an increased incidence of epilepsy.

In over 90% of patients, no physical "cause" of epilepsy can be found. Even at autopsy, individuals with long-standing epilepsy may have perfectly "normal" brains, and elaborate chemical studies often are equally normal. Thus, epilepsy is only an electrical "storm" that may be initiated by psychological stress, as seen in the case study on this disorder.

ENERGY ANALYSIS OF EPILEPSY

(M y s s)

From the perspective of energy, an epileptic seizure is an internalized explosion of violent and enraged feelings that are ignited when an individual is frightened or threatened. In spite of the out-of-control nature of a seizure, my sense is that epileptic seizures frequently are "irrational" control mechanisms. They are a form of releasing emotion that a person is incapable of expressing directly or consciously. This is not meant as an unsympathetic evaluation of epilepsy; rather, it is an interpretation of "seizures" that indicates a person is overwhelmed by intense emotions and is unable to cope through normal channels of expression.

AL

(S h e a l y)

Diagnosis: Idiopathic Epilepsy.

Al is a twenty-nine-year-old man who has had epilepsy since age two, shortly after the birth of his sister. He has never lived away from his parents or held a job because of his tremendous dependency on his parents, now in their sixties. Elaborate neurological testing, including CT and MRI scans and EEG's, all indicated normal brain functioning.

In a consultation with Caroline, she associated Al's seizures with the birth of his sister, suggesting that her birth caused Al to feel so emotionally insecure that he created the response of epilepsy. This disorder continued into adulthood, resulting in Al's overly dependent relationship with his parents. Caroline further suggested that Al's parents insist that he find a job, even if that job were part-time.

I related this reading to both Al and his parents, all of whom were in my office. Immediately following the disclosure of this information, Al had a very severe generalized grand mal seizure, lasting several minutes. He was dazed for five to ten minutes afterward.

His parents informed me that in dozens of previous test situations, including hospitalizations, Al had never had a seizure in front of a physician or nurse. His seizures seem always to be precipitated by power struggles with his father or other threats to his extreme dependency upon his parents.

ENERGY ANALYSIS

(M y s s)

It was immediately clear to me that Al was enraged over having to share his emotional territory with another human being. Obviously, as a two-year-old, he lacked any ability to communicate his feelings, or even to understand them. His fears took control of his emotions and this resulted in his developing epileptic seizures.

My suggestion that his parents *force* him to get a job meant that he take a step toward becoming independent. Logically, if he were able to handle a part-time job, eventually he would be able to work full-time. And that would mean he would be able to move out on his own. This was so threatening to him that he created a seizure. For Al, becoming healthy and able is far more terrifying than remaining an epileptic.

MULTIPLE SCLEROSIS (MS) AND
AMYOTROPHIC LATERAL SCLEROSIS (ALS)

(S h e a l y)

These "degenerative" diseases of the nervous system, although rare, will serve for this brief discussion as major examples of the "great unknowns." Medical science frankly admits that many illnesses have no proven etiology.

Interesting correlates with MS are climate, dietary intake and personality type. Long-standing suspicions about the cause of these diseases include some infectious agent ranging from spirochetes to viruses. It is believed, however, that some auto-immune mechanism is involved; that is, the body's immune system *attacks* the nervous system itself, which is, symbolically, a very self-destructive act.

Of some interest is Edgar Cayce's comment that MS represents a situation of the "entity meeting itself." He was referring mostly to what Cayce interpreter Mary Ann Woodward has called "cash karma"—that is, paying the penalty for cruel and selfish behavior. Cayce also included references to patterns of behavior held over from previous lives in his analysis of people with this illness.

Most physicians dealing with multiple sclerosis patients notice specific patterns of behavior. There seems to be a great deal of suppressed anger in people who develop MS. These patients tend often to be socially polite and nice while simultaneously having a tremendous problem of passive-aggressive behavior and resentment toward a family member, usually a parent figure.

Interestingly, after these patients develop multiple sclerosis, they often begin to behave in an immature and child-like fashion. They become very dependent upon someone to take care of them. Often, the particular individual who needs to take care of the patient is someone who has been previously very supportive.

Obviously, these are generalizations and there are certainly strong exceptions. I have known patients with multiple sclerosis who appeared to have an extremely loving relationship with parents or spouse. They did not seem to have an abundance of suppressed anger or passive-aggressive behavior.

What, then, is the difference in that patient with multiple sclerosis and another who is obviously psychologically disturbed? Why does multiple sclerosis tend to occur more commonly in a colder climate? Why is it related to dietary fat intake? These are the questions that medicine has not been able to answer to this point.

ENERGY ANALYSIS OF MULTIPLE SCLEROSIS

(Myss)

Most commonly, multiple sclerosis is created as a result of a warehousing of resentment and fear regarding how well an individual feels he or she has been prepared for the demands of living as an adult in the world. Dependency is a major issue; specifically, the individual has not completed the dependency phase of childhood and is overwhelmed at the prospect of taking responsibility for his or her life.

This illness can develop at any time during a person's life; that is, it does not necessarily emerge simultaneously with a person's entering adulthood years, which might be a logical conclusion given this description. Certain emotional conditions need to be present in order for this illness to form. These conditions are usually a combination of a situation that demands greater responsibility from the individual coupled with feelings of inadequacy that are much stronger than ordinary insecurities. What occurs, from my perspective, is that the demands of the situation cause the person to retreat into his or her emotional territory created during childhood, thus unlocking all of those unresolved feelings of dependency and inadequacy. This causes the adult mind to confront the child mind. The adult mind resents the child mind for its immaturity and childlike fears, and thus begins the process of attacking oneself. The pattern of neglect experienced during the years of childhood is thus now repeated with oneself as the target of neglect and resentment.

As Norm pointed out, there are exceptions to this pattern in which the individuals who develop this illness have no history of emotional resentment left over from childhood. Yet, one pattern that is present in those individuals whom I have encountered is a pronounced fear of failing in their adult responsibilities. The feelings of inadequacy are just as dominant, even though these individuals may have had supportive childhoods.

I can only speculate on the questions concerning the tendency of the illness to develop more frequently in people who live in a colder climate or who have a high intake of fat in their diets. My sense is that cold climates are more demanding living environments than are warmer regions and, as such, could provide one more threatening factor for someone who is already fearful of taking care of oneself. High fat foods are, likewise, heavily consumed in colder climates and contribute a chemical stress to a person's body that can encourage the development of states of depression and fear.

KATRINA

(Shealy)

Diagnosis: Multiple Sclerosis.

This thirty-five-year-old lady, the wife of a prominent attorney, had a six-month history of progressive neurological difficulties. These included slurred speech, double vision and difficulty in walking. Neurologically, she showed nystagmus (jerking of the eyes), slight difficulty with speech, problems with coordination of finger-to-nose and ataxia (a broad-based unsteady walk). She also had a positive Babinski response; the big toe involuntarily extends when the bottom of the foot is scratched. This indicates damage to the corticospinal tracts or motor system between spine and brain.

She was very frustrated and had wanted a career of her own, which she had postponed in order to help her husband build his career. Katrina had a great deal of unresolved anger over this which she had attempted to work through using meditation and yoga. She was treated with an intense biofeedback, autogenic counseling session for two weeks, and that helped her to gain some positive insights about her situation.

During the following two years, however, she degenerated to the point of requiring a wheelchair and, thus, needed a considerable amount of attention from her husband who, incidentally, had to alter his professional demands in order to accommodate her illness.

She eventually underwent treatment with hyperbaric oxygen, one of the most controversial treatments in multiple sclerosis today. She made a striking improvement following that and, over the next eighteen months, Katrina has improved and stablized. Her neurological problem is only about 10% as bad as it was originally. Her children are now grown and out of the house. She and her husband seem to have a better relationship than they have ever had before.

ENERGY ANALYSIS
(Myss)

Katrina's case study is particularly impressive because of the fact that multiple sclerosis is so often considered as an illness with an inevitably grim outcome.

In marrying her husband, Katrina found a person with

whom she could form a very dependent relationship. Even though she saw herself as creative and as having a need to develop her own talents, it is important to note that she also saw her personal development as intimately linked to and dependent upon her husband's attention and approval.

As his career demanded more and more of his energy, she received less support and attention. This caused her to feel isolated and abandoned, which awakened her fear of being responsible for herself along with her feelings of inadequacy. It is important to note that the anger she experienced was more self-directed than aimed at her husband. Note, too, that Katrina wanted to be released from her limitations and her childlike dependency on her husband. As her husband's attention returned, so did her health.

AMYOTROPHIC LATERAL SCLEROSIS—ALS OR LOU GEHRIG'S DISEASE

(S h e a l y)

Similar to multiple sclerosis in the destruction of the corticospinal tract, ALS destroys only that system. It occurs most often in individuals at the prime of life, thirty-five to fifty-five years of age, and is almost invariably fatal within five years.

ENERGY ANALYSIS OF ALS

(M y s s)

The spinal column is the conduit of the life force system into and through the body. In this disease, the body gradually loses all mobility. What remains active is the brain, intelligence and perception.

This illness develops in response to the need for a person's focus to expand beyond the physical connection to life and incorporate other planes or dimensions of thought into one's reality. Specifically, this is a substantial challenge to reevaluate the quality of one's inner life. This description by no means negates the terror of losing one's physical body bit by bit; however, what is apparent in terms of the dimension of energy is that this disease can serve the purpose of expanding a person's awareness and, through that inner process, heal an imbalance that exists within one's perceptions of reality and spirituality.

The finest example I can offer of this process is illustrated in the life of British physicist Stephen Hawking. Famous for his development of the Black Hole Theory, Hawking is considered to be the most brilliant physicist since Albert Einstein. He is also famous for medical reasons in that he has, since his early twenties, suffered from ALS. He has lived with this disease for almost twenty-five years, dramatically exceeding the five-year estimated life span for ALS. Not only has Hawking lived with this illness, he has produced all of his work and research while simultaneously losing his physical mobility. He has worked totally from a wheelchair for more than a decade and travels the world extensively, sharing his research. His wife Jane commented in a private interview that she feels that Stephen "created" this illness to insure that he would complete his life's work by making certain that he would not be distracted by anything physical.

There is purpose to all that we create, even when what we create is a private mountain that only we can climb.

OSTEOARTHRITIS

(Shealy)

Since osteoarthritis affects 100% of human beings to some extent, its cause is of considerable interest. The diagnosis of osteoarthritis is made most often by examination of x-rays of joints, which show irregularities we call osteoarthritis. There is little inflammation, in most cases, but considerable slow build-up of calcium deposits in damaged cartilage, a condition present in every person to some degree.

Rarely crippling, osteoarthritis is nevertheless quite painful to some individuals. Medically, virtually nothing is known of its cause. Commonly thought to be degenerative or wear and tear, it is clearly to some extent genetic and occasionally the result of specific joint trauma.

There is considerable suspicion that there is a metabolic cause of osteoarthritis, ranging from disturbances in calcium metabolism to acid-base balance (acid vs. alkaline diet). Other nutritional etiologies believed by some are consumption of red meat, excess grains and nightshades, namely potatoes, tomatoes, peppers and eggplant.

ENERGY ANALYSIS OF OSTEOARTHRITIS

(Myss)

All forms of arthritis are created in response to feelings of irritation, frustration and anger. In general, the causes generating these underlying, irritable feelings have to do with issues of control. These range from minor power confrontations that occur in daily life to major situations in which a person becomes obsessed with controlling another person or consumed in resentment over being controlled. How serious the condition is depends upon how intense and/or chronic the stressful emotions are inside of a person.

Osteoarthritis is rooted in irritation and frustration, like small deposits of "energy grit" that get caught in the joints of the body. Interestingly, the specific joints that are affected are strong symbolic indications of the source of the stress, as is illustrated in the following case report. It is impossible, of course, to get through one's life, start to finish, without experiencing irritating encounters with other people. When these irritating experiences accumulate, however, the "grit" in the joints builds to the point of pain and swelling.

GERI

(Shealy)

Diagnosis: Osteoarthritis.

This fifty-five-year-old woman presented with severe hip pain and marked degenerative disease in the left hip. We attempted working with her through intense biofeedback and autogenic training, but she simply was unwilling and unable to do the autogenic training or visualization, and one year later, she underwent surgery for a total hip replacement.

Six months after the hip replacement, she separated from her husband of thirty years because of an ongoing feeling of a total lack of love in the relationship. She has done very well since that time.

ENERGY ANALYSIS

(Myss)

Geri's energy revealed that she had become obsessed by her anger over her empty relationship with her husband. Unable to express her anger, she internalized it to the point that it destroyed her hip joint.

Why the hip joint and not her hands? My sense is that Geri's "grit" settled into her hip joint because she had felt for so long that her husband was not someone who cared about her needs. Rather, he cared that she took care of his needs. She felt trapped in the relationship for reasons of financial security. In other words, Geri felt that she could not physically "walk away" from her marriage, even though emotionally she wanted a divorce. Given the duration of the marriage, thirty years, it is obvious that this emotional pattern of neglect and resentment developed gradually and was, indeed, chronic in their relationship.

Geri's decision to leave her husband is symbolically represented in her surgery in that she had made a choice to regain her movement, symbolically, emotionally and physically.

OSTEOPOROSIS

(S h e a l y)

This is a condition in which the breakdown of bone tissue (loss of calcium in the bones) occurs more rapidly than replacement. It is referred to as bone deterioration. Osteoporosis is a major cause of fractured hips and death in elderly people. Again, this is a degenerative process, largely of aging, increased by the following: cortisone therapy, physical inactivity, post-meno-pause, high meat and high fat diet, low calcium intake and high phosphorus diet. This disease is largely absent in those who eat a vegetarian diet and obtain adequate physical exercise.

ENERGY ANALYSIS OF OSTEOPOROSIS

(M y s s)

This disease is brought about through the gradual diminishing of the energy required to generate life. The business of living becomes more and more demanding and exhausting. Eventually, all movement, both inwardly and externally, is brought to a halt. More than anything else, this illness is associated with feeling that life is just "too much of an effort," and, as such, the physical body begins to feel and act as though it were chattel needing to be hauled. Becoming immobile is a natural response to this type of exhaustion.

RHEUMATOID ARTHRITIS

(S h e a l y)

Rheumatoid arthritis is an autoimmune disorder in which the body attacks the joints themselves. A moderate genetic pre-disposition sets the stage for the development of this potentially crippling disorder, which is often precipitated by major stressful events in a person's life. Treatment often consists of drugs that create more damage than the disease itself.

ENERGY ANALYSIS OF RHEUMATOID ARTHRITIS

(Myss)

This illness is generated by a combination of chronic anger and resentment. Specifically, these emotions are generated because a person feels controlled by the emotional and/or psychological needs of someone with whom they are closely involved. Usually, the patient perceives the controlling source as a person who is emotionally very dependent, and, for that reason, the patient feels unable to challenge the imbalanced emotional dynamics of the relationship. In one sense, the patient often feels as though he or she is being held in emotional bondage with no alternative available for emotional release other than to internalize it. The patient perceives that his or her own movements are being restricted due to the demands of another person.

JANE

(Shealy)

Diagnosis: Rheumatoid arthritis.

At least some degree of "reversibility" is exemplified in Jane's case. She came to see me for treatment of painful rheumatoid arthritis, following unresponsive results from cortisone and gold shots.

She entered our two-week intensive workshop and, on the seventh day of training, she told me that she no longer had rheumatoid arthritis. On the twelfth day, she said,

> I want to tell you the cause of my rheumatoid arthritis. I've been married twenty-eight years and my husband has been unfaithful since we were married. I found out about it when our third child was three years old.
> I decided to stay in the marriage until our children were grown. When our third son was eighteen, he was drafted and sent to Vietnam along with his two brothers.

I couldn't divorce their father while they were in Vietnam. That's when I developed rheumatoid arthritis.

When our boys came home safely, I couldn't divorce their father because I was an invalid. Who would take care of me? I kept saying to myself, 'If it wasn't for that S.O.B., I wouldn't have this disease.'

What I realized during this intensive is that my husband did not create my disease—I did, through my attitude toward him.

With that insight, Jane got well. Her blood tests became normal and she decided that she wanted to remain with her husband because she loved him, despite his problem.

It is important to note that physicians discount reports such as this. And they ignore evidence that depressed patients develop positive rheumatoid blood tests that go away when the depression is successfully treated. Of course, depression is correlated with as many illnesses as is smoking, so its effect is a more generalized one and not the specific "cause." Indeed, depression has multiple causes, some of which are chemical. But most certainly, the majority of depressions are primarily emotional and attitudinal.

ENERGY ANALYSIS

(Myss)

Jane obviously perceived herself as being totally victimized by her husband. She projected onto her husband her own inability to take charge of her life, and she grew to resent herself as much as her husband. The point of particular interest in Jane's case is that she had abdicated her own power of choice to her situation, to her sons and to her dependency on her husband. Without a realization that one has choice, the person can only feel victimized and unable to challenge situations that generate such intense negative feelings. Jane internalized all of her anger and resentment toward not only her husband but also herself and her weaknesses in handling the situation.

Once she realized that her anger was directed at herself, her capacity to retrieve her power of choice returned, as did her health. Thus, she could return to her marriage feeling that it was on her terms.

RHEUMATOID SPONDYLITIS

(Shealy)

Rheumatoid spondylitis is a specialized form of rheumatoid arthritis that primarily affects the spine and occurs more commonly in men than in women. This disease can lead to total fusion of the spine. Rheumatoid arthritis, on the other hand, is more common in women.

ENERGY ANALYSIS OF
RHEUMATOID SPONDYLITIS

(Myss)

It is essential for most individuals to feel that their lives reflect choices they have made regarding the appropriate and satisfactory use of their energy. The actual job or career one has is irrelevant. The important consideration is that no matter what one does, he or she finds value in it.

The absence of this element of choice often results in the feeling that one is "stuck with doing something" that he or she has not "chosen" and that, consequently, both the task and the individual are worthless.

Rheumatoid spondylitis is created as a result of the frustration and anger that accompany the belief that Life somehow assigned to a person his or her circumstances without the element of choice. This belief causes all sense of creativity and the capacity to try something else to disintegrate. A person is left feeling permanently "assigned" to a situation while believing he or she can do nothing to change it. It is an illness that thrives on self-pity, and that attitude is key to the development of this disease.

The life force, that is, the vital life-giving energy that runs along the spinal column, gradually diminishes in strength, and the spine responds by developing an illness that reflects the belief that one is forced to remain as is.

CHARLES

(S h e a l y)

Diagnosis: Rheumatoid Spondylitis.

This forty-one-year-old man was seen for generalized spinal pain that he felt was due to a fall six years earlier when his pain first began. He had seen several physicians who considered him to be a hypochondriac. However, it was quite obvious upon physical examination that he had severe rheumatoid spondylitis with total fusion of the spine from the neck to the sacrum. Charles smoked one and one-half packs of cigarettes per day. He worked as a lawn maintenance person. He was placed in a program of intense autogenic training and biofeedback. Within one week, he had his pain totally under control. He quit smoking at the same time. His pain has now been controlled for three years.

ENERGY ANALYSIS

(M y s s)

Charles exemplifies the trauma of feeling that one has allowed all of the opportunities in life to pass one by. As he hit his mid-thirties, Charles began to reevaluate what he was doing with his life and what his present situation meant in terms of his future. He concluded that he had let the better part of his life, meaning his "youth," slip by and that as a thirty-five-year-old man, there was little he could do to improve his skills and change his life's direction.

This frustration grew to the point of Charles developing very negative feelings about himself and his life's work. As he looked ahead to his future, he saw himself only diminishing in potential rather than developing potential. As a result of his continuing focus on his own limitations of movement and creativity, his spine began to absorb this tension, causing the development of rheumatoid spondylitis.

During the two-week intensive retraining program, Charles began to realize that his attitude had anesthetized his creativity and his power of choice. Even his "choice" to quit smoking represented his taking charge of the direction of his life. In a very real sense, what increased his healing process was that Charles was able to experience hope and optimism once again in his life, thereby opening up his future in a way he had not been able to see previously.

CLARICE

(Shealy)

Diagnosis: Rheumatoid spondylitis.

This thirty-three-year-old former actress had a history of progressive back and pelvic pain for some twenty years. A diagnosis had not been made clearly earlier, although she had somewhat suspected the problem. As a child, she attempted to excel in dance and had wanted to become a professional dancer. She repeatedly injured her back and had to release her ambitions as a dancer. She turned to acting as a career and even there had been frustrated because of her continuing back pain.

Clarice comes from a wealthy family. Her father divorced her mother when Clarice was ten years old, leaving her with a feeling of rejection by her father.

Clinically, the diagnosis of rheumatoid spondylitis was obvious when we examined her. She had no movement whatsoever in the lumbar spine and an x-ray revealed that the spine was fused with the typical changes of rheumatoid spondylitis.

ENERGY ANALYSIS

(M y s s)

Similar to Charles, Clarice is someone whose dreams and ambitions, as she saw them, would never come to fruition. With the obvious conclusion to her dreams of becoming a successful dancer followed by her thwarted efforts to become an actress, Clarice's creative vitality evaporated. Without either of these professions, she could not envision moving forward with her life. Whatever she would do from this point on was less than meaningful, the remains of her unfulfilled ambitions. She felt angry, cheated by life, full of self-pity and victimized.

Her relationship with her father was yet another influential factor in the development of this illness, as Clarice sought to win her father's approval by becoming an "outstanding" talent in the field of dance. The lack of support from her father was no doubt a major contributing stress to the root cause of the number of back injuries she began to experience during her early years of training.

LUPUS ERYTHEMATOSUS

(S h e a l y)

Another of the autoimmune disorders affecting collagen throughout the body, lupus is a "first cousin" of rheumatoid arthritis and is potentially fatal. Treatment of this disease is likely to be more risky than treatment of rheumatoid arthritis.

ENERGY ANALYSIS OF LUPUS
ERYTHEMATOSUS

(M y s s)

Lupus originates in continual and intense feelings of self-hate and disappointment in oneself. Specifically, these negative feelings toward oneself emerge out of an inability to challenge one's own weaknesses, specifically weaknesses that relate to major life patterns, such as being controlled by the expectations of a parent or never being able to take a risk and follow one's dreams. One lives in a continual cycle of repeating the same frustrating situations because these patterns of artificial boundaries or limitations exert more control over a person than his or her capacity to break through them.

SCLERODERMA

(S h e a l y)

Commonly fatal, this disease is another of the connective tissue disorders in which the entire body, from skin through deep organs, turns rigid. There is no significant standard medical treatment.

ENERGY ANALYSIS OF SCLERODERMA

(M y s s)

This disease is created as a reflection of a person obsessed with inflexibility and rigidity. The factor of obsession is crucial, since most people experience some level of inflexibility in their lives.

In the case of scleroderma, however, the individual maintains an attitude of inflexibility out of fear of everything and of every person. Judgmentalism and a highly critical nature most often accompany this illness and these qualities promote "stiffness of mind." The negativity that these attitudes create literally causes the natural softness of the body to disintegrate as a reflection of the absence of softness or openness of the heart.

POLLY

(S h e a l y)

Diagnosis: Scleroderma.

This sixty-two-year-old woman was brought to the clinic by her husband because he wanted to try alternative therapy for scleroderma. Polly had been diagnosed at Mayo Clinic and had only 15% kidney function. She informed me immediately that she would not consider any diet change, that she hated vegetables and would not give up ham. She had a particular obsession with the need to eat ham.

She was unwilling to consider any of the usual alternatives we recommend for scleroderma: enemas, a largely vegetarian diet, castor oil packs to the abdomen. She agreed to participate in our biofeedback-Biogenics® training program with counseling, and she even began to smile a bit. The greatest problem seemed, from perceptions offered by our staff, that Polly was consumed in a chronic power struggle with her husband.

ENERGY ANALYSIS

(M y s s)

Polly became inflexible and highly irritable gradually during her life. Her husband was a domineering individual and they had a relationship in which Polly's role was to support his choices and attitudes. Support was not a reciprocal part of this marriage. Since Polly's need to have a determining voice in the marriage could not be satisfied through healthy, normal, couple dynamics, she became stubborn and unyielding in areas that her husband could not challenge, such as her *compulsive need* to eat only certain foods. Her stubbornness surrounding her choices of personal habits was intensified by her anger in having no power over larger issues.

In regard to suggesting that she consider a healthier diet, I have little doubt that she was clinging to her compulsive eating habits as a reaction to being manipulated and controlled by the advice of others. Though this advice was meant for her own good, perhaps her husband had used the "for your own good" approach to her many times in order to have his own way in decisions. Her inflexibility had become her defensive mechanism and, unfortunately, Polly could no longer discern sincere help when it was offered to her.

DIABETES MELLITUS

(Shealy)

Diabetes is one of the most common disorders. When its onset occurs prior to age thirty-five, it is also called juvenile diabetes. It is thought that these individuals must take insulin the rest of their lives, although we have seen a few patients who seem to have been able to come off insulin or avoid it even though they had juvenile diabetes.

The pancreas, located in the center of the upper abdomen, is both an endocrine gland, producing "hormones" or chemicals that go directly into the blood, and an exocrine gland, producing critical digestive enzymes released into the small intestine to assist digestion of fat, protein and starch. The pancreatic "endocrine" is *insulin*, which helps regulate blood sugar. In diabetes, either inadequate insulin is manufactured or there is a block to the metabolism of insulin.

The most common form is adult onset diabetes which seems to be primarily the result of overeating, excess sugar or too much calorie intake with generalized obesity. It can almost always be controlled with adequate diet and physical exercise, although many of the patients are not motivated enough to do that.

ENERGY ANALYSIS OF DIABETES MELLITUS

(Myss)

Diabetes is a disorder related almost entirely to issues of responsibility. These issues have multiple forms. All of the following qualify as potential causes of diabetes:

- Resentment over having to take responsibility for another person. This may be because that individual refuses to mature or because the person denies being irresponsible, thus causing the more responsible person to compensate.
- Children who resent the demands of one or both of

their parents to "parent" them. When the actual parent
lacks the emotional maturity to give a child the care
and attention that is required, but rather expects the
child to understand and compensate for the ineptitude
of the parent, the child becomes filled with resentment
over the role reversal and the obvious premature ending of his or her childhood years.

- Resentment over having to take responsibility for oneself, expecting that someone else should do this task.
This is a way of postponing or completely disregarding
one's own natural process of maturing.

- Preventing someone else from growing into his or her
natural role of personal responsibility as it threatens
the control one has over the other person.

- Continually making excuses for the irresponsible behavior or attitudes of another. When this happens, the
person making the excuses ends up on the receiving
end of emotional energy that is meant to be directed to
the primary source.

All of these issues of responsibility attack the pancreas. The
reason is that the pancreas is like a fuel tank in a car. It contains
just enough fuel for one driver. In other words, insulin is energy
and the body produces sufficient energy for the appropriate
tasks of only one person. The energy of resentment is a signal
to the body that the allocation of a person's given ration of energy
is being used in ways that are inappropriate. This resentment
signal throws off the production of insulin (or energy) in response to this signal.

EUGENE

(S h e a l y)

Diagnosis: Juvenile Diabetes.

This young man came to the clinic at thirty-one years of
age with acute diabetes. His blood sugar was 350. His difficulties
began shortly after he lost his job and fell into a deep depression.

His mother came to visit him and fixed all of the desserts he had enjoyed as a child. Essentially, he gorged himself on pies and candies. He was diagnosed as having acute diabetes requiring insulin. He was treated with intense biofeedback, autogenic training, systemic relaxation and counseling. It was recommended that he eat a high carbohydrate and high fiber diet, and begin a regular exercise program. He was given six tablets of Myo-Inositol per day and six tablets per day of Brewer's yeast.

Not only did his blood sugar return to normal, but his cholesterol count dropped from 300 to 188. He has been able to control his diabetes entirely.

ENERGY ANALYSIS

(Myss)

It is certainly symbolic that upon losing his job, Eugene's mother came to visit her child to "baby" him back to health. His emotional response to being released from his job ignited all of his issues about fear of taking responsibility for himself. This episode that resulted in an attack of diabetes was just like taking an emotional journey back to childhood. Indeed, it was very much a living out of how Eugene felt privately to himself, in spite of his age of thirty-one. Emotionally, Eugene still wanted to be at home and be cared for. He wanted his mom to "make his problems all better for him," which she tried to do with sugar. Obviously, some part of him experienced an automatic conflict as he attempted, even briefly, to return to his emotional childhood state. The need to take a look at what he was doing that caused him to lose his job had a collision with his desire to return emotionally to his childhood. The result was the eruption of his pancreas and an acute attack of diabetes.

POLYNEUROPATHY

(Shealy)

Polyneuropathy is an unusual and potentially serious illness. The most common measurable cause is diabetes, and often polyneuropathy begins up to ten years before diabetes even is diagnosed.

Polyneuropathy is essentially the death of or severe damage to a variety of nerves outside the spinal cord and can lead to severe numbness and weakness. Other causes are thyroid disorders, lead poisoning and other heavy metal poisonings, viral infections and the great "unknown" or "idiopathic." This means, as in my personal experience, that we cannot find a detectable cause in at least 50% of these people. Vitamin deficiencies, such as vitamin B_{12} deficiency, may also lead to peripheral neuropathy.

ENERGY ANALYSIS OF POLYNEUROPATHY

(Myss)

This disorder is similar in cause to diabetes in that it relates to the fear of taking charge of one's own life. The additional factor is the fear of being alone, or abandoned, which causes the dependency aspect characteristic of this illness. Frequently, individuals who develop this illness have experienced themselves as being their only support system, regardless of whether or not they were married or single. It seems that the fear of being abandoned is like a permanent lens implant through which they see and experience the world.

KAY

(Shealy)

Diagnosis: Polyneuropathy; severe obesity.

This forty-five-year-old woman came to me with a three and one-half year history of severe fatigue, with left-sided weakness and numbness and a feeling of choking, as well as a loss of hot-cold sensation in her throat, slurred speech and intermittent blurring of vision with some double vision.

She had been seen by twenty-one physicians. On examination, she had a marked decreased gag response, minimal deep tendon reflexes, absent ankle jerks, and decrease in vibration sensation and severe decrease in pin-prick sensation, especially in the right leg and most of her right side up to the top of her head. An EMG confirmed that she had severe generalized polyneuropathy. The patient weighed 297 pounds at 5'7" in height.

The patient has responded well to intense biofeedback training, autogenic training, acupuncture and counseling. She then went through a rather traumatic divorce without relapsing.

ENERGY ANALYSIS

(M y s s)

Kay's relationship to her husband was obviously the central source of her stress. In marrying, Kay thought she had resolved her fear of taking rsponsibility for herself. In actuality, she was plagued by fears and insecurities constantly. Her own creativity was stifled and she blamed her relationship with her husband for her inability to express herself.

Obesity is often the result of the inability to express one's creative energies or to bring one's ideas into full physical manifestation. Creative inspiration and ideas are energy, and energy expands. It must have a channel through which to come into physical form. When no channel exists, the energy becomes congested in the body, causing the body to retain additional fats and calories that it would otherwise burn up through the creative process. Certainly, one's calorie intake is also a major part of weight gain, but this emotional counterpart is an equally valid factor. Kay became obese as a response to feeling incapable and inadequate as well as emotionally abandoned. The combination of these factors resulted in her numerous dysfunctions, including polyneuropathy.

SPASTIC COLON

(Shealy)

Spastic colon is a clinically interesting disorder in which individuals vary between having diarrhea and constipation, both of which are associated with abdominal cramps, gaseousness, indigestion and general discomfort of the abdominal area of the body. No known etiology exists, although it is generally thought to be primarily present in people who eat a low fiber diet and are nervous and anxious.

ENERGY ANALYSIS OF SPASTIC COLON

(Myss)

A spastic colon is created as a result of the stress that accompanies a lack of self-confidence, self-esteem and personal power. That particular area of the body is the third chakra and, as described in Chapter Four, this region corresponds to one's personal sense of well-being.

People prone to spastic colons tend to be easily intimidated by others and find expressing their ideas and opinions extremely difficult. Public speaking is a perfect example of a situation that would engage a spastic colon in such a person.

SARAH

(Shealy)

Diagnosis: Severe spastic colon.

This thirty-seven-year-old lady was suffering from severe fatigue, weakness and diarrhea. She has had intermittent episodes of diarrhea and constipation since childhood. She has a history of having used marijuana fairly frequently but has been using it rarely more recently. She also used mescaline once in the past. She has had multiple evaluations of the gastrointestinal tract and no abnormalities have been found. The diagnosis of severe spastic colon has been the only major medical diagnosis.

The patient responded exceptionally well to castor oil packs, intense biofeedback, counseling and autogentic training.

ENERGY ANALYSIS

(Myss)

Sarah's energy reading revealed that she has suffered severe stress all of her life caused by feelings of inadequacy. These dominated her consciousness, and thus, dominated all of her life's feelings. For Sarah, everything was a potential trigger for a spastic attack, from meeting new people to trying something new in her life. Her exhaustion was the result of continually feeling highly anxious and nervous, which is essentially counterproductive to rest and relaxation. She had a poor self-image and little confidence that she possessed anything that was special or unique.

Her response to the training in biofeedback, autogenic training and counseling provided Sarah with the opportunity to challenge her insecurities in an environment that was supportive. That was essential for her since she was emotionally very fragile.

HEPATITIS

(Shealy)

Hepatitis is diagnosed whenever there is any inflammation of the liver, which leads usually to jaundice and a variety of abnormal liver enzyme tests. It is most commonly diagnosed as the result of a viral infection, Hepatitis A, which is rampant in India and other countries where sewage is poorly handled. Hepatitis B, another virus, is more often found in homosexuals or drug addicts and can become a very chronic and contagious disorder. Transmission of the B virus is primarily by fecal or blood contamination.

Mononucleosis and a wide variety of non-viral agents may also cause hepatitis. Alcohol and many drugs are toxic to the liver and can lead to hepatitis or cirrhosis, a severe, chronic scarring of the liver.

ENERGY ANALYSIS OF HEPATITIS

(M y s s)

Hepatitis is created as a direct result of not being able to process emotional toxins, specifically fears and insecurities. Whereas kidney malfunction relates to "hot" toxins, such as anger and rage, the liver is more responsive to emotional issues related to fears concerning finances and feelings of physical security, such as job or home security. Often, anxiety over feeling powerless in these areas is present.

One characteristic of people who are most susceptible to hepatitis is that they never want to hurt anyone's feelings and, thus, they find that they cannot discuss matters that are upsetting to them. They keep matters to themselves, even though this keeps them in a constant state of emotional stress. Their perception of kindness, in other words, is often self-toxic.

CHRIS

(S h e a l y)

Diagnosis: Post-hepatitis electrical dysesthesia.

Chris is a fifty-year-old man who had hepatitis at age eighteen. Following that, he suffered from constant electrical tingling in every part of his body *except the genitalia*. He has been examined and evaluated by numerous experts and no abnormalities can be found. He has tried dozens of therapeutic approaches to heal, including acupuncture, TENS, homeopathy, Biogenics training and counseling, all without success. Despite his frequent seeking of a cure, he functions quite successfully as an outstanding college teacher.

ENERGY ANALYSIS

(M y s s)

Chris is a classical example of a gentle soul who cannot successfully express his emotional concerns for fear of causing controversy. The tingling sensation that he constantly must cope with is his emotional current moving though his body *without any productive outlet*. In other words, his desire to keep his emotional perceptions to himself has effectively created an energy seal around his own body in which, according to his choice, he keeps his emotional electricity only to himself. His fear of sharing has blocked off the natural energy dynamic of give and take. Without this process, his energy becomes stale, like the air in a sealed basement. Obviously, the only channel through which he feels comfortable expressing emotions is sexually, since that is primarily a physical act that "does the expressing for him."

CONCLUSION

(S h e a l y)

Some physicians have stated, rather tongue in cheek, that the clue to a long life is to acquire a chronic disease and then take good care of it. Osteoarthritis and spastic colon, for instance, rarely shorten life, but all chronic illnesses lead to some degree of pain and suffering. Some chronic diseases, such as scleroderma and ALS, shorten life considerably.

The study of chronic illnesses is the study of our own chronic negative patterns. No doubt, each of the people we have discussed could have avoided some degree of suffering had they had the wisdom to know what they were creating through the choice to give in to negativity and fear.

CHAPTER NINE

Chronic Pain

(S h e a l y   a n d   M y s s)

CHRONIC PAIN SYNDROME

(S h e a l y)

E veryone experiences pain from time to time. Acute pain is commonly felt when there is either tissue damage or a threat of tissue damage—cuts, bruises, abrasions, sprains and fractured bones. We may have a problem of pain that may last anywhere from a few hours to a few weeks, depending upon the injury. With healing, the majority of the time, the pain disappears. Unfortunately, between 5% and 10% of patients, depending upon the specific injury and whether it is surgical or some other type of injury, develop a chronic pain syndrome for which no apparent "physical" cause can be found.

In our society today, the most common problem that in-

capacitates individuals and causes them to become invalids who
are no longer able to perform their usual activities, is chronic
back pain. Prior to 1939, back pain was diagnosed generally as
a back strain or sprain or as lumbago. With the advent of the
myelogram, an x-ray technique in which a material is injected
into the spinal canal to provide density contrasting to bone or
nerve, neurosurgeons and orthopedists began to diagnose ruptured discs with increasing frequency, and, indeed, today most
often the diagnosis is either back strain or a ruptured disc. Theoretically, when there is a truly ruptured disc, there should be
not only nerve root pain, but numbness and weakness involving
a specific nerve root. The majority of people operated for a so-
called ruptured disc do not have a ruptured disc. They may have
a bulging or degenerated disc but not a disc truly ruptured and
pressing on a nerve root. In 1972, I reviewed two hundred and
fifty original operative notes and myelograms and could be sure
of a ruptured disc in only twenty-two cases.

Prior to the last ten years, a myelogram was performed
using iodinized poppyseed oil injected into the spinal canal. One
fourth of those patients who had a single myelogram developed
arachnoiditis or an inflammatory scar of the spinal nerve roots,
which in itself is quite painful. Even when there is a ruptured
disc, the best statistics generally state that 70% of patients improve significantly following surgery.

One study by an orthopedist in Portland, Oregon reported
that only 39% of Workers' Compensation injured patients who
underwent a lumbar laminectory, or back operation, for a ruptured disc returned to work within two years, and even then,
of course, not all of them would have been free of pain.

Even when the surgery is indicated and there is a truly
ruptured disc, removal of the disc does not necessarily mean
that a patient will wind up free of pain. I think it is fairly safe
to conclude that a *maximum* of 50% of patients who undergo
back surgery wind up virtually free of pain following surgery.
Post-operative scarring, scarring created by the myelogram, or

settling of the vertebrae with the facet joints developing an arthritis stress syndrome are common physical causes of postoperative lumbar back pain.

About 50% of those people who are operated on for a lumbar disc have some kind of compensation-related problem; that is, the so-called injury to the back occurred on the job or in an accident. The other 50% of people may just walk across the room or get up off a couch and suffer the onset of their acute, disabling pain.

It is my impression that about 70% of people who have severe back pain, with or without sciatica, have a problem that I call a facet joint syndrome; namely, the tiny joints on either side of the spine, present at each vertebral level and overlapping like the shingles on a roof, have become "stuck" in an abnormal position and are not moving properly. They may be physically rotated from their normal position of alignment.

In these individuals, proper attention with osteopathic manipulative therapy, or a nerve block done under fluoroscopic guide, will lead to an excellent resolution of the back pain. Probably at least 20% of the time, the problem, instead of coming from the facet joints, comes from a rotation of the sacrum causing a sacroiliac joint syndrome. This particular diagnosis is virtually unknown by most allopathic physicians, and probably not more than 10% of osteopathic physicians recognize it and treat it. The proper treatment, in the first few weeks at least, would be good osteopathic manipulative therapy. Once the sacrum has been rotated for six months to a year or more, it is highly unlikely that it can ever be mechanically put back into the right position. At that time, desensitizing nerve blocks would be the treatment of choice.

The real problem in chronic back pain, as in other forms of chronic pain, is that there usually seems to be some kind of physical precipitating problem that is treated sometimes appropriately, sometimes not. When the pain does not respond within the first few weeks as is generally expected, physicians begin to be puzzled and start trying tranquilizers or continuing narcotics;

and this leads to a vicious cycle of more and more depression, increasing physical inactivity and more and more pain. Finally physicians decide that the patient is a "crock" and that the pain is all in their head. This leads to a power struggle between the patient and the physician that often involves a third-party—an attorney or insurance company—as well.

Patients who smoke are twice as likely to have ruptured discs and/or acute or chronic back injuries as are those who do not smoke. The statistics suggest that if a patient smokes and has a back operation, they are nine times as unlikely to recover from it as a non-smoker. Other major contributors to both acute and chronic back pain are poor physical condition, especially with weak abdominal muscles, and poor posture.

In acute lumbar pain, most patients can be adequately treated with acupuncture. Interestingly, Sir William Osler, the father of American medicine, wrote as late as 1912 that the treatment of preference in lumbago was acupuncture. His practical experience demonstrated the benefit of acupuncture.

Acupuncture is the treatment of preference in many cases of acute low back pain. If that does not work, transcutaneous electrical nerve stimulation (TENS) should be applied, and the patients should then be taken to x-ray the following day to have a local anesthetic injected into an appropriate spot on the affected facet joints. Osteopathic manipulative therapy (OMT) should be considered as early as possible, but muscle spasm sometimes prevents manipulative correction. Thus, quieting the irritation with acupuncture, TENS or a nerve block may make OMT easier and more effective.

In my experience, this will take care of about 99% of acute lumbar pain problems, and if patients are treated rapidly and appropriately in this way, I think we will wind up with 99% less back surgery and probably an equally decreased number of chronic back invalids.

Ruptured discs in the neck are also a not infrequent diagnosis and surgical procedures on the neck are the common approach. If patients do not get well with immobilization in a collar or use of cervical traction within a few weeks, they usually end up having a myelogram and going on to surgery. Even here, I believe that a majority of the time, the pain is due to facet joint difficulties rather than to truly ruptured discs.

In all types of pain, fear is a major factor that may make pain more intense or more prolonged. Fear that *something is wrong*, that serious physical harm has occurred, is common. Fears that one will be unable to work, to be financially secure, to function sexually, are also part of the initial and continuing emotional reaction to pain. Many minor "accidents," which initiate pain, occur when individuals are preoccupied with outside worries or anger with someone closely connected to them, such as a boss, fellow employees or family members. This mental preoccupation leads to inattention or carelessness, which precipitates accidents. Most individuals blame the accident, or the employer, for the pain. It is consciously, and subconsciously, easier to say, "My back hurts" than it is to admit, "my marriage or my job hurts."

Physical pain is considered more *real* than emotional pain, and physical complaints are more socially acceptable. The increased attention derived from pain may provide nurturing that is otherwise missing. This nurturing may "condition" the patient to continue hurting in order to receive "love," extra nurturing or special privileges.

Pain-reducing medications and tranquilizers often cause depression, further complicating a difficult social problem aggravated by financial concerns when one is unable to work. Habituation and addiction to *prescribed* drugs are major aggravators of an invalid pain state.

Only when psychological, social and drug problems are resolved is chronic pain likely to improve. Major marital, family and vocational counseling is often required before patients with chronic pain can recover.

ENERGY ANALYSIS OF CHRONIC PAIN

(M y s s)

Chronic pain is the area of my work that is both the most fascinating and the most frustrating. Chronic pain, according to energy analysis, develops as a result of having chronically negative attitudes and/or unconscious emotional response mechanisms that keep a person continually in stress. Chronic attitude problems are particularly difficult to deal with by virtue of the fact that they *are* chronic, meaning that these patterns are so much a part of a person's self-image that he or she *does not recognize them as separate* from his or her personality. Rather, chronic patterns tend to fall into the category of "that's just the way I am," with the assumption being that we cannot change the way we are. We are born with certain character traits and tendencies and these, so we tend to believe, are permanent.

Unconscious emotional response mechanisms are behavioral characteristics that develop in response to chronic attitudes. For example, a very common unconscious emotional response is to become defensive or emotionally closed down when we are threatened. Frequently, we are not even aware of how our attitude and body language change when we shift from feeling secure to insecure. Yet, from the moment our insecurities are activated, we automatically begin to behave in ways to protect ourselves. Often we are not consciously aware of these patterns of protective behavior. These patterns that are automatic are chronic.

Chronic negative attitudes are equally automatic. The tendency to complain constantly or to have a pessimistic outlook on life may be so habitual for a person that he or she is unaware of these negative attitudes. Other people can usually spot a person's chronic negative attitudes immediately.

Chronic negative patterns, attitudes and behavior create chronic pain. Whether it is a tendency toward criticizing others, or a habit of always responding in anger when one is upset, or whether the negativity is present in an overall attitude of pessimism and distrust of others, these chronic ways of being produce continual currents of stress that disrupt the emotions and the physical body.

The invisible nature of chronic patterns cannot be overemphasized. Nothing is more difficult to identify than our assumed "natural" ways of being in the world that, in fact, are essentially patterns we have developed to help us cope. Much of the difficulty rests with the fact that we frequently confuse our motivations and our needs with our behavior. We believe our motivations to be honorable, so how can our behavior indicate anything else?

There are certain parts of the body that are especially susceptible to chronic negative patterns and, thus, chronic pain: the spine (which includes everything from the shoulders and neck down to the base of the spine), the stomach (as in ulcers), and the head (headaches or migraines). From the perspective of energy, this location of chronic pain makes a great deal of obvious sense.

The spine appears like a thermometer that regulates the flow of energy up and down the spinal column. Symbolically (and perhaps literally), the spine represents our capacity to stand up for ourselves, to carry our own weight and responsibility. Virtually everything we deal with, from the time we become adolescents through the remaining adult years of our lives, revolves around ourselves in relationship to the external world. Can we make it on our own? Can we take care of ourselves and other people? Can we earn a living? Can we handle the demands of our lives, our professions and our relationships?

All of these questions and their consequent pressures affect our physical bodies—in particular, our spinal column. We use several expressions that refer to pressure building up in the cranial area: "to blow one's top," to "lose one's cool," to be driven "crazy" by something or someone. These forms of expression should be recognized as *literal descriptions* of how an external situation is affecting the flow of energy within someone's body because, literally, this imbalance of energy is the source of migraines and neck pain. The energy flows up the spine and becomes congested in the cranial area, causing immense pain.

Ineffective emotional and psychological patterns can be challenged and they can be altered, but it takes a substantial amount of awareness to see oneself clearly and to separate one's patterns of behavior from the deeper self that is alive inside each of us.

The following case reports are all chronic pain cases. In all of these cases, the individuals were living out patterns that were nonproductive and pain inducing, yet they saw their motivations as positive.

ROBERT

(S h e a l y)

Diagnosis: Chronic post-surgical back and neck pain.

This fifty-year-old physician has had difficulties with both neck and lower back pain since age seventeen when he had his first of a series of accidents, a football injury. He underwent two lumbar laminectomies for ruptured discs, one in 1967 and another in 1968, following which he developed post-transfusion hepatitis. His final lumbar operation was a fusion from L3 to the sacrum done in 1976.

In 1973, he had an anterior fusion at C5-6. In 1982, he had an anterior fusion at C4-5. This actually increased the pain in his neck, and he has been intermittently incapacitated with severe neck pain and muscle spasms, leaving him out of work up to 50% of the time. He has responded extremely well to our intense two-week treatment program, including massage, transcutaneous electrical nerve stimulation, autogenic training and biofeedback. He is now working a reasonable schedule, though not his previously attempted sixty plus hours per week regimen.

ENERGY ANALYSIS

(M y s s)

Robert's energy system revealed that he was motivated by chronic "responsibility-itis," so much so that he was incapable of relying on other people or of trusting other people. In his mind, if he did not handle the responsibilities, surely the whole system would break down. Moreover, because of his need to see himself as the central authority figure, he became critical of other people's actions and motivations.

In keeping with the invisible nature of chronic patterns, Robert believed that how he was and what he did and said were all acceptable because his motivation was *to be fully responsible for his patients*. Thus, it was difficult for Robert to look at himself and wonder if he was thinking or acting in ways that contributed to the stress he was physically experiencing. The source for his pain, consequently, had to be *external* (in other words, someone else's fault) because, from his point of view, his motivations were beyond reproach. He was not able to look beyond his obvious motivations and into his fear and insecurities which made it impossible for him to trust or appreciate another person (the motivations behind the motivations, so to speak). His inability to "lean on" others caused continual patterns of stress and strain on his spine that began during his teenage years and continued through the rest of his life.

When Robert finally entered a two-week intensive program, he had to confront his own patterns and his own ways of seeing others and reacting to the stimuli from the outside world. He was able to begin to realize how easily threatened he was by the notion of sharing authority, which he viewed as relinquishing control.

MARY BETH

(S h e a l y)

Diagnosis: Chronic post-surgical back pain.

This fifty-nine-year-old woman has had pain throughout her back for at least twenty-six years. She underwent her first lumbar laminectomy for presumed ruptured disc in 1960. She had a repeat one in 1968 coupled with a fusion. She had continued to have many episodes of low back and, at times, upper back pain. She has also had high blood pressure, hypothyroidism (for which she takes 3 grains of thyroid) and many episodes of severe agitated depression, for which she has had multiple psychiatric hospitalizations.

She now rarely complains of severe lumbar back pain and has responded intermittently to nerve blocks, acupuncture, biofeedback and autogenic training, sometimes going for a number of months with a decrease in her pain before having a flare-up requiring further therapy.

ENERGY ANALYSIS

(M y s s)

Mary Beth is an individual who has wrestled her entire life with challenges revolving around who is in control of her life and her "structure." The breakdown of her thyroid represents her struggle over the development of her own willpower (refer to the material in Chapter Four on the Fifth Chakra). She has never found it easy to assert herself and has consequently felt that the movement in her own life was controlled, and therefore limited, by the demands of others.

High blood pressure is indicative of emotional responses of anger and frustration. Depression is a condition frequently brought about through feeling that one's power of choice is either absent completely or totally eclipsed by the demands of one's situation. Mary Beth felt that her power of choice was eclipsed by her situation.

In learning alternative methods, such as biofeedback, Mary Beth developed coping mechanisms that provide her with alternatives to releasing her frustration other than through back pain and depression, even though she has occasional relapses into her older and more familiar patterns.

MIGRAINE HEADACHES

(S h e a l y)

Perhaps as many as 50% of patients who suffer from severe and incapacitating headaches have migraine. Migraine headaches are vascular headaches. They tend to occur more in women, are sometimes associated with menstrual cycles and are occasionally aggravated by taking birth control pills. They are frequently associated with a variety of food allergies, including red wine, cheese, chocolate and sometimes common foods such as wheat, corn, milk, citrus and eggs.

Abnormalities of serotonin metabolism have been demonstrated and a number of enzymatic biochemical abnormalities are present in patients with migraine. The mechanism for the headache seems to be first a vasoconstriction, a narrowing of the blood vessel created by some electrical-chemical disturbance, followed by dilation or enlargement of the blood vessels at the base of the brain, which leads to a headache.

Interestingly, about 90% of patients with migraine tend to have very cold hands, especially during a headache attack. This finding results from a reflex disturbance in the autonomic nervous system that constricts blood vessels in the hands while dilating blood vessels at the base of the brain. The dilated blood vessels inside the skull cause the headache. Although there are numerous drugs that are partially or temporarily effective in treating migraine, 84% of the patients with migraine can have them totally brought under control with temperature biofeedback training in which they learn to raise the temperature of their hands. This can be accomplished without any other psychotherapeutic approach. Nevertheless, most physicians recognize that migraine sufferers tend to be compulsively neat and perfectionistic. Headaches also respond well to resolution of this need to be perfect.

ENERGY ANALYSIS OF MIGRAINE HEADACHES

(Myss)

Migraine headaches develop in response to an attempt to control one's emotional reactions of anger, frustration, rage or other emotions containing the same quality of energy. By control, I am referring to someone trying to prevent an emotional explosion from occurring externally and, thus, it occurs internally. The need to control is the major characteristic of people prone to migraines. This need may be directed toward controlling themselves, other people or circumstances.

As mentioned in the opening segment on chronic pain, the energy of anger, for instance, is rapid in movement. The person's body can literally start to shake when anger-filled. As the energy begins to "race" up and down the spine, it is seeking a means of expression. As this energy bombards the brain, it forces a person's reasoning capacity to go on overdrive in an attempt to cope with the external source of the stress. When one's reasoning powers fail to cope with the emotional tension, an explosion of some sort becomes inevitable.

It is not surprising that migraines are more common in women, since women tend to be more aware of their emotional energy and more prone to internalize their reactions. Also, women are more likely to feel that their "options" in terms of changing situations are more limited then men's, and that is a crucial factor in understanding the prevalence of migraines in women.

KATHERINE

(S h e a l y)

Diagnosis: Migraine headaches.

This young lady came to the clinic at age sixteen with intractable migraine headaches that she felt were due to severe stress and tension. The headaches had been a problem for about three and one-half years. They were brought under total control through counseling, biofeedback and autogenic training.

ENERGY ANALYSIS

(M y s s)

Katherine's situation was very typical. She felt emotionally alone, very misunderstood and frightened about growing up. She felt that she had no outlet for her feelings and, in particular, for coping with her insecurities. Her migraines began shortly after she entered puberty and were connected to the increased emotional sensitivity brought about through the menstrual cycle.

For Katherine, the counseling was especially healing since it provided her with a means of discovering that she was more normal than she realized, and that what she was finding confusing in her life represented what *every* teenager found to be confusing.

PHANTOM LIMB PAIN

(S h e a l y)

Pain of an incapacitating nature, perceived by the patient as being in the actual limb which has been totally amputated, is one of the more frustrating and interesting chronic pain problems. Prior to our work with biofeedback training, we had found no effective treatment for phantom limb pain.

Loss of any body part has obvious self-esteem implications.

In a society where physical beauty and physical power are highly regarded, only a remarkably strong individual can adjust to the loss of a limb, or a breast. Physical mutilation of any part of the body may lead to great anxiety and loss of self-esteem, even in individuals who were previously coping well. Effective therapy must include thorough analysis of emotional conflict created by the grief of physical loss.

ENERGY ANALYSIS OF PHANTOM LIMB PAIN

(Myss)

Phantom limb pain is created as a result of the person not coping with or accepting the reasons why the amputation occurred in the first place, and it is also a substitute for the more authentic issues that arise, which are vulnerability and inadequacy. This type of pain is fairly clear evidence that "cutting away" the problem does not resolve the cause of the problem.

LOUANNE

(Shealy)

Diagnosis: Phantom limb pain.

This sixty-six-year-old nun presented with a twenty-six year history of severe phantom limb pain as a result of a leg amputation. Actually, the difficulty began in 1942 when she had surgery on her knee for a chronic arthritic problem. She then underwent an attempted fusion of the left knee that failed. Following that, she had amputation of the leg.

She also underwent a cordotomy (cutting of the anterior half of the spinal cord) in 1950, which did not relieve the pain. Her pain was brought totally under control with the use of acupuncture, local nerve blocks, autogenic training and biofeedback. She has been able to wear a prosthesis since that time and has functioned well for five years.

ENERGY ANALYSIS

(M y s s)

Sister Louanne's stress was deeply connected to her living situation within the confines of the convent. The controls and demands for obedience, standard to the religious life, created an enormous amount of resentment in this woman, coupled with her fears related to dependency. First, this created her arthritis located in the knee, an indication of the mounting and, literally, crippling degree of stress in this woman's life.

The surgical treatment for arthritis did not include counseling. Therefore, the condition of stress persisted, resulting in the amputation of her leg. Physically, Sister Louanne became as crippled as she felt emotionally.

The phantom pain continued for twenty-six years. During these years, she was incapable of successfully challenging her feeling of being vulnerable and therefore controlled. Note that these feelings were chronic in Sister Louanne. She no doubt had issues with dependency prior to her entering religious life. Her situation as nun served as a circumstance in which her inadequacies surfaced.

Her therapeutic treatment was effective primarily because her emotional suffering was acknowledged and recognized as an authentic stress.

MYOFASCIAL PAIN

(S h e a l y)

One of the more frustrating forms of pain is a problem called myofascial pain, a painful condition involving primarily the muscles of the back.

It tends to occur in individuals who are not sleeping well or who have stage four sleep interrupted. This is the deep or restorative form of sleep, and stage four sleep is severely interrupted by almost all tranquilizers, especially the Valium, benzodiazepine, group of drugs, and by almost all sleeping pills.

Interestingly, individuals who get a great deal of aerobic exercise almost never develop myofascial pain and seem to be able to get by without the type of myofascial pain coming from inadequate sleep.

ENERGY ANALYSIS OF MYOFASCIAL PAIN

(M y s s)

This dysfunction is rooted in the need to block the signals from the unconscious mind coming into the conscious mind. During normal and healthy sleep patterns, much of the day-to-day tensions are "processed" through dreams. This is Nature's way of providing a daily maintenance system for stress management.

When a person blocks this function, it is indicative of the fact that the individual does not want to deal consciously with the tensions occurring in his or her life. The block creates pain through the back or along the spinal column. In the language of energy, all of the chakras along the spine become congested through the desire *not to address the reasons for the build-up of tension in one's life*. It is a pain state created through denial of difficulties and through fear of having to face the reasons why the difficulties are present.

CHARLENE

(S h e a l y)

Diagnosis: Scoliosis and myofascial pain.

This forty-five-year-old individual had a problem with both scoliosis and myofascial pain. Charlene considered herself to be in good health until May 20, 1984, when she was involved in an automobile-truck accident. This exacerbated a long-standing, recurrent neck pain problem. She had been having some difficulty for at least twenty-three years with neck pain which required some chiropractic treatments. The accident occurred when the car she was driving had stopped to turn and was rear-ended. Following that, she developed severe pain in the neck and between the shoulder blades. The major problems seemed to be a mild scoliosis and a severe myofascial pain syndrome. She does not smoke. She has responded only modestly to intense physical therapy, biofeedback and autogenic training.

ENERGY ANALYSIS

(Myss)

Charlene's energy field revealed that she had chronic difficulty with issues of assertion and self-responsibility, which created continual obstacles for her in terms of her daily work activities and her personal life. Her sense of inadequacy drove her to push herself mentally without much attention to her emotional wear and tear. She felt stifled in her creativity and unable to live up to her expectations of herself. She was plagued with tension that could not abate as she was incapable of relaxation.

For me, the fact that Charlene had an "accident" is a significant piece of her situation. From the perspective of the manner in which we create reality from our energy systems, Charlene had become a system of frenzied energy. She was no longer able to process her stress in a productive or clear-thinking manner. Frenzied energy creates accidents as a way of halting the activity of fragmented thought.

Even with therapy, Charlene was not able to release her internal stressful processes, believing instead that if she learned to relax, her entire world would fall apart.

FRANK

(Shealy)

Diagnosis: Myofascial pain.

This is a thirty-year-old business executive who developed right shoulder pain following a tennis match. Over the next couple of months, this spread to involve his entire upper body, including the chest, shoulder and arms. He developed extremely cold hands, and a diagnosis of sympathetic dystrophy was made by some physicians. When we saw him, however, there was no evidence of dystrophy, which means that the skin has actually had severe changes from restriction of the blood vessels to the hands. He did have cold hands, but this would come and go. While his hands were sweaty, there were no actual tissue changes. He was extremely unresponsive to all the usual modalities of therapy in a chronic pain clinic. Interestingly, there were some very severe psychological problems involving a potential marriage.

From my perspective, his greatest problem seems to be an existential crisis resulting from the absence of any reference point for spirituality in his life.

ENERGY ANALYSIS

(Myss)

Frank gave the appearance of being a highly qualified overachiever. Underneath his appearance, however, was a man fraught with insecurities about actually achieving and competing in the outside world. His qualifications had led everyone in his world to develop high expectations of him.

Because Frank had so many obvious skills and talents, he focused all of his attention on his external life. He gave little thought to deeper considerations, such as questioning and developing his personal and spiritual values. In short, he may have looked good from the outside, but inside he was hollow. The more that was expected of him as he took on the full magnitude of his adult life in terms of professional and personal responsibilities, the more Frank began to collapse under the weight of his insecurities.

His lack of internal development revealed an existential crisis in which Frank had to confront the fact that he had no idea why he was doing what he was doing, what motivated him, what his values were, what the source of meaning was in his life. In fact, so unskilled was he at introspection that he found it difficult to even recognize that this was the root of his crisis.As Norm described, his pain continued regardless of all forms of treatment.

POST-SURGICAL PAIN

(S h e a l y)

Post-surgical pain, persisting for months or years after surgery, can occur following any type of surgical approach. Such pain may occur even after very minor surgery. There is some physical component to post-surgical pain; sensory nerves are damaged, upsetting the normal balance of proprioceptive nerve fibers (those that tell us that our body is okay). Individuals who have major pre-existing social and/or psychological problems seem to be more likely to develop persisting pain, and they are often more compulsively preoccupied with pain than almost any other type of pain patient.

ENERGY ANALYSIS OF POST-SURGICAL PAIN

(M y s s)

In my experience, I have seen post-surgical pain develop as a result of some form of emotional/psychological incompletion concerning the surgery itself. Specifically, this incompletion may be the result of residual fear from having to undergo surgery in the first place. It also may occur as a result of not feeling a sufficient level of trust in either the necessity of the surgery or in the medical team itself. Or it may be the result of removing or correcting the physical manifestation of the stress without any consideration paid to the underlying emotional or psychological tensions.

As we continue to learn more about the subtle levels of the human being, perhaps some light will be shed concerning the necessity to humanize surgery itself. Because we have yet to

recognize the reality of the "energy" level of the human being, much less appreciate it, there is no awareness of the requirements of the energy level of the human being in terms of
surgery.

Imagine, for the sake of discussion, that we were already
twenty-five years in the future and that we had developed a
sensitivity toward the reality and consciousness of energy fields.
We would recognize that anesthetizing the body does not put
the spirit to sleep. Rather, it alerts and involves the spirit in the
activity of surgery.

A ritual, if you will, or a recognition that the patient's inner
being needs to be included within the activity of surgery, should
occur *prior* to the actual surgical event. A meditation with the
surgical team and patient is perhaps one means of accomplishing
this.

Certainly, what has been realized about the "consciousness" of patients in coma stands as a level of evidence that the
spirit remains alert regardless of the limitations of the physical
body.

MARIA

(Shealy)

Diagnosis: Post-surgical abdominal pain.

This thirty-nine-year-old lady has had severe upper abdominal pain for some twelve years, following a diagnosis of
congenital atresia (severe narrowing) of the bile duct. She had
several surgical procedures to correct this before we saw her.
Even though the narrowing of the bile duct was corrected, she
was left with severe pain and has had great difficulties since
that time with drug habituation and addiction to narcotics. On
several occasions, the pain has been markedly reduced through
autogenic training, biofeedback, acupuncture, counseling and
withdrawal from narcotics.

More recently, intravenous Colchicine has given her a noticeable decrease in the pain. (Colchicine is usually used for gout but also is a powerful anti-inflammatory drug.)

ENERGY ANALYSIS

(M y s s)

The energy reading on Maria revealed that the root cause of her stress surrounded her inability to cope with the very essential demands of life, beginning with providing a secure physical life for herself. Maria's tension was like a twisted ball of yarn, revealing that she had little, if any, effective support system in her life. She was a chronic "worrier," never able fully to trust in herself or in others. Chronic worry destroys the second and third chakra areas of the body; it forms a congestion that grows and grows, feeling like an endless lump in the gut.

Maria was unable to challenge and finally release herself from her chronic condition of worry and stress. Regardless of the surgical procedures, her emotional health remained unhealed and, therefore, her pain continued for years.

TEMPOROMANDIBULAR JOINT SYNDROME (TMJ)

(S h e a l y)

Temporomandibular joint pain is one of the more common causes of both earache and headache. It occurs because of chronic severe muscle tension in the jaw muscles with grinding of the teeth and irritation of the joint that we use in speaking and in chewing. This is the junction between the mandible and the maxilla and occurs just in front of the ear. Often these patients have ground down their teeth rather significantly and have multiple dental procedures as well. They always have some degree of emotional tension.

ENERGY ANALYSIS OF TMJ

(M y s s)

The causes of stress in the jaw muscles are multiple, though they all stem from tension resulting from blockages concerning the use of one's willpower and self-expression.

One source of this stress is the inability to articulate verbally what one needs to say. Whether this block is caused by a fear of rejection, criticism or insecurity rooted in the fear of losing one's physical base of security, the experience of physical tension and teeth-grinding is the same.

Another source of this stress is that the grinding of teeth, like fingernail-biting or gum-chewing, becomes a habit one does unconsciously as a release of tension. Yet another source is that the jaw area becomes the receptacle for the energies of anger and frustration, holding the "words" one would like to say to someone but cannot, for whatever reasons.

Any time a person's power of choice, personal development in terms of self-expression, or creative expression is stifled, there is negative residue and this can lodge in the jaw as well. This dysfunction is remarkably common because the issues that create it are remarkably common.

JULIE

(S h e a l y)

Diagnoses: TMJ and myofascial pain.

This forty-two-year-old lady had generalized thoracic spine, neck and head pain which had come on slowly over a period of several years. She is a very intelligent lady, happily married, and a perfectionist in her work as a college professor. Although her thoracic pain responded well to biofeedback training and an intense pain treatment program, the headaches did not respond until she was given a dental appliance, specifically a plastic mold to wear in the mouth at night. This prevented her from grinding her teeth during sleep.

ENERGY ANALYSIS

(M y s s)

Julie's tension was almost totally connected to her struggle for recognition and authority in her professional position. She found herself holding back her comments and opinions as a result of a basic insecurity over the loss of her position or, at the very least, risking the loss of tenure and promotion. While Julie was certainly professionally qualified, she had to face job politics and a degree of unsupport due to her being a woman in a highly competitive academic environment.

CONCLUDING REMARKS

(S h e a l y)

Patients with chronic pain remain one of the most frustrating problems for the average physician. It is estimated that there are at least twenty million Americans who suffer from some degree of chronic pain. At least two million of these are individuals with incapacitating back pain.

Others tend to be less incapacitated but, nevertheless, suffer pain to a greater or lesser extent. They may have arthritis of various kinds or other types of pain due to post-surgery or post-injury. The ideal approach to these patients from a medical point of view is to send them to a comprehensive pain clinic facility if they do not respond within a maximum of four weeks to conservative physical therapy and the usual individual approaches.

At a comprehensive pain clinic, patients will have the benefit of an integrated team approach that will include well-trained therapists in physical therapy, counseling, acupuncture, transcutaneous electrical nerve stimulation, massage, postural correction, osteopathic manipulative therapy, biofeedback training, a drug withdrawal program and nutritional supplementation.

Of the patients who go through the comprehensive pain

program at our clinic, 90% improve during a two-week intensive session, though some of them do not continue to follow through with what we have taught them. Nevertheless, 70% of the people who have been invalids, sometimes for many years, improve remarkably and remain improved when followed up, even as much as three years later.

CHAPTER TEN

Primary Mental and Emotional Disorders

(S h e a l y   a n d   M y s s)

UNDERSTANDING MENTAL AND EMOTIONAL STRESS

(S h e a l y)

In general, so-called mental or psychological disorders are considered neurosis or psychosis. Neurosis is a disorder not accompanied by any apparent physical change in the nervous system and with symptoms of hysteria, anxiety, obsession, compulsions and most depressive disorders.

Psychosis, on the other hand, is a much more serious mental derangement in which patients lose touch with reality and the usual cognitive functions. These include those things which are usually called "insanity": schizophrenia; manic depressive psychosis; involutional melancholia; paranoia; and senile psychosis.

Disorders falling somewhere in between psychosis and neurosis are called psychoneurosis, or moderate maladapted behavioral problems, in which there is a minimal loss of contact with "popularly accepted views of reality." Even psychoneurotic patients often recognize that their reactions are inappropriate. At the end of the list of psychoses is psychopathia; individuals who have no conscience, do not learn from experiences and commit crimes without concern.

Increasingly, it is being discovered that there are biochemical abnormalities in patients with various mental or psychological disorders. Ordinarily, for instance, in patients suffering from depression, the adrenal glands would slow production of cortisone. In some depressed patients, however, the glands continue to produce cortisone and "adrenalin." This keeps them in a constant state of alarm, which is the primary reaction to stress.

Similarly, some patients with manic depressive or bipolar depression do not have the normal response to thyroid-stimulating hormone, which means the thyroid gland and pituitary gland are "running" independently of one another.

Most significantly, depressed people whom we have measured are very deficient in beta endorphins, the body's natural narcotics. On the other hand, those individuals who were depressed and also severely agitated had a very high level of beta endorphins. Low levels of serotonin and high or low levels of norepinephrine are other common findings in patients with depression. Serotonin is a chemical that facilitates transmission of information between nerve cells. Deficiencies of serotonin, found in 40% of chronic pain patients, lead to depression, insomnia and even pain. Tryptophan, an essential amino acid, and the cornerstone for producing serotonin, is deficient in 79% of chronic pain patients. Another group of chemicals, catecholamines, is involved in the primary stress reaction. This group includes dopamine (elevated in people with panic and severe anxiety), norepinephrine, which races the heart and raises the blood pressure, and epinephrine ("adrenalin"), which also speeds up heart rate and increases blood pressure. High levels of catecholamines are reactions to stress. Low-level readings indicate that a person is burned out, or depressed.

I was taught in medical school that 99% of all patients who had sexual impotency had a psychological disorder. Interestingly, however, about ten years ago a paper appeared in the *Journal of the American Medical Association* indicating that 78% of men with impotentia had hormonal disorders ranging from low testosterone levels and abnormalities of thyroid function to high levels of prolactin, the chemical ordinarily associated with increasing milk in the breast. (One can only speculate upon the metaphysical meaning of such inappropriate physiology.)

A month after this report was released, the *Journal of Clinical Hypnosis* ran an article reporting that patients who had such endocrine disorders were restored to normal, both in their potentia and in their normal hormonal levels, through the use of hypnosis. In no place is the interaction among the mind, body and biochemistry more obvious than it is in psychological and mental disorders.

And in no area of modern medicine is there greater controversy than in this whole field of "emotional" illnesses. The challenge to physicians is that of accepting emotional disorders as "real." Perhaps only when this is fully accepted by physicians will we recognize that you cannot "cure" emotions with drugs or surgery. You can anesthetize, you can suppress and repress emotions with drugs and surgery, but you cannot cure the basic disorder. Of equal importance is the fact that there is an emotional component, either as a precipitating factor or as an aggravating emotional distress in *every* disorder.

For instance, even the healthiest individual may have an "accident" in which a leg is broken. How that leg heals will depend, among other factors, upon the person's emotional strength, fortitude and health. If the individual tends to be depressed and negative or worried and excitable, there is some possibility of the fracture not healing or of developing prolonged pain despite normal healing.

Physicians have accepted for many years that peptic ulcer is a physical disorder when there is actually a "hole" in the intestinal wall. An increase in gastric acidity with discomfort is considered mostly a stress reaction. Actually, peptic ulcer is generally considered to be rooted *more* in stress than in strictly physical causes, except in a very few individuals in whom there is a familial predisposition to this particular disorder.

Rheumatoid arthritis is another disorder in which the significant mental and emotional disturbances are strong precipitating factors. Yet once a patient develops this potentially crippling disease, with positive blood tests indicating the rheumatoid factor, the disease is accepted as more "real" than just the pain without the "proof" of chemical changes.

But is there any difference between an elevated rheumatoid factor, high blood sugar and pain as "real" disorders? Physicians generally accept a high rheumatoid factor as being a "legitimate" abnormality. Similarly, in diabetes, initially the only "finding" may be an elevated blood sugar. Diabetes is considered a "real" disease. In other words, high blood sugar is indicative of genuine distress occurring in the body. While this disorder can result from smoking, drinking coffee, a major accident or a shot of cortisone, high blood sugar can also be caused by emotional distress.

Even though cold hands are not necessarily a disease, cold hands do provide evidence of a "stress reaction," a response of the nervous system requiring the autonomic system to go into an alarm mode. Elevated rheumatoid factors, elevated blood sugar and cold hands represent reactions to emotional stress.

Certainly the elevation of blood sugar does not "prove" that the patient has diabetes. Nor do cold hands "prove" that the individual had a significant physical injury; and, likewise, an "emotional attack" on the heart does not become legitimate until the heart truly malfunctions. Unfortunately, in the case of a heart attack, for instance, by the time a major artery has been occluded, either a serious incapacity or even death can result.

At that point, the attention of the medical profession is focused largely upon doing the heroic to save the patient's life.

Even more unfortunately, it appears that a great deal of the time, even after such massive interventional approaches as coronary bypass surgery, all too little attention is paid to the emotional strain that created the illness in the first place. Given that the heart disease was also brought about by a combination of genetic predisposition, diet, weight, lack of exercise, or smoking, an extremely important contributing factor is always the emotional component. Treating such major disease as coronary occlusion with bypass surgery without then doing significant education and counseling is almost as bad as trying to treat the fever of meningitis with aspirin to suppress the fever without curing the infection with appropriate antibiotics.

In no area of medicine is the influence of stress more ignored than in the management of chronic pain. Pain often creates changes through the sympathetic (autonomic or "automatic") nervous system in blood flow to skin and in the general distribution related to the internal organs.

Sir Charles Scott Sherrington, one of the great physiologists, demonstrated back in the 1920s that there are viscero cutaneous reflexes and cutaneo visceral reflexes, that is, strong electrical connections between the internal organs and the skin and vice versa. These are "real" but they are electrical/chemical. They are changeable, meaning that the electrical/chemical connections are not necessarily physically permanent. When there has been damage to an area, either in the skin or in one of the internal organs or internal structures, then that electrical/chemical reflex disturbance may become long-lasting and be very difficult to reverse.

When individuals have significant trauma to the body, whether it is a small fracture or a huge crushing injury, not uncommonly, the autonomic nervous system becomes very dysfuctional. Most often, extremely cold areas occur on the skin that can become discolored and rather bluish; but also abnormally warm areas can develop. During the past two decades, a technique called thermography has been widely used to demonstrate such temperature changes. Unfortunately, both attorneys and physicians who are not adequately educated about neuroanatomy and neurophysiology tend to miss the significance of interpreting thermograms.

What a thermogram shows is changes in blood flow, usually areas that are decreased in blood flow (cold areas) but, occasionally, those areas that have an increase in blood flow (hot areas). Both of these changes in skin temperature are physically real. They can be palpated with the naked hand. They can be measured with electrical thermometers (called thermisters) attached to the skin or they can be photographed with a thermogram. These temperature differences indicate *emotional* stress responses affecting the physical body.

The interpretation of thermogram data done by some physicians and lawyers has led to claims that these data represent nerve root injury. Actually, one could never interpret a thermogram as meaning that there is unequivocal "injury" to nerve roots. What *can* be said, however, is that they show disturbances or reflexes of distress focalized in those places where the skin is unusually warm or unusually cold. Mostly these are aggravations created by emotional distress and, probably, focal emotional concern about the area of injury.

These reports are as real as elevated blood sugar counts or a minor electrical abnormality on an electrocardiogram. Physiological changes are *real*, but they are subject to change and they are potentially reversible. As in all illnesses, such changes are also significantly influenced by chemical stress. But the bottom line is that all illness is the result of stress, though the *reactions* to stress may be emotional, chemical or physical.

When physicians begin to accept the reality of emotional distress as a pervasive influence in every illness as well as the legitimacy of emotionally based physiological (electrical/chemical) changes in the body, we will truly enter a new era of understanding in medicine.

ENERGY ANALYSIS OF
EMOTIONAL DISORDERS

(M y s s)

The area of mental and emotional disorders is, by far, the most complex. This area is also the most challenging to the traditional medical "model" of the human being. What takes place "behind the eyes" of a person is largely subjective territory. Aside from the quantifiable influences of genetics, neurological as well as physiological and chemical imbalances, injuries, accidents or known abusive experiences, the remaining factors that influence a person's mental and emotional well-being have to do with the unquantifiable dimension of emotional needs and personal beliefs.

Contemporary analysis of the origin of a psychological disorder and its "meaning" as well as effective therapeutic treatments vary in unlimited number, from traditional analysis to Gestalt therapy and so on. There is no one psychological school of analysis and interpretation that is recognized as the central, acceptable authority for and by the entire profession of psychology and psychiatry. What is recognized amongst all of the different psychological approaches are theories and techniques that have "validity" to them, but none is considered the standard "most accurate truth."

Why is this? When so much can be agreed upon in terms of physical medicine, why is there such variety and discrepancy in the area of mental and emotional disorders?

My sense is that both the patient and the therapist exist in subjective worlds. In other words, just as most patients choose a form of therapy that suits their needs, beliefs and personalities, so also do therapists become involved in a school (or schools) of psychotherapy that reflects their personal beliefs. A therapist who believes in past lives, for example, would hardly become a Freudian analyst.

And what about the "reality" of spiritual crises—of actual mystical suffering? The ancient and classic work of Saint John of the Cross entitled *The Dark Night of the Soul* outlined in the twelfth century the inner psychological pitfalls a person would experience automatically during the pursuit of his or her divine connection.

Spiritual crises have not been given fair representation in the classical world of psychoanalysis. Indeed, they have been discredited and even considered a psychosis unto themselves. Traditional analysis paralleled the development of traditional medicine in its approach to be scientific and clinical. Spiritual crises, therefore, belonged inside a spiritual organization, which, by the way, did not mean they were recognized as legitimate human suffering. After all, to recognize the spiritual crisis as real presumes the "official" recognition of a Divine Principle at work within this Universe and the validity of the soul. These two criteria are simply not scientifically provable.

Personally, when I began this work, I could not accept the influence of past lives. I considered that every mental and emotional disorder originated in this lifetime and was a complex weave of childhood experiences, environmental influences and the quality of one's beliefs. While I believed in the validity of the spiritual crisis, I assumed that only those who were consciously involved in their spiritual lives, such as those in religious communities, were candidates for a genuine "spiritual crisis."

My work has brought about the reshuffling and expansion of my perceptions. I now totally accept that a person can have a deep and very real inner crisis that may well have its origin in a lifetime other than this one. While I remain hazy about exactly how that influence finds its way into this lifetime, nonetheless I have, at times, perceived images and information in the course of doing thousands of readings that suggest to me that we do indeed exist within an ongoing process of conscious evolution that includes the experience of multiple lifetimes.

My understanding of who qualifies for a spiritual crisis has likewise been completely reconstructed. The perception that only those within the world of the religious life could experience a "dark night of the soul" has shifted to the point where I now assume that the proverbial "dark night" will enter into each person's life, at some point, without exception.

Whereas I once believed that a person had to enter into a religious community to encounter such an experience, I now realize that what opens the door for this process is not the physical building one steps into or the potency of taking religious vows, but the questions one has the courage to ask mentally, emotionally and spiritually: What is the meaning of my life? For what purpose was I born? Is there a God? Why am I involved in the struggles that fill my life? Why can't I seem to find love?

For me, these are not ordinary questions. They are depth charges that unlock the rumblings of the soul. And in my experience, I have yet to meet the person who has not wondered about these matters, albeit appropriate to the context of his or her life. As people who exist in a culture in which the spiritual crisis has minimal regard, the "suffering of the soul" is the last place either a patient or a therapist would look for root causes of distress. Though this is beginning to change somewhat with the advent of the more spiritually focused therapies, still we have a long way to go before the spiritual crisis is seen as legitimately as the crisis, for example, of parental rejection.

On a less etheric note, discussions of mental and emotional disorders always include the recognition of the influence of repressed and/or damaged emotions, in particular, anger, guilt and fear. The language of psychology describes syndromes in terms of repression, suppression and disassociation—all of which communicate particular behavioral characteristics.

In the language of energy, these are described as "energy blocks" which indicate that a "congestion" is occurring within a person's consciousness. The normal condition of processing emotional and psychological data is being interfered with or is being conducted in such a way that the blockages are causing distress within the physical body. From the perspective of energy, the connection between the congestion and the physical distress is clearly evident.

While these two descriptions may seem to be indicating

identical frameworks, there are differences worth noting. From an intuitive perspective, the sensitivities that a person may have to light or sound or to other people's energy fields are, first of all, actually apparent and, secondly, they are noted as "legitimate" dysfunctions that indicate electrical imbalances in a person's energy field that cause very genuine internal stress.

While conventional psychology may address itself to the neurosis that results from these types of sensitivities, it would also tend to view these sensitivities as the *result* of a neurosis and not the *cause* of the neurosis.

Many times I have seen that a person's energy field is contaminated with environmental pollution, such as toxic air or water or even pesticide intake. These physical pollutants actually affect a person's nervous system and, more significantly, they constantly raise anxiety and stress levels in people. These factors, however, are not officially recognized as "emotional toxins" (meaning there is no way to quantify the effects of these pollutants), and thus the abnormal behavior they generate would have to be credited to a source other than toxic pollution.

This is the same as the realization that depression and many other inner sufferings are very often rooted in *chemical* imbalances and are *not* always the result of an external tension or a personality abnormality.

Another difference worth pointing out is the contribution intuition offers by studying even more directly the effects of intense emotions upon the physical body. Specifically, I am referring to identifying the variations of emotions (anger, fear, etc.) and their intensities and how these factors contribute to the formation of specific diseases.

Norm has pondered numerous times, for instance, why anger causes cancer in one patient and neurosis in another. What are the factors involved in the two different outcomes? Is it possible to identify the "quality" of emotions to such a fine degree that we could clearly determine what certain emotions are capable of creating? And, at what "rate"?

In Chapter Six, we mentioned the case of Mark, a man who

developed and eventually died of cancer of the colon. I could "clearly see" that he was developing cancer prior to the cancer actually becoming physically present in his body and, later, I could "clearly see" when he would die. I based my analysis and prediction of Mark's fate on my *technical* understanding of energy from which I drew my data, and not on an intuitive "vision." Energy has variations of density to it, and the more "dense" or "heavy" it feels, the closer that energy is to fully merging with physical matter.

Predictions are nothing more than the capacity to identify and then interpret the natural cause and effect of patterns of energy that a person sets in motion through personal choices. The nature of human energy, as I hope we may one day realize, is a science unto itself. Indeed, it is the science of creation. The contribution that intuition can make to the study of the creative powers of emotions and their connections to disease is potentially enormous.

The following case studies are but a very small sampling of primary mental and emotional disorders.

GLORIA

(Shealy)

Diagnosis: Rectal and perineal pain—unknown causes.

This sixty-six-year-old woman was suffering from severe rectal, perineal and suprapubic pain. This began in 1965 when she underwent a left mastectomy for cancer of the breast followed by removal of the ovaries. Although the cancer has never recurred, the patient has had severe and incapacitating rectal pain since that time.

Gloria later underwent a hysterectomy, an exploratory laparotomy and even a temporary colostomy, all in an attempt to relieve her pain. She has been on Valium for many years and, more recently on Xanax.

In her personal life, Gloria has many marital problems. She has had a great deal of difficulty accepting her husband's preoccupation with his work rather than with her illness. She refused to take anti-depressant drugs and would not come off Xanax. She showed minimal response to acupuncture, transcutaneous electrical nerve stimulation, biofeedback and autogenic training.

Although we could have included this case in the chapter on Chronic Pain, it appears to me, after working with more than five thousand chronic pain patients, that those patients who have severe genital or rectal pain have unusually dominant psychological problems.

ENERGY ANALYSIS

(M y s s)

Gloria is an individual obsessed with both the need to control and the need to punish. Her body produced one dysfunction after another in the areas of her first, second and third chakras— all of which indicate that she felt compulsively insecure about taking responsibility for herself and that she feared abandonment. Thus, she became ill in order to control her husband through guilt and need. The more guilt and sympathy Gloria could create, the more she calmed her fears about her husband abandoning her.

It is no wonder that she would not cooperate with any form of self-training or self-healing techniques. For Gloria, becoming healthy was a very threatening proposition. It meant the releasing of all control mechanisms and, emotionally, this was not acceptable to her.

PATRICIA

(S h e a l y)

Diagnosis: Excessive uterine bleeding due to fibroids.

This thirty-eight-year-old lady suffered from severe uterine bleeding. She had a diagnosis of a tumor of the left ovary fifteen years earlier. She has had two previous D&C's for uterine bleeding. The second time she was seen, she had been bleeding very intensely for two days. She does not smoke. She has used a variety of drugs and marijuana in the past but not in about eight years. She is currently married to her third husband. Because of severe bleeding, the patient was referred to a gynecologist. She had a very enlarged uterus, her hemoglobin was approximately 50% normal and she underwent a total hysterectomy to "cure" the bleeding.

This patient and her husband were unwilling to work with us at the clinic. In my opinion, Patricia's problem was primarily severe psychological distress.

ENERGY ANALYSIS

(M y s s)

While Norm lists Patricia's problem as severe psychological distress, I interpret it as severe psychological abuse. Her energy analysis indicates that she has a history of being emotionally battered and, at times, physically battered. So successfully has her self-esteem been destroyed that she no longer controls any aspect of herself.

In my opinion, her physical problems, all located in her female organs, indicate that, emotionally and psychologically, this woman feels like a constant victim of rape. She is totally controlled by the men in her life, and despite her multiple divorces—all due to abuse—she still has yet to deal with her victim consciousness and her intense lack of personal power and self-esteem.

DANIEL

(S h e a l y)

Diagnosis: Neurasthenia.

This forty-four-year-old man complained of a weakened nervous system and an inability to function sexually. This began concomitant with a divorce seven years earlier. His divorce occurred because he was feeling unhappy with his life, and he stated that he and his wife of eight years were heading in different directions.

He became involved with another woman and became even more discontent with his life. He had a very unpleasant divorce and admitted to having been depressed due to feeling extremely guilty about his divorce.

Though he was able to become sexually aroused, he felt that even sexual arousement left him feeling exhausted. If he actually had sex and an orgasm, he was totally depleted and unable to function.

ENERGY ANALYSIS

(Myss)

Daniel's energy reading revealed that he felt a deep resentment toward women, believing that women were "takers" and always manipulative. He felt taken advantage of in his marriage and emotionally dominated by his wife.

In leaving the marriage, Daniel had to confront his own weakness and dependency on women. He exists in a continual power struggle with women which manifested both physically and symbolically in his sexual dysfunction.

SANDY

(Shealy)

Diagnosis: Torsion of sacrum with intractable back and vaginal pain.

This thirty-nine-year-old woman complained of severe pain both in the buttocks and in the vagina. She was (and still is at this time) totally unable to have sexual intercourse because of excruciating pain. Although other physicians have found no cause for the pain, this lady does indeed have a torsion of a portion of the sacrum that apparently has been present for at least ten years following a fall on her buttocks. It is probably not physically correctable. She has had intense therapy in the pain clinic through manipulative therapy and desensitizing nerve blocks, yet she continues to be moderately incapacitated because of her pain.

ENERGY ANALYSIS

(M y s s)

Sandy's energy revealed that she had been molested as a child and, still, as an adult, remained unable to cope with that memory. Her experience with being sexually violated caused her to equate any act of sex with pain and loss of self. In my opinion, the only way Sandy will ever become totally free of pain is through intense therapy in which she finally releases both the memory and the emotions of anger that have lodged in her vaginal area.

WILLIS

(S h e a l y)

Diagnosis: Workers' Compensation Neurosis.

This is a classic case of Workers' Compensation neurosis. Willis had a minor injury at work through falling. This occurred while he was working as a counselor at a state facility in California. He received a long-lasting disability as a stress psychoneurotic reaction. He showed no interest in ever returning to any form of productive work and complains steadily about the abuse he has recieved from the system. I pointed out to him that that same "system" supports him well while he refuses to work.

ENERGY ANALYSIS

(M y s s)

Willis was (and still is) a man who absolutely refuses to take any responsibility for himself. From the time he was a child, he was an underachiever (in his own eyes) who failed to attain his goals. He blamed these failures on a series of people, from his parents to his teachers to his professional authorities.

I found it interesting that he worked in a state facility because in his own mind, he was very much a prisoner of his own nature. He frequently had violent thoughts toward others, while at the same time, fantasizing that he had great potential as a leader and an authority figure.

He believed that if only given a chance, he would prove himself to be an authority. The problem with Willis, however, is that he never wanted to work for what he fantasized accomplishing. He had great dreams and only mediocre ambition. But his greatest difficulties were his attitudes about what the world owed him. He resented the achievements of other people and constantly held a negative and suspicious mental outlook toward others.

Since the world owed him a living anyway, Workers' Compensation was a perfect way for him to deal "successfully" with his nonsuccessful life. It afforded him a legitimate reason not to work and never to challenge his own limitations.

WARREN

(S h e a l y)

Diagnosis: Depression; homosexual obsession.

This thirty-six-year-old man has been severely depressed for much of his life. His father was a Fundamentalist minister. The patient has severe problems with inability to function in society. He has never held a job for more than a few months. Although he is married and has four children, he has homosexual fantasies and probably has had at least one homosexual affair about which he has considerable guilt. Extensive counseling and anti-depressant medication have led to no improvement.

ENERGY ANALYSIS

(M y s s)

It's obvious that the source of Warren's depression is his sexuality and his inability to accept himself for who he is. His case is important not because it is complicated, but because his situation is so remarkably common. Warren has no self-esteem and no love of self. Without these qualities, even in the slightest degree, healing is almost impossible.

His inability to hold a job, that is, to feel successful financially, is directly connected to his inability to accept himself sexually. As discussed in Chapter Four, the second chakra, which is located in the sexual region of the body, relates to issues of power, sexuality, money and control. This chakra relates most directly to Warren's inner struggle and, therefore, all of the issues of this chakra (money, power) are present in his life. And, more interestingly, the lack of self-esteem Warren feels is reflected in each of these areas in that they are all deficient: lack of earthly power, lack of financial success and lack of sexual acceptance.

RENEE

(M y s s)

Diagnosis: Depression and vaginal bleeding.

This is a woman I met during a workshop. She was shy and withdrawn and commented that she had severe vaginal bleeding that did not seem to have a physiological reason.

In doing her reading, I received the impression that something was trying to take her children from her. I asked her about this, and she said that she and her husband were practicing members of a religion that expected all the participants to release their children to the training program of the organization when the children reached the age of five.

She and her husband have three children, ages seven, five and two. They had agreed to this practice in entering the religion several years ago, prior to having their own children. When her eldest turned five years of age, she convinced her husband to let him stay at home with them until his younger brother reached the age of five, at which time both siblings could be sent together.

The truth was that she did not want to send any of her children to the organization. She felt that her children were being "ripped away" from her. She noted that she had had several conversations with her husband about her feelings, but he felt that since they had attained a level of stature in the organization, they had to fulfill this commitment as part of setting a proper example. Her frustration and her feeling that she had no choice in determining the fate of her children resulted in the creation of vaginal bleeding, symbolically a very powerful illustration of her emotional trauma.

I later met with both Renee and her husband and explained the origin of Renee's stress. We discussed the very crucial need for the children to remain at home and we also discussed the nature of spiritual commitments. The parents then agreed to keep their children at home.

ALZHEIMER'S DISEASE

(S h e a l y)

This is one of the more common problems of aging although it can occur in younger people as well. Basically it consists of degeneration of the brain, especially in the part of the brain associated with memory (the hippocampus). It has been found that there is a high concentration of aluminum in the brain of patients with Alzheimer's syndrome. It is not known whether that is an excess from toxicity or if it is an indirect effect of the aluminum deposited in damaged tissue.

Some scientists have thought that there is a type of slow virus or chronic viral infection associated with Alzheimer's syndrome. There is no known medical treatment, although some therapists believe that a series of chelation therapy is beneficial in 50% of patients with Alzheimer's. Chelation consists of giving intravenously EDTA, a chemical which, according to some therapists, is supposed to chelate out, or filter, heavy metals such as cadmium, arsenic and aluminum as well as taking calcium deposits out of the arteries. Large doses of lecithin and a vitamin supplementation program may help a few patients with Alzheimer's syndrome. This has not been confirmed in a double-blind study.

Alzheimer's disease is one of the more frustrating and moderately feared illnesses. When I was in medical school, we were taught that it was a disease that was very rare; and to make the diagnosis, it had to come on usually before the patient was sixty years old.

ENERGY ANALYSIS OF ALZHEIMER'S DISEASE

(Myss)

We are a tribal species. By that, I mean that up until the end of the last century when individual mobility increased, we remained, in general, closely tied to our families. As more and more people moved away from their family settings, the breakdown of the natural order of family caretaking occurred.

Suddenly, the elderly members of our families faced abandonment in the later years of their lives, along with the loss of rank and privilege in the family and the loss of their value as people once their income-producing years ceased. They went from being the respected heads of the family to physical and/or financial burdens, with independent family members arguing over who is responsible for their care. In many cases, the abandonment is even more severe as the separation of the family unit often breaks the bonds of the heart due to the absence of familiarity between generations.

In my opinion, diseases such as Alzheimer's are directly related to the breakdown of the family unit and the dissolving of familial bonds of security that once extended naturally from birth to death. Fears of providing for oneself in one's old age and the demand to remain strong, productive and financially secure until the last day of one's life have caused an entirely new dimension of stress to enter into the experience of aging within a society that is not geared toward coping with its elders.

With the more traditional structures disintegrating, the values once associated with the elderly tribal members have been discounted completely. As our values have changed to revolve so intensely around remaining young, financially secure and vital, aging has become a negative—something to be postponed as long as possible. The elders, who were once considered to be the keepers of wisdom within a tribe, have now become the elderly—dependent family members whose needs greatly interfere with the life structures of the nuclear or single-parent family.

Alzheimer's disease has grown in proportion to these changing patterns of our society. The withdrawal of the conscious minds of our elderly family members is an indication to me that the pressure to remain young, and financially and physically independent, coupled with the devaluation of the significance of the aging process, has resulted in an inability to cope with the expectations demanded by the breakdown of our tribal structures.

The fear of rejection, of having continually to prove one's value and self-worth during the golden years when such should be a given, is the primary root cause of the need to become unconscious and completely dependent. Thus, if the elderly face their future in institutions, the process of being and remaining institutionalized and abandoned occurs unconsciously.

It is my opinion that this disease, as well as others in our society, should be looked upon as diseases of the collective unconscious of our society. The pressures of aging as described above filter into each of our lives, regardless of our individual family units. In other words, even if a parent is surrounded by loving children, the society itself exerts a sufficient amount of pressure by virtue of these societal values-at-large, which often eclipse the emotional security of the single-family unit. Therefore, the desire to prove one's self-worth as one ages is just as real a stress in a loving family as it is for someone who is aging miles away from the nearest family member. We, as individuals, do not and, in fact, cannot exist apart from the ills of our social/ physical environment or our society. We are one and the same.

Consider also that the rising number of divorces and the subsequent multiple marriages have created the additional pressure of several elderly per family unit. The family lineage has been, in most cases, diluted to the point where the bonds of blood run thin. Children and grandchildren grow up in environments in which the family members change frequently. How, then, is deep bonding and blood loyalty to develop? Relationships, as these children learn all too quickly, come and go easily. One set of grandparents begins to look much the same as another, and the cycle of bonding and separation results eventually in no bonding at all.

Yet another social crisis is the paradox created by the need to prolong life technologically to its absolute last possible breath, which is directly in conflict with the fact that we do not value the lives being prolonged. We applaud our technological breakthroughs, yet we are faced with the financial cost of this enterprise within a society that does not know how to cope with the end product—more elderly people.

Norm mentioned that there is the possibility that Alzheimer's disease is brought about by a slow-growing virus. My experience has taught me that viruses develop in people whose sense of safety and well-being is threatened. Under threats of insecurity, a person's defensive mechanisms are constantly at work and under stress. Feeling defensive is not only a conscious sensation that a person undergoes within a business or personal relationship, or in a street fight; it is also, and usually, a chronic condition that permeates a person's consciousness to the point at which feeling unsafe becomes second nature. People are no longer able to realize that the underlying motivation for most, if not all, of their activities is chronic insecurity and the need to prove self-worth until the day one dies.

In my experience, chronic insecurity breaks down and

eventually destroys the immune system. Thus, the possibility that Alzheimer's is rooted in a slow-growing virus is highly likely, particularly since the process of aging and the fears inherent in the process are also "slow-growing."

What about younger people who develop Alzheimer's? There are cases of individuals developing this illness who are in their forties. I maintain that the same pressures exist as the root cause, regardless of one's chronological age. It is no different than other unusual situations in which diseases more prone to strike in middle or later years, such as heart attacks, have been known to occur in individuals in their twenties.

From my perspective, the "cure" for Alzheimer's may someday be found in a vaccine, but a vaccine will not cure the stress behind the illness, nor the increasing numbers of elderly who are finding the pressure of remaining young while simultaneously aging impossible to cope with. Likewise, getting drugs off the streets of our communities will not solve the greater problem, which is: How do we heal our children who have been fragmented and splintered because of the breakdown of the tribal unit?

There is also a more metaphysical interpretation of Alzheimer's that is appropriate to mention. From a metaphysical point of view, Alzheimer's, as well as other mental disorders such as forms of schizophrenia, catatonic states, coma and autism, is considered to be a form of an altered state of consciousness. Certainly, this is not the same type of altered state that is brought about through hallucinogenic drugs or through mystical experiences. Nevertheless, this position is valid from the perception that these states of consciousness exceed the definition of what is considered "normal" functioning awareness.

As such, the metaphysical question that arises is, "Why would an individual withdraw awareness from his or her 'normal' state of consciousness and enter into an altered state?"

Consider that even altered states of consciousness are systems of perceptions. That the individual cannot communicate normally is a given, but does the communication breakdown necessarily indicate that the capacity to perceive data coming from external and internal stimuli is dysfunctional? The question is, "Does this shift in consciousness allow the individual to receive data and stimuli from channels not readily accessible to the normal human awareness?" If that is possible, then what forms of stimuli are being perceived and for what purpose?

One can only speculate about these states of consciousness, but we must recognize that, at the very least, much about the nature of the human unconscious remains an unknown. It is understandable that assumptions are made that the quality of consciousness is severely lacking in individuals with mental disorders. These individuals very often cannot function independently and, in some cases, their behavior can be harmful or even dangerous to others.

Yet, as in the cases of Alzheimer's, coma and autism, the possibility might also exist that a process related to one's spiritual growth is occurring and that this process is such that it eclipses "normal" consciousness. Similar to the manner in which one must close down normal consciousness in the form of sleep in order to enter into the dream state, perhaps in some of the cases of these types of disorders, the individual withdraws his or her normal consciousness in order to have access to processes of spiritual development that we, as yet, know nothing about. And thus, we only can assume that the state of consciousness that the person is in is dysfunctional and seemingly without "purpose" as we understand purpose. These states have no "functional purpose" to be sure, but what if the purpose served by withdrawing from one's association with ordinary consciousness is spiritual in nature?

That this possibility has not been seriously considered, at least not by traditional clinical professionals, does not mean that it may not be a possibility worthy of serious exploration. Bear in mind that the entire dimension of spirituality and spiritual experiences has not been given any legitimacy in clinical psychological and psychiatric analysis and, thus, these possibilities have never been pursued. Perhaps as we come to know more about our spiritual natures, explorations into this dimension will unfold.

The following case reports on Alzheimer's disease require no individual explanation as they are all variations on the same theme.

LEONA

(S h e a l y)

This forty-year-old lady had problems of severe memory loss. A CAT scan showed mild to moderate generalized cerebral atrophy. A diagnosis of Alzheimer's disease was made on the basis of her memory loss and the CAT scan. Actually, over the next two years, she has had very little further progression of the disease but is not able to function and has been unable to work.

PAULINE

(S h e a l y)

This seventy-five-year-old lady presented with severe memory loss. She has a long-standing history of over thirty years of severe psychological disorders and depression. She has had numerous anti-depressant drugs with minimal benefits. She has had at least two series of electric shock therapy treatments in the past. She has had, over a two-year period, a rapid loss of memory and ability to function and has progressed at this time to a state in which she is incontinent and totally confused and has to be taken care of like a baby.

CLARENCE

(S h e a l y)

This seventy-six-year-old man was brought in by his daughter who was concerned that he might have Alzheimer's disease.

Basically, he shows severe loss of memory but only minimal atrophy on his brain scan, even though his memory loss has been going on for several years. From a clinical point of view, one suspects Alzheimer's but is not able to confirm the diagnosis.

ALCOHOL AND DRUG ADDICTION

(S h e a l y)

Anne Schaef, in her bestselling book, *Co-dependence*, has emphasized that society, as a whole, is addicted. Consider the various types of addiction: nicotine (at least 25% of adults); alcohol (15% of adults or more; most also smoke); narcotics (10 to 15% of Americans); sugar (15 to 50% of Americans). Then consider the number of people addicted to television and other forms of non-stimulating habits.

It appears that at least 15% of Americans have *severe* addictive problems that are believed by psychiatrists today to be an inherent metabolic defect or disease. These individuals simply "can't stop" once they start drinking, smoking or taking narcotics. Extensive behavioral training and psychotherapy are essential for these people. They need continual reinforcement of non-addictive behavior, such as the *12-Step Program of Alcoholics Anonymous*.

ENERGY ANALYSIS OF ADDICTIONS

(M y s s)

Addictions are the strongest experience we can have of something external exerting control over us. Addictions are a study in personal power and the development of the strength of one's willpower. We form addictive patterns in response to emotional experiences that are painful, intimidating and particularly challenging, such as sexual or mental abuse.

In these situations, we withdraw to protect ourselves from what we are experiencing, largely because it is so difficult to know how to respond effectively when the trauma happens. Learning to respond in a productive and healthy manner usually occurs *after* we have amassed traumas that need healing. Once we realize that we *have been hurt and need to heal ourselves*, then we are able to learn how to make choices that lead to empowerment and not more abuse.

In between the traumatic experiences and the path of empowerment is the dimension of addictions, where painful memories, low self-esteem, and feelings of guilt, anger, fear and self-hate are anesthetized by cravings for substances, habits and relationships that create the illusion of self-control and safety.

In reality, addictions are statements people make regarding what they *cannot cope with*. And in my experience, the majority of addictions are rooted in emotional traumas that have resulted in serious damage to a person's sense of self-esteem and self-worth.

I personally believe that far more than 15% of Americans are severe addicts. That may be an accurate figure in terms of drug and alcohol addiction, but these are not the only forms of addiction that should be considered as serious problems.

Negative thought and behavioral patterns are also forms of addictions. We can become addicted to losing control of our tempers, for instance, because the release of anger in that fashion temporarily feels empowering. We can become addicted to certain patterns that allow us to think we are in control of other people. The forms of addictive behavior that we can create are virtually endless. In this category of addictions, I would surmise that most people have an addiction or two.

It is not surprising that the healing of addictions is a massive undertaking for the addict. It would seem practically impossible to give up an addiction without a support system that recognizes the emotional damage the individual needs to confront in addition to an effective method for developing self-love, which is certainly the greater challenge.

ANDY

(S h e a l y)

Diagnosis: Addiction to narcotics.

This thirty-four-year-old physician consulted us for assistance in overcoming a fifteen-year history of addiction to street drugs and narcotics. He had completed a drug treatment program earlier and almost immediately began again to smoke marijuana and to take Darvon. We worked with him for two weeks, teaching him self-regulation and insight techniques. Within a month, he relapsed again. Over a year later, he returned for another two-week session and has now been free of drugs for about one year.

ENERGY ANALYSIS

(M y s s)

More and more, we are realizing in our society that addictions and physical and sexual abuse are not products of low-income situations, as has been previously assumed. Andy's situation has become typical in our culture.

Andy found coping with stress to be overwhelming long before he became a physician. He developed his addictions when he was a student in order to keep up with his studies. The fact that taking drugs was also socially popular contributed to his use of them.

The reason Andy found stress so difficult to handle was because the source of his stress was his fear of not meeting expectations and of failing in a very competitive field. He needed to project an image of self-confidence, and drugs assisted him to achieve this, and to convince himself that he had everything under control. In truth, Andy had everything under "anesthesia" and not under control.

Andy managed to kick the narcotics addiction because he was finally able to face the fact that he had a problem with his emotional well-being. As he learned to recognize what he was feeling, he was then able to learn to respond to his feelings with authentic inner control and challenge his need to drug himself in order to cope with life's stresses.

PANIC ATTACK

(Shealy)

Panic attacks are among the most "popular" topics today in medicine. Indeed, if you look at the state of the world, it is easy to conclude that everyone *should* panic at how sick society is. Those individuals who suffer incapacitating panic attacks have marked increases in dopamine, which seems to trigger overwhelming feelings of inability to cope. Panic represents the ultimate anxiety—anxiety that is totally out of control and without obvious "reason."

ENERGY ANALYSIS OF PANIC ATTACKS

(Myss)

Consider the demands placed upon each of us, either directly or implied, that are present in our society. Through various channels, by the time we are teenagers, we all receive the very clear messages that to be successful, one must be: thin, rich, attractive, powerful, sexually active and sexually open, self-confident, invulnerable, able to cope with all forms of personal and professional challenges and have an exciting profession. Nowhere on that list are the values of wisdom, integrity, a loving nature, nonjudgmental attitudes, clear thinking skills and concern for the well-being of others.

Individuals who become unable to cope when their inner resources are not strong enough or well-developed enough to maintain a healthy capacity to challenge one's fears. In other words, in a panic attack, one's fears become more real than one's ability to recognize them as fears and thus challenge them with inner resources. It is a type of "circuitry overload" that is becoming alarmingly common in our society.

Panic attacks can come on suddenly, without any warning and without a previous history of anxiety. In one case, a woman with no prior encounters with panic awoke in the morning emotionally panic-stricken and would not leave her house. She remained in her home for the next four years. She eventually made contact with a therapist who specialized in people with panic disorders and re-learned how to enter the world again. It was a gradual process of "reentry" that included exercises such as walking to and from the corner and making a trip to the grocery store. For people with panic disorders, these incredibly simple exercises represent major challenges as the feelings of vulnerability and fear of potential harm to oneself are paralyzing.

As this woman regained her inner balance, she commented that, in her opinion, she had never realized how much her fears consumed her every action. She described the source of her panic attacks this way: her unconscious self had achieved "control" over her conscious mind and, suddenly, no matter how much she tried to remind herself that she was safe, her emotions continued to react as though her life were in danger. Unconsciously, she had always felt that her safety was threatened, and when her capacity to keep these feelings under control became exhausted, her fears took over.

BRUCE

(S h e a l y)

Diagnosis: Panic attacks.

This fifty-four-year-old man came to the clinic because he was experiencing moderate panic, high blood pressure and neck pain. He had had an anterior cervical fusion for the neck pain, but it did not help. His blood pressure was not well-controlled, despite a variety of medications.

After two weeks of intensive biofeedback and self-regulation training, as well as follow-up counseling over a period of six months, all of his symptoms returned to normal. He no longer has any panic attacks, his blood pressure is under control and his neck pain is alleviated by frequent massage.

ENERGY ANALYSIS

(M y s s)

Everyone can expect to enter into a process of personal reevaluation anywhere from the mid-forties through the fifties. Often called the "mid-life crisis," this process is real and not just the realization that one is getting closer to the end of one's life than the beginning.

During these years, the signs of the aging process become apparent in terms of diminishing physical stamina and changes in the physical body itself. This is a time in which individuals naturally begin to re-prioritize how and in what way they are investing their energies.

Frequently, a sense of inadequacy arises, particularly in men, because of the competitiveness of the business and corporate world, with middle-aged executives being commonly replaced by lesser paid, younger people.

Bruce is a man who experienced panic attacks as a result of feelings of inadequacy in terms of keeping pace with the demands of his life. His *fear* of losing control became the *experience* of losing control. All of the insecurities that had motivated him during his twenties, thirties and forties seemed to explode into his consciousness at once, leaving him emotionally distraught.

The six-month period of counseling, coupled with the learning of self-regulated management of the body, allowed Bruce gradually to regain his self-confidence as well as to accept this phase of his life. The couseling provided him an opportunity to complete a process of reevaluation so that he could feel good about himself and his life once again.

CONCLUSION

Our society has many ills. It seems incomprehensible that we could separate the intense pressures of our fragmented lifestyles from the diseases we produce which so thoroughly indicate that we have an inability to cope with the demands of our contemporary world.

Diseases such as Alzheimer's, AIDS, drug addiction, massive depression and other widespread ills are ills of our collective consciousness. Successful treatment begins with realizing the source of the dysfunction. Our lifestyles, for the most part, have become too stressful for the creation of maximum health.

Healing the ills of the collective unconscious of our societies and our world is probably more of a dream than it could ever be a reality. The most we can realistically strive for is to heal ourselves and, thus, heal our own corner of the earth. We will no doubt always confront challenges, and yet, let us at least strive for worthy challenges. So much of the pain and suffering that is a part of our human experience is *unnecessary*. The struggle for human rights, for example, continuing for so many centuries, is an unnecessary suffering. We can strive for equality amongst all peoples.

Starvation is unnecessary. Drug addiction and alcoholism, child abuse and violence, are unnecessary. These are obstacles that are able to be conquered.

And, many diseases are unnecessary. As we learn more about the physical effects of emotional stress, we will have it in our power to free ourselves from optional pain.

STRESS: THE COMMON DENOMINATOR

CHAPTER ELEVEN

Conflicts of Sex and Sexuality: The Roots of Low Self-Esteem

(Shealy)

C onflicts of sex and sexuality provide the roots for most societal problems. Low self-esteem initiated by these conflicts leads to physical and economic competition, oppressive political power, unequal pay for women, rape, divorce, prostitution, crime, drug-abuse and disease.

Irresponsible and unwise responses to sexual feelings may be the most critical factor in every power struggle, both in primitive society and in our most civilized countries. And feelings of sexual inadequacy are rampant in men and women.

In examining sexual power conflicts, I am primarily interested in encouraging you to think about the consequences of conflicting values and behaviors, repressed desires and covert actions.

For at least five thousand years, males have dominated and repressed virtually everything feminine and have competed amongst themselves to be the strongest and most powerful. The majority of world religions have denigrated women, while exalting a male God and empowering males to dominate family, church, society and government—all seats of power, in other words.

These "macho" attitudes have led to widespread sexual repression, sexual frustration and the double standard of sexual behavior. There is a hypocritical code of sexual behavior that society espouses in church and civil law. Our legal and religious laws have proclaimed:

- Males are *superior* to females and should be masters of business, government, church, home, wife and children
- Sexual contact is acceptable only:
  a. with someone of the opposite sex, or
  b. in the marriage union
- Masturbation is evil or unhealthy.

These three "laws" provide the roots of virtually all hypocrisy as well as social and personal distress. Let us examine concept number one: Males are superior to females and should be masters of business, government, church, home, wife and children.

HYPOCRISY NUMBER ONE

From the moment of the decision to reproduce, a majority of women and men pray for a boy. Kingdoms and marriages may topple if the wife fails to produce the highly desired male heir. The woman is blamed if a girl is born, even though it is the male's sperm that determines the sex.

From the moment of birth, a girl is made to feel inferior and a boy is revered as more powerful and more useful than any woman, including his mother. Thus, sons are expected to express the fantasies and unfulfilled life goals of the wife-mother who has no value except as a servant to her "superior" husband and son. Even the most well-adjusted couple live in a society where these collective concepts lay the foundation for poor self-esteem in both sexes.

Freud's contribution to the perpetuation of this notion is substantial. He felt that a woman could only be brought "unlimited satisfaction by her relationship to her son." Through her son, she could "transfer to her son the ambition" she had not been able to satisfy (because of male domination). He also felt that no marriage was secure "until the wife had succeeded in making her husband a child."

Throughout history, women have been paid little and always less than men for equal work. Husbands have determined whether their wives could eat, dress, create or communicate. Women have been denied education since their primary role is nursemaid and servant. They have been denied the right to vote, even for many years after black male slaves were "freed" and granted the power of the poll.

Women have been raped and then accused of being the seducer. Prostitutes have been jailed while the males who support them are just considered "good ol' boys sewing a few wild oats." Men have fostered the notion that a victim of sexual aggression (rape) has actually brought it upon herself by teasing and enticing men. Women who have been raped have been said by men to experience great sensory pleasure from it. It is unlikely that any man would find physical force, especially to the genitalia, pleasurable.

The Church has been run by men who demand that men be masters of the home, who have murdered women who committed adultery and spared men, who preach that God is a man and who murder in holy wars those who do not worship as the Church decrees. For hundreds of years, the Catholic Church was exclusively run by men who were supposed to be celibate but who often fornicated extensively or practiced the even more forbidden sin of homosexuality. The advent of Protestantism has not significantly changed such repression, and the issue of celibacy in the Catholic Church remains, at the very least, controversial.

Competition among males is inevitable and strongly encouraged. Competition is the guiding principle of moral, intellectual, economic, creative and sexual behavior. Male superiority must be proved again and again, year after year. Society demands the impossible of every male: to be superior to all other men and women.

Since they are presumed from birth to be superior and powerful, men are not allowed any self-doubt nor must they show any indication that they are less "male" than any other man. This competitiveness prevents men from developing close interpersonal relationships with either men or women. The aspect of competitiveness is the result of societal conditioning and not one primarily hormonal in nature.

Marc Fasteau, in his book *The Male Machine*, makes several revealing observations about men that are rooted in the climate of hypocrisy that exists so strongly in our society, for example, "The male machine is a special kind of being, different from women, children and men who don't measure up."

Fasteau's insights into male behavior and the social problems resulting from it are unexcelled. He says, for instance, that males are tremendously task oriented, always in a competitive mood, always on guard. Wilhelm Reich, one of the greatest psychiatrists of all time, created the concept of armoring, i.e., muscle tightness is used to protect one's vulnerability. In this respect, the male is virtually a complete coat of armor, blocking every personal feeling.

According to Fasteau, male relationships with other males are distant, respectful of power and authority, never intimate. The idea of intimacy of one male with another is abhorrent. Male esteem is maintained only by one-upmanship or by power plays to attract female attention or male domination.

Women, he says, are servants who shower the male with love and devotion, if not worship, and provide him sexual release. Publicly, men are paragons of virtue and respect for the "weaker sex" but they tolerate virtually no questioning from either women or from men of inferior power status.

The result all this research shows is a shallow, hollow, personal life for men, leading many to repeated existential crises.

In other words, men attempt to avoid confronting their fears by bantering, rough play, sports, alcohol, marijuana. They avoid at all cost self-exposure of even the faintest weakness. Men compensate at all levels of life with "my theory tops your theory."

The greatest taboo of most men, says Fasteau, is being vulnerable—under no circumstance can they express weakness or personal need. Sex, however, is the one experience in which men can and do exhibit some emotion—mostly lust and a macho pretense to be interested in every attractive woman who passes within imagination.

Rollo May has stated that "sex is a need, but eros is a desire." The eros part of sex is the sensuality that is almost totally missing from most men. Rollo May further finds eros as "the experiencing of the personal intentions and meanings of the (sex) act." Many men are unable to relate sexually to women and to participate as equals in the initiation of the pleasures of sex.

Boys are taught almost from birth that the male is superior. Many girls want, for a time, to be boys, but very few boys want to be girls. And in fact, if boys exhibited such feelings, this would be recognized as a problem. The major male-female differences seem to be almost totally ones of societal conditioning.

For instance, researchers Money and Ehrhardt reported on a pair of identical male twins, one of whom lost his penis in a circumcision accident and was "reassigned" as a girl through a process of surgical reconstruction. Her behavior was "in remarkable contrast to the little boy behavior of her identical twin brother."

These researchers concluded that after eighteen months, "influence and conditioning on gender identity is so strong that it is possible to reassign effectively the sex of a child raised as a member of the other sex, regardless of the child's genetic, gonadal and hormonal situation."

Work becomes the major societal proof of masculine power after a man concludes his teenage years. Football, boxing and wrestling are the prized sports in adolescence, and professional athletes in these areas earn huge rewards. War is also connected to the need for males to prove themselves. Indeed, males seem to be fascinated by violence. Toughness and productivity are driving forces of what Fasteau calls "the male machine."

The male sex organ is the ultimate symbol for power. And as in every other aspect of male life, competition for size and endurance is strong. Thus, penis size is a major factor for insecurity and anxiety among males. Virtually all men worry that their penis is too small. Indeed, this may be "man's greatest fear."

This fear is based upon inadequate understanding of physical facts. In Kinsey's reports, 30% of white males had an erect penis less than six inches in length and 54.4% were less than 6.25 inches (average was 6.14 inches in whites and 6.44 inches in blacks). Ninety-eight percent of whites had penises less than 8 inches in length with only 0.8% over 8 inches. Despite these facts, most pornographic literature, even much of the "soft porn," has implied that the penis is two feet long, hard as steel and can perform all night long. Such fantasies are caricatures that feed male inferiority fears and spark competition.

It is also obvious that men have a great deal of distrust of women, even when they may have positive relationships with women and hold them in high esteem. This ancient problem dates back at least to the biblical times. For instance, Eve is supposedly made out of Adam's rib and, therefore, could not have come into existence without the man. This seems to be an attempt by men to gain some control over the birth process, proclaiming themselves as both father and mother of women.

Woman is then given, in the Old Testament, a curse to "bear children and sorrow." Then this moral anarchy goes on to make woman the original sexual temptress, plunging humanity into misery by tempting Adam to eat at the tree of knowledge.

Freud, among his other perverted views of sex, emphasized that men got more pleasure than women from sex. How he could have known this is impossible to fathom since he seems to have had no major intellectual conversations with even remotely well-adjusted women. And of course, it was Freud who produced the theory that women suffered from "penis envy." What was never released until thirty plus years after his death was that Freud had a gay lover, and it appears that he was the one suffering from penis envy.

Women have always been exploited in the work force. They are paid approximately 60% of what men are paid for the same output. Child and female labor were introduced during the earliest stages of the industrial revolution when men were more employed in crafts. This differential persists today.

The medical field has also perpetuated remarkable other hypocrises and attacks upon women. There is even one surgeon who performed numerous clitoridectomies on women to prevent sexual excitement, which he was convinced caused, "insanities, cataplexy, hysteria, epilepsy and other diseases."

In the 1950s, a major group of gynecologists, obviously dominated by men, proposed that every woman over childbearing age should have a hysterectomy, and there have been some gynecologists who have certainly worked hard to do more than their share of accomplishing this. I wonder how many men would be willing to have their testicles removed after they have passed through the childbearing age.

One of the early male spokespersons for women was George Bernard Shaw who wrote,

> If we have come to think that the nursery and the kitchen are the natural sphere of a woman, we have done so exactly as children come to think that a cage is the natural sphere of a parrot because they have never seen one anywhere else. I will not go so far as to affirm that there are theological parrots who are convinced that imprisonment is the will of God because it is unpleasant. Still, the only parrot a free-souled person can sympathize with is the one that insists on being let out as the first condition of its making itself agreeable.
> The sum of the matter is that unless woman repudiates her womanliness, her duty to her husband, to her children, to society, to the law and to everyone but her-

self, she cannot emancipate herself. For women to be able to achieve equality, a whole basketful of ideals of the most sacred quality will be smashed.

In *The Psychology of Power*, published in 1966, Ronald V. Sampson argued that "an inequality of power between people wholly distorts the life of both the dominant and submissive parties, thereby making any form of justice or decency impossible. Dominance is inseparable from pride or arrogance and is accompanied by resentment, consciously or unconsciously."

We give at least an occasional amount of credit to John Stuart Mill who, as early as 1880, argued that "all moral deficiency of the greater society would not be abolished until men and women are treated completely equal." He further argued that men were corrupted as despots because of their absolute power, a statement for which he was attacked and ridiculed.

Anne Schaef has written in *Women's Reality* of this "white male system" that surrounds us and permeates our lives, its myths, beliefs, rituals, procedures and outcomes affecting everything we think, feel and do. She outlines four great myths of the white male system. These are:

- The White Male System is the only thing that exists.
- The White Male System is innately superior.
- The White Male System knows and understands everything.
- It is possible to be totally logical, rational and objective.

Says Schaef, "These very assumptions, of course, denigrate intuition and subjectivity. The White Male System has made a religion of the 'scientific method' which leads only to statistics and numbers, which are used to support its mythology."

Interestingly, Schaef insists that women "normally do not like or trust one another." She thinks that they feel safer attacking women than they do attacking men. She feels that there is a basic philosophy of women which is "the original sin of being born female, which means that you are 'tainted', that there is something wrong with you from the moment of conception, that it is impossible to change that wrongness and that women's birthright is one of innate inferiority."

As with other intelligent therapists, Schaef states, "I have met very few women who really wish they had a penis. What women want is a birthright of innate superiority, power and influence which comes from being born male."

As a result of this discrimination, intimidation and maltreatment, Schaef reports that women experience a feeling of emptiness which they describe as a "hole, pit, nothingness, a void, a black space, a cavern located within the solar plexus." She considers this void or cavern an essential part of the identity and wholeness of women. "It is in the solar plexus area where women carry their original sin of being born a female. This leads to women feeling as if they have to be sick, bad, crazy or stupid not to buy the whole male line."

It is no wonder that women are angry. Interestingly, within this backdrop, it is not surprising that women have learned very little about their own sexuality, because even women's sexuality has usually been described only by men who hardly know what they are talking about since they don't listen to women long enough to find out.

However, in general, women are not likely to judge other individuals on their sexuality or to assume that all interpersonal relationships are sexual, as men seem to do. As with almost all individuals who have discussed needs and preferences, Schaef feels that "intercourse and orgasm are far less important than touching, holding, stroking and cuddling. In fact, it appears that women often participate in sexual intercourse only because it is the only way they can get touching and holding."

Perhaps one of the reasons that men do not like touching is that it appears, not only in people but even in apes, that when two people encounter, the first person who touches the other gains power and control over the situation.

Schaef disagrees with the concept that in the perfect marriage, the woman becomes a mother because she feels that in the "Public Perfect Marriage, the man is the parent and the woman is the child. The man takes care of the woman." She does, however, admit that in the privacy of a marriage, the man is treated by his wife as a child, for she feeds him, clothes him and picks up after him.

Adding to woman's resentment is the fact that as soon as she bears a male child, the woman is supposed to teach that child that he is an innately superior being (over mother and women, at least). Obviously, mothers have to have a great deal of repressed rage and hostility beneath their natural mothering, nurturing instincts. In our society, women are "validated" only when they have been able to have children. An infertile woman is considered almost as bad as a barren sow.

It is amazing that any love relationship could continue to exist in this area of open and suppressed hostility. Of course, children respond to the many painful and humiliating experiences of such a society. Because of the conflict between men and women, children are often pawns in the open or suppressed battlefield between their parents, and this certainly promotes fear and anger. It also means that love has an impossible time being the dominant force in an individual's life because there is much conflict. And, of course, children are exposed to the sexual stereotypes and role models from birth.

Dorothy Sayers is quoted in *Masculine/Feminine*, edited by Betty and Theodore Roszak in 1969, saying

> Probably no man is ever troubled to imagine how strange his life would appear to him if it were only assessed in terms of his maleness. If everything he wrote, said or did had to be justified by reference to female approval; if he were compelled to regard himself, day in and day out, not as a member of society but merely as a *virile* member of society; if the center of his dress consciousness were the cod-piece; his education directed to making him a spirited lover and meek paterfamilias; his interests held to be natural only insofar as they were sex-

ual; if he were vexed by continual advice on how to add a rough male touch to his typing, how to learn without losing his masculine appeal, how to combine chemical research with education, how to play bridge without incurring the suspicion of impotence. Suppose a man were told, 'and why should you trouble your handsome little head about politics?'

Sayers, interestingly, emphasized that women had much more power and equality in medieval times, for women controlled many industries including, "spinning, weaving, baking, brewing, distilling, perfumery, preserving, pickling," in which they worked with their intellect and hands, as well as commanded a domestic staff.

At least some increased competitiveness began to appear when men took over these jobs by industrializing virtually all of them. The "empty head and idle hands" status of women created by this change made men both envy their leisure and despise them at the same time.

Almost all authors have emphasized that for a woman, the sexual relationship is more of a spiritual rapport and it is its own reason for being. Long after the male sex act is completed, the woman's relationship to the man continues. Women have a much greater interest in attractiveness, personality, home, family and other people, while men are much more interested in safety, physical fitness, money and sex.

At least some women are aware that the usual "missionary position" in sex is also one of domination by the male. Some women have argued that marriage itself is a tremendous vehicle for perpetuating this male domination of women.

Of course, Masters and Johnson have demonstrated that one place that women strongly outperform men is in their ability to have multiple orgasms. Of equal devastation to the male ego is the fact that the most intense orgasms experienced by women who were research subjects were produced by masturbatory manual stimulation and far less intense orgasms were experienced during sexual intercourse.

The idea that female sexuality and orgasm were vaginal, perpetuated by Freud, helped to make women sexually, economically, socially and politically inferior to men since even the smallest clitoris, the female counterpart of the male penis, was not considered important to women having orgasm. As with most other Freudian comments about sex, it was totally wrong.

To this point, most of the discussion has related to the male perspective on sexuality. It is worth noting that women are more concerned with caring and genuine love than they are with the physical aspects of sexual intercourse itself. Even in this day of so-called womens' liberation, a majority of women do not seem to be as interested in a promiscuous, quick relationship as appears to be true with men. It seems that women stray into extramarital relationships primarily because of lack of love and a lack of a feeling of communication with their spouse.

HYPOCRISY NUMBER TWO

Let's examine the second greatest hypocrisy: Sexual contact is acceptable only with someone of the opposite sex or with one's marriage partner.

The concept of exclusive heterosexuality is another societal lie. Alfred C. Kinsey provided the first scientific study of hetero-bi-homosexual arousal. He asked men to rate themselves on a scale of 0 to 6 in relation to capability of sexual arousal. Zero means capable of arousal *only* by someone of the opposite sex. Six means capable of arousal *only* by someone of the same sex. By age fifteen, 70% of males have indulged in some homosexual activity. *This is the norm.*

And the evidence is overwhelming that, under deprivation conditions such as the military or prison, homosexuality becomes the "choice" of a huge majority. Furthermore, even in "normal" society, 37% of post-adolescent men have actually had at least one homosexual experience. Thus, unless this urge is suppressed by adult society, homosexual interest is more likely than not to occur. And a significant plurality (37%) of adults actually engage in homosexual acts. Obviously, a huge majority (70%) are *capable* of being bisexual.

The "requirement" of society that individuals avoid sex until marriage is so universally ignored as to be ludicrous. At least 75% of teenagers in this country experiment, often regularly, with sexual intercourse. Teenage pregnancy and abortion are unfortunate by-products of our open, sexual culture.

The religious and legal requirement of monogamy is almost equally subverted. At least 58% of men, and presumably women, have extramarital affairs. Probably as a result of civil and religious law, most marriages suffer from such affairs. Thus, despite the 58% preponderance of behavior, the most common cause of divorce is infidelity.

In human beings, the power to create has been overshadowed by the power to dominate. Wisdom is almost totally lacking in the human species in relation to sex and sexuality. What should be obvious is ignored; that is, there are virtually no classes in the American school system that prepare young individuals for parenthood. If we ever hope to achieve a sense of balance and health in terms of sex and sexuality, we must have an educational system that prepares young people from kindergarten through college for their role as parents, teaching them the responsibility of parenting and a healthy respect for sex and sexuality.

THE THIRD HYPOCRISY

The third great societal hypocrisy is that masturbation is evil or unhealthy. This law denies the most basic aspect of human nature and sexuality, which is a natural tendency to explore one's own body and to indulge in feelings that are pleasant.

Male babies are usually born with an erection and females with vaginal lubrication, indicating sexual arousal. The pleasure of sexual sensation is so obvious to any human being that the infant's tendency to fondle its genitalia should be considered natural. Even Boy Scout manuals, at least through the 1940s, lied openly (as did much of society) in claiming that masturbation leads to all types of illnesses, including blindness and insanity.

Most modern scientists consider masturbation healthy and desirable. Some even believe that no individual can satisfy someone else sexually unless they can satisfy themselves.

At least 98% of males admit to practicing masturbation post-marriage, especially if the wife is pregnant, ill or away. A majority of women masturbate at some time in life but seem less preoccupied with sexual sensation than are men.

From a detached, philosophical viewpoint, sexual maturity includes a personal ego-strength that allows one first to develop an ability to enjoy one's own sexual response freely through masturbation. When that personal ability is adequately accomplished, an individual is likely to meet, from time to time throughout life, other persons to whom one is strongly attracted.

Sometimes that attraction is physical, sometimes it is emotional or mental and, rarely, it is spiritual. Of the thousands of persons one encounters, a very small number will be so compatible that the possibility of strong sexual attraction exists.

Theoretically, such an attraction might be with persons of either sex and it is conceivable that sexual sharing, the purest form of spiritual communion, might be "normal" with either sex. If done at that level of spiritual exchange, it may be natural. Indeed, sexual expression without true love, respect and caring, whether heterosexual or homosexual, is itself hypocritical.

In fact, women who tolerate sex with a despised husband may be committing a greater spiritual conflict than is a paid prostitute. At least with prostitution, the terms are openly understood.

Similarly, homosexual promiscuity with dozens of partners per week is impossible to comprehend from a spiritual perspective. If sex is a real spiritual communion, it deserves the same care that goes into meditation and devotion.

Edgar Cayce emphasized the spirituality of sex in discussing sexual intercourse outside of marriage (A26)2, M.33): "For thy body is the temple of the living God. Do not desecrate same in thine own consciousness."

CONCLUSION

As you will recognize by now from the extensive discussions related to stress and disease, the wide variety of conflicts represented by society's attitudes toward sex provides a natural breeding ground for the root of all illness—poor self-esteem. Until we honor all males and females, empowering each with unique and equally valid attributes, all of us individually, and society as a whole, will suffer.

As in every other aspect of life, sexual health requires the acknowledgment of the spirit as a guiding principle. In no area of behavior is the Golden Rule more needed. If society and individuals develop spiritual-sexual behavior, then the foundations for health become solid.

As a way of examining your attitudes toward sex, consider the Sexual Attitude Inventory test in Chapter Thirteen. Perhaps you'll understand yourself and the roots of your self-esteem issues more easily after taking that test.

In relation to the eight patterns of dysfunction discussed in Chapter One, consider the following:

- Societal and personal sexual conflicts are a frequent cause of unresolved stress.
- Negative beliefs: women are not as good as men; men must be super-macho and well-hung.
- Sex is tied to "love" by women but not by men.
- Male preoccupation with minor sex concerns (size of penis).
- Women are put down at all levels of society.
- Sexual expression is unhealthy in many individuals.
- Society's requirements of the super male and put-down of women lead to low self-esteem and lack of meaning.
- Women are supposed to be the good little women; men are supposed never to cry.

CHAPTER TWELVE

Psychosomatic Health

D r. Elmer Green of the Menninger Foundation has emphasized that if there is such a thing as psychosomatic illness, there must also be psychosomatic health. Unfortunately, the term psychosomatic has tended to be interpreted both by the medical profession and by the lay public as a primarily psychological "defect, a basic personality flaw which one purposefully chooses." Since 95% of people in the United States are born physically healthy, we have to assume that they are also born mentally healthy.

Pessimism, for example, is largely the result of being born into a family where circumstances create that personality complex early in life. Thus, if pessimists or optimists are "made" or created by the home environment, it should be possible at any age to convert a pessimist into an optimist. The evidence is overwhelming that health is the result of a positive attitude and the choices we make in relation to lifestyle.

Personally, I prefer the concept of Stress Illness rather than psychosomatic illness. Hans Selye, the greatest research scientist in the field of stress, has demonstrated that a variety of chemical changes accompany stress. More importantly, he has proven that a stress reaction results from excess physical, chemical or emotional pressure.

Whenever the body is chemically, physically or emotionally overloaded, it causes a state of *alarm* that results in a complex interaction which I call the stress cycle:

THE STRESS CYCLE

STRESS

Blood Pressure, Pulse Go Up

Brain Releases ACTH (Stimulates Adrenal Glands)

Liver Releases Stored Blood Sugar

Beta-Endorphin (Natural Narcotics

Sympathetic Nervous System Releases Norepinephrine

Prostaglandin E1 (Natural anti-inflammatory)

Adrenal Glands Release Epinephrine (Adrenalin) Cortisone

Serotonin (Speeds up Ability of Nerve Cells to Communicate)

This is the "fight or flight" cycle. If we react physically to "burn up" the stress chemicals, relatively little harm is done. If we fail to dissipate the stress chemicals by physical exercise or deep relaxation, which also acts to decrease blood sugar, epinephrine and norepinephrine, then the cycle continues:

Pancreas Releases Insulin

Either Insulin or Resulting Lowered Blood Sugar Lead to *Stress*

Selye demonstrated that the alarm reaction can be elicited by:

Chemicals such as
> Nicotine
> Alcohol
> Caffeine
> Sugar
> High Fat Diet
> Poisons (Smog, DDT, etc.)

Physical Stress, especially
> Physical Inactivity
> Accidents
> Barometric Pressure Changes

Emotions
> Fear
> Anger
> Guilt
> Depression
> Anxiety

He also demonstrated that individual small levels of stress that do not cause an alarm reaction are *additive*. For instance, one cigarette elicits an alarm reaction but a few puffs don't. One cup of coffee elicits an alarm reaction but a few sips don't. One martini elicits an alarm reaction but one gulp doesn't. However, combining a few puffs of a cigarette, a few swallows of coffee, plus a small amount of martini all at once *will* produce an alarm reaction.

When the same stress is repeated frequently, we *adapt* and respond less intensely; *but* this adaptation lowers our tolerance for new stress. Thus, we may adapt to coffee, sugar, alcohol and nicotine; but then we become less able to tolerate emotional or physical stress. Repeated adaptation leads to mal-adaptation or illness.

As we focus our attention in this chapter upon emotional stress, it is important to remember that our total stress is additive and that how we react emotionally is influenced constantly by chemically induced stress (coffee, sugar, etc.) and by our level of physical exercise.

In *Cancer, Stress and Death* (edited by Gene Tache, Hans

Selye and Stacey B. Day, a Sloan Kettering Institute Cancer Series Book), Selye concludes that exposure to a variety of stressors can induce malignant growth, especially in those people who are predisposed and under the right (or "wrong") conditions of chemical stress. The authors, writing from the most publicly recognized, mainline establishment in cancer research, emphasize that although not scientifically "proven beyond any reasonable medical doubt, evidence suggests the assumption that systemic stress can influence" production of cancer. They also say "it is clear, therefore, that from historical and circumstantial evidence—and in more recent times through experimental data and in vitro assays—that a direct link between abnormal immune responses, the growth of malignant tumors, and various forms of emotional disturbance and stress exist." In other words, stress is a major cause of cancer.

In *The Role of Medicine: Dream, Mirage and Nemesis*, by Thomas McKeown, a professor of social medicine and an outstanding physician, he emphasizes that in all developed countries it is personal behavior "in relation to diet, exercise, tobacco, alcohol, drugs" which "is now even more important than provision of food and control of hazards." Few diseases are determined irreversible at the time of conception. Dr. McKeown emphasizes that in the future it will be modification of health habits rather than interventions in disease mechanisms that will lead to further health and longevity. "The treatment of established disease, although important for patients, does not usually restore them to a life of normal duration and quality; and the modern improvement in health is due to prevention of disease rather than to treatment that had occurred." He considers the role of medicine to be "the prevention of sickness and premature death and the care of the sick and disabled."

In 1986 Carla A. Kubitz and co-workers demonstrated a marked difference in salivary IGA (one measure of immune function) in relation to high levels of stress over which individuals feel that they have no control. Interestingly, she also found that at the premenstrual phase, women had lower IGA levels, suggesting that at that time they have a lower immunity and lower resistance to stress. Coupled with the fact that women tend to be emotionally more volatile at that time, normal hormonal cycles are also prime contributors to so-called "psychosomatic illness."

Research over the last decade has demonstrated convincingly that the brain is capable of regulating all body functions and that this regulation is capable of being brought under voluntary control. Thus, the central nervous system (mind) is now increasingly implicated as a major contributor to disease. Most people, including physicians, don't want to accept this fact because "if the brain has such power over what happens in our bodies, *then we might have to watch our attitudes if we wish to be helped.*" (Emphasis mine.)

It has now been demonstrated quite conclusively that certain antibody levels are diminished by the need for power and domination, and enhanced by love, intimacy and affiliation. Perhaps one of the most striking paradoxical denials of the effect of attitude upon health is a 1987 article in the *Journal of Preventive Medicine* in which the authors conclude that a positive attitude has no statistically significant influence upon longevity in people who have had heart attacks; but lifestyle habits such as smoking, drinking, inadequate exercise and poor diet do. *I find the "attitude" of the authors absolutely incomprehensible because it is precisely the patients' attitudes that determine whether or not they will change those life-threatening habits!*

It is important to recognize that it is not stress itself but the reaction to stress or the feeling that stress is uncontrollable that makes stress harmful. Many authors have emphasized that it is hard to "give tuberculosis, a cold, or infectious hepatitis to someone." Even carcinogenic agents (chemicals that seem to induce cancerous changes in cells) are inadequate in and of themselves to produce the disease unless there are *co-factors. Total stress and attitude are the major co-factors.* Disease is not so much the effect of noxious, external "bugs" or germs but of the internal factors that regulate homeostasis or balance of metabolism. The mind and behavior are common contributors to disease.

Stuart Wolf, one of the best-known researchers in stress illness, has suggested that "disease is a way of life," the end result of reaction to life's problems.

Numerous studies indicate that approximately *half* of all illnesses and *two-thirds* of all "can't cope" days result in illness in about *one-fourth* of individuals, those with the greatest stress. In other words, individuals who are "dissatisfied and discontented" have many more illnesses than others. The frequently sick have a lower morale that has long since preceded their illnesses and job dissatisfaction. They also tend to perceive events in their lives, both at work and at home, as much more stressful than those who are not frequently sick.

In an outstanding study at Harvard Medical School, pediatricians Roger Meyer and Robert Haggerty studied sixteen families containing one hundred individual persons over a one-year period. They found that both streptococcal illness and other respiratory diseases were four times more common after episodes that the families identified as stressful. Cognitive and emotional factors, both mentally induced, are equally implicated in the activation of viruses.

Individuals who have trouble coping are likely to have raised levels of rheumatoid factor and antinuclear antibody as found in rheumatoid arthritis. Indeed, individuals who are depressed are also likely to produce rheumatoid factor. When the depression is adequately treated, the rheumatoid factor, an immune complex found in the blood, goes away.

When American Indians were forced onto reservations, the death rate from tuberculosis and other illnesses shot up, even though bureaucrats felt they were providing a "higher standard of living." It is not the stress of change but the feeling of *having no control over their lives* that seems to have been a major debilitating factor. Individuals who migrated from Portugal to Canada, for instance, convinced that their move meant new jobs and an improved future, actually had improved health.

As early as 1910, Sir William Osler discussed "angina pectoris as related to stress and strain." Many individuals, of course, remain healthy even under extreme stress. Whether or not stress causes illness seems to be largely the result of how we view the troubles or react to them. A sense of control in our lives can keep our stress chemicals from becoming imbalanced enough to lead to illness. A feeling of openness to change and an attitude of involvement enhance our resistance to stress and disease, whereas a sense of helplessness depresses the immune system. The belief that we must have power and dominance also adversely affects our immune system. Hostility, distrust and cynicism contribute to the risk of both atherosclerosis and heart disease. Hostility and anger lead to an increased output in both "cortisone" related hormones, which alter the immune system, and serotonin, a major chemical involved in sleep, mood and pain.

Worry produces a chronic disturbance of the homeostatic neurochemicals. Hans Selye often emphasized the story of a drunk who showers you with insults even though he or she doesn't know you. If you choose to become angry with the alcoholic, your blood pressure goes up and your whole nervous system is in a state of alarm, which could make you a candidate for a heart attack. Under these circumstances, who is responsible for your heart "attack": the drunk, his insult or you by "choosing the wrong reaction"?!

Suzanne Kobasa and Salvatory Maddey, of the University of Chicago, have worked extensively with the differences between the helpless and the hardy. Approximately half of two hundred business executives at Illinois Bell Telephone Company had numerous symptoms, but the other half evidenced very little reaction to stress. *The healthier individuals considered change as an opportunity for growth and a new experience. Those who felt that it was a threat to security were the ones who became ill.*

Those individuals who have a sense of personal control and challenge as their commitment to life have a sense of meaning, direction and excitement and survive most "stresses." Those who have a sense of importance and value in what they do and a sense of purpose have far fewer symptoms and illnesses. If, on the other hand, we see stress as "inevitable" and a challenge as a negative experience, then the challenge becomes a stress and has a more adverse effect upon the body.

According to Kobasa and Maddey, "belief and control, commitment and challenge" are the keys to "psychological hardiness." The sense of personal control is essential to effective coping and remaining healthy. The most powerful control is actually cognitive, that is, the ability to appraise mentally a bad situation in such a way as to reduce stress. By choosing our *reaction* to hostile events, we control the power over us of those events and, therefore, diminish any harmful effects. Thus, we need to learn to interact with events and the harmful effects by thinking about them optimistically.

Effective coping or psychosomatic health means viewing problems optimistically and thus decreasing the stress or alarm reaction from them; taking positive action to change or adapt to the problem; and decreasing the stress reaction by physical exercise and deep relaxation.

At Vanderbilt University, it has been shown that basic ego strength is the most powerful predictor of how long individuals remain sick and even whether or not they become sick under given stresses. The most basic of our immune reactions, the ability of our lymphocytes and antibodies to maintain normal activity, is strongly affected by how we view stress opportunities. "A good attitude and ability to get along with other people" are associated with less illness. Even reviewing prisoners of war, not everyone breaks down physically and emotionally. Viktor Frankl, psychoanalyst and author of *Man's Search for Meaning*, emphasized that the loss of meaning in life was more important than both starvation and typhus, one of the most serious of infections.

In undergraduate students, the response to immunization for flu is different in those who cope poorly with stress. Those who cope well had significantly greater, natural killer cell response (a major measurement of immune competency) than those who had high levels of anxiety and depression. Thus, anxiety, distress, anger and depression all further compromise the immune system. In addition, individuals who want to dominate the scene have a higher incidence of respiratory illness and lower levels of salivary IGA, another measurement of the immune system. It is the *chronic reaction to stress with prolonged elevations of norepinephrine, "adrenalin," and "cortisone" or glucosteroids that compromises the immune system.* The T-cells, as well as the natural killer cells, are depressed by anxiety and a need to dominate others. The more we perceive ourselves as being hassled, or the greater pessimists we are, the lower and more abnormal will be our T-cells, natural killer cells. In other words, every function of the immune system is inhibited by negative stress.

Robert Good, Founder, President and Director of Memorial Sloan Kettering Cancer Hospital, emphasized that "a positive attitude" and "a constructive frame of mind" enhance our ability to resist infections, allergies, cancer and autoimmune disorders, while depression weakens this ability. It has been shown that norepinephrine, the major stress chemical, or "adrenalin," blocks the ability of our white blood cells to kill tumor cells. People who are cynical and hostile have a greater degree of atherosclerosis and a higher incidence of heart attacks. At the University of North Carolina, physicians who have a "higher hostility score" are four times more likely to have a heart attack and six times more likely to die of it than those who block that negative influence. And Duke University scientists found that hostility, anger, cynicism and mistrust lead to a greater mortality rate. Those persons with the highest hostility scores had a death rate 6.4 times those with the lowest hostility score!

Thus, health is controlled by our brain, our mind or our attitude, which, in turn, control the chemicals mediating stress. Both excessive norepinephrine from anxiety or decreased norepinephrine from depression are harmful. An excess of dopamine, the precursor of norepinephrine, is found in schizophrenia and in panic attacks; deficiency of serotonin is found in depression. Many significant neurochemical abnormalities occur in depression. Interestingly, chronically heavy drinkers and alcoholics who tend to be highly depressed also have high levels of cortisol production, which leads to both abnormal fat distribution in the body and high blood pressure, as well as a weakened immune system. Other neurochemicals that are out of balance in almost all diseases include acetylcholine, the basic chemical of the parasympathetic nervous system, which is deficient in certain nerve cells in Alzheimer's disease. Low levels of serotonin or its by-product are found both in suicide patients and in alcoholics.

Diet and nutrition, too, strongly influence mood. Tryptophan, an essential amino acid, is the precursor for serotonin. Inadequate amounts of tryptophan can lead to lowered levels of serotonin, agitation, insomnia, depression and even spontaneous pain without a physical cause for it. Tyrosine and phenylalanine, other amino acids, are essential for production of dopamine, norepinephrine and epinephrine. Interestingly, inadequate amounts of these may lead to either high blood pressure or depression. Deficient phenylalanine may adversely affect memory, learning and motivation. Glutamine, another amino acid, also has a beneficial effect upon memory and concentration and may help those who are addicted to alcohol and tobacco. An excess of phenylalanine in the diet, however, can lead to a deficiency in tryptophan and thus a resultant decrease in serotonin levels. Increased amounts of tryptophan are helpful in treating depression, insomnia and chronic pain.

Manic depressives tend to have abnormalities in acetylcholine production with overabundance of receptors for acetylcholine. Lithium is a mineral that is markedly helpful in people with manic depressive disease and may be a regulator of many neurochemical processes. It is also essential in the conversion of tryptophan to serotonin.

A typical American junk-food diet, high in fat, sugar and salt, and deficient in fiber, vitamins, minerals, complex carbohydrates and essential fatty acids, can lead to a variety of mental changes, including hostility and hyperactivity, as well as depression, but also can lead to marked weakness of the immune system. It is of some interest that we have found that individuals who are both agitated and depressed have a marked increase in the natural narcotics, beta endorphines, which can cause a diminished immune response and faster growth of tumors, if cancer is present, or make one "susceptible" to cancer.

The quality of our relationships has much more to do with how often we get sick than do genes, diet, environment and basic physiology. For instance, the highest rates of tuberculosis are found among those of the poorer social status, that is, with the lowest level of social support. Individuals who sense a lack of internal control or external support have much higher rates of both accidents and mental illnesses. In England, civil servants with the highest death rate from heart attacks are those who have the least social contact with neighbors, relatives or friends.

A sense of permanence and continuity, attachment to home or religion, diminishes the effect of negative experiences and promotes well-being. Those individuals who have many social ties, including marriage, friends, contacts with relatives and participation in church affairs, have lower death rates and higher health rates. Women who are socially isolated have a much higher risk of dying of cancer. Even support from supervisors and co-workers has been identified as enhancing health and reducing the incidence of heart disease, ulcers, chronic respiratory disease and even skin rashes.

Those who have a strong attachment to church have less heart disease, emphysema, cirrhosis, high blood pressure and even abnormal Pap smears. In Israel, men were found to be twice as likely to have angina pectoris if they did not have a feeling of a loving and supporting relationship in their marriage. Even such adverse factors as high blood pressure and high cholesterol levels were not as important as the love and support of a wife.

In the case of women under high stress, they have one third less complications in pregnancy if they have a good social support system and a happy marriage. A strong social support system enhances the immune system. Even such simple factors as visits received in a retirement home three times a week have produced an increase in people's T-cells, thereby reducing the chance for infections and other illnesses.

In women, a good marriage is significantly associated with enhanced immune function. And those women who have happy marriages are less depressed and have a more competent immune system. Having a support system with animals seems to be of some benefit. Those individuals who have a high sense of personal power or internal control and see themselves as being capable of altering or influencing a situation, rather than being at the mercy of it, actually create and make better use of their social support than those who do not.

Allen Langer, a psychologist at Harvard, and Judith Roden, a psychologist at Yale, have demonstrated that the death rate of those individuals who exercise strong self-responsibility and have a positive outlook is only half the mortality rate of those who do not. The sense of an internal ability to control our lives diminishes the effects of many other forms of stress. This feeling of internal control is highly correlated with both psychological and physical well-being. In over thirty-five controlled situations, scientific studies have demonstrated that increased emotional support and relaxation training and exercises decrease hospital stay, enhance recovery and lead to lower blood pressure and fewer complications after hospitalization. Of course, those patients with chronic pain who are training to have a positive internal dialogue have a marked decrease in pain compared with those who continue with negative thinking.

Many people, even those who have the AIDS virus, never manifest symptoms, *and it is now increasingly believed that emotions, attitudes and beliefs are major factors in determining whether individuals exposed to the AIDS virus develop the illness.* Those who develop AIDS have been found to have a higher level of unresolved, stressful events just prior to the onset of their disease. A significant correlation has been found in AIDS patients between survival and a sense of internal control. Survivors of pneumocystis carne pneumonia, a major cause of death in AIDS patients, are much more optimistic and sought more help from others in solving their problems. Those who died were more passive and helpless. Those patients with greater anxiety and a sense of helplessness had lower levels of white blood cell counts and lower T4/T8 ratios (critical factors in immune competency). Those who had a feeling that they could do something to help themselves seemed better able to ward off progression of the disease. Some health professionals believe that those individuals who develop AIDS already had some level of immune depression before they developed AIDS. Other contributors to diminished immune competence are amyl nitrite, a street drug for getting "high," hepatitis B, cytomegalic virus diseases, and venereal herpes, as well as candidiasis.

The fact that no illness, infectious or otherwise, can be explained strictly on the basis of a germ or some other single agent, has left medicine without an adequate theory for disease. Thus, medicine has not been able to answer the question of who is at risk of having a particular disease and under what circumstances predisposed individuals will develop that disease. The field of medicine, as a whole, largely ignores psychosocial influences and thus is largely responsible for the current crisis in health care. We continue to expand technology, which increases costs, while ignoring root causes, such as poor self-esteem, smoking and overall attitude.

Hostility or giving up, a feeling of helplessness, weakens the immune system and increases the risk of illness. This passive victim pattern is what researcher Joyce Solomon has called the "Immunosuppression-Prone Personality." Studies on cadets at West Point have indicated that those individuals who have a positive attitude are less likely to develop mononucleosis. Those who are overachievers and strive too hard were shown to be more susceptible to mononucleosis. Overstriving increases catecholamine or adrenalin production, as well as cortisone production, and weakens the immune system.

Even those individuals who have repeated attacks of herpes simplex, or fever blister, have higher incidences of anxiety and guilt. Interestingly, in that illness as in many others, the virus can be activated to produce a fever blister by suggestion during hypnosis. Students, of course, have an increased incidence of "cold sores" during exams. Those individuals who have a much higher incidence of episodic negative, unhappy moods or depression have many more cold sores.

Extensive health diaries kept by five hundred and eighty-nine adults in Detroit showed that "bad moods consistently triggered physical problems." Loneliness and stress in general are the major problems. Venereal herpes, a first cousin of fever blister, also occurs much more commonly in individuals who have negative moods and lack of a social support system. Poor functioning of the essential T-cells is consistently found in cases of depression, stress, anxiety, hostility and fatigue. Both latent bacteria, as well as viruses in cancer, may be activated by negative moods and such stress reactions. Even dental caries has been found to be increased in individuals who feel that they are under chronic stress, and the bacteria in saliva decreases when they relax.

In medical students taught relaxation techniques, T-cells increased, and the level of increase in T-cells could actually be predicted "by how frequently the students practiced relaxation." The shock from the death of a spouse markedly weakens the immune system, with the survivors having decreases in the activity of lymphocytes for over a year after the death of a spouse. And, of course, we know that Pasteur, on his death bed, is reported to have stated that it is not the germ but the "soil" or culture medium on which it falls that determines whether or not an individual develops a disease when exposed to various germs or bacteria.

The majority of individuals in our culture, if tested, would show a positive skin test to tuberculosis, and antibodies to the hepatitis virus, even though they have never developed either disease. This indicates that under ordinary circumstances, individuals who are not under great stress can develop a protective immune response and avoid having a serious clinical illness.

Even during flu epidemics, those who are more psychologically stressed with lower morale have a higher incidence and more severe episodes of flu, as well as longer duration of illness.

The degree of satisfaction that we derive from work and home life influences our health. Those who are less happy with work and home life smoke more, drink more and experience greater stress and, of course, have more illness.

Those individuals who adopt the expectations of the Male Machine have greater distress and dissatisfaction with life. This is because these individuals have difficulty expressing feelings and are thus more restricted emotionally. They have limited expression of affection, tenderness and nurturing and are much more preoccupied with success while neglecting interpersonal relationships and family commitments. Individuals who have those masculine role values and beliefs were significantly predisposed to experience distress and dissatisfaction in the face of high stress. On the other hand, those who have more favorable and positive attitudes are consistently more healthy. Work satisfaction is even a predictor of how long we live as well as how healthy we will continue to be.

Even in identical male twins, the individual who has greater satisfaction with childhood experiences, education and achievements in life is less likely to have a severe heart attack. Similar findings have come from studies of many thousands of American workers at all levels of life. Those who go through life trying too much, in a constant state of stress or alarm with little joy, are more likely to be unhealthy. Unfortunately, only 30% of the population in 1980 said that they were happy, and in 1987, 90% wanted to make a major life change.

There is excellent evidence, in the case of unexpected or sudden death, that those individuals who have "decided that life is unbearable enough to commit suicide" tend to have been depressed for a week and up to several months. Of course, psychiatrist Eric Berne has emphasized the importance of life script—that individuals set the age and cause of their death, often before they are even ten years of age! This problem of helplessness, depression or "giving up" is found in about 80% of individuals suffering from a wide variety of illnesses ranging from colitis to multiple sclerosis to cancer. Even a cold may be the reaction to a reactively weak, giving-up attitude. *Some scientists have concluded that 70-80% of all illnesses are largely related to or proceeded by the giving-up syndrome.* This mental state obviously is not constant. It comes and goes and waxes and wanes, but the predominant theme is one of helplessness brought on by perceiving that there is no solution to a problem. In diabetes mellitus, it has been found that a sense of helplessness and hopelessness is related to both the onset and exacerbation of this illness. *Considering the current high suicide rate in children under ten years of age,* even "juvenile" diabetes probably is associated with some degree of giving up.

Many studies have confirmed the influence of helplessness and giving up as major contributors to illness. It is important to recognize that it is not just a question of taking personal responsibility. Those individuals who become depressed and ill often tend to blame themselves. Yet it is not a question of taking responsibility for doing something about it that seems more important. Those individuals who are basically pessimistic have a much higher incidence of cancer associated with lower immune function in both the T-cells and the natural killer cells. In women who have mastectomies for cancer, those who take control of their behavior and lifestyle by changing their habits and developing a more positive attitude have a higher survival rate.

The syndrome of giving up, depression and helplessness is related to many illnesses and, of course, as with most other factors, begins in childhood. Individuals who lose their mothers before age eleven have a much higher risk of depression later in life than they experience from any other loss.

Even watching an inspiring movie improves immune function. Students who watch a movie of Mother Theresa have an enhanced salivary IGA response. Individuals who have close intimacy with another human being also have higher levels of IGA antibodies and have less serious illness. Individuals who seek friendship and interpersonal relationships are generally more healthy. Individuals who are "in love" have fewer colds and a more active immune system. They also have higher levels of endorphins and have less awareness of pain. Even rabbits who are talked to and petted have less atherosclerosis on a high fat diet than those who are not pampered. Women who have just a minimal amount of tender, loving care by nurses leave the hospital sooner and recover faster after surgery than those with no care. Some people have suggested that "love is more important than healthy living." This effect seems to come through enhancement of the immune system. In older individuals, "love of others and being loved" seems to be a key factor in the length of life. Those individuals who live to be one hundred or more have a greater eagerness about life, a greater sense of purpose, a greater drive and greater general happiness. Such simple things as having a nice view out of the hospital room will enhance the ability of individuals to recover faster after surgery and to require less narcotics for pain control.

Even individuals who smoke, overeat and practice other unhealthy habits have a decreased risk of illness if they have a strong support system. There is indeed considerable evidence that "love is more important than healthy living." In my own study of one hundred retired nuns, sixty-eight were over the age of eighty and about eighteen were over the age of ninety. All but one of them seemed to be in reasonably good health and she was one hundred. These individuals tended to be over-weight, under-exercised, and to have a high affinity for caffeine, chocolate and sugar. However, they were extremely content with their lifestyle and obviously outliving many outside the convent. Being enthusiastic rather than cynical and hostile is important. Individuals who live longer have a greater sense of hope, order, control and meaning. But *a positive mental attitude and hope can be cultivated through training*. Even in patients who have cancer, there is a significant increase in longevity if they develop a strong sense of optimism and hope. Those who are optimistic have a decreased risk of dying, even in the face of "objective" laboratory tests showing them to be in poor health. Individuals who tend to "believe" that their health is excellent have only one-third the risk of those who think that their health is poor.

In another study, the mortality rate among "health pessimists" was twice as great as that of those who are "health optimists" in men, and the difference is five times as great in women! The sense of optimism also increases recovery after surgery. Positive attitude and optimism are associated with a good or improved marriage and, as we have indicated earlier, marriage satisfaction is a significant predictor of physical, psychological and immune system health. As one popular slogan goes, "happiness is an inside job." Happiness seems to result from optimism, a relative lack of cynicism, a feeling of meaning in life and a feeling of personal control over circumstances.

Those individuals who have a higher involvement with religion also have a reduced risk of premature dying. Of course, this is best exemplified in the Mormons and the Seventh Day Adventists, both of whom also practice better than average health habits.

A sense of humor also enhances health. Those individuals who laugh regularly have an increase in IGA antibodies, and individuals who ordinarily use humor as a method of coping with stress have a higher concentration of antibodies. Some individuals have found that laughter is as effective as biofeedback training in reducing stress; and of course, Norman Cousin's well-known book, *The Anatomy of an Illness*, has emphasized his recovery from a serious illness, one somewhat like rheumatoid spondylitis, using high doses of intravenous vitamin C and laughter. Even Freud had a better view of humor than he did of sex! He felt that humor could "take the sting out of bad situations." Raymond A. Moody, a major researcher on near-death experiences, has emphasized that humor enhances our "will to live."

THE PLACEBO FACTOR

Perhaps the most exciting aspect of psychosomatic health is placebos or "sugar pills," which are not supposed to do anything. Dr. Herb Benson of Harvard has demonstrated that not one single treatment for angina pectoris is truly more effective than a placebo. And in some studies in which the physician had a strong belief in a particular therapy, up to 80 or 90% effectiveness was achieved even though when impartial, controlled, double-blind studies were done, the treatment was found to be only as effective as a placebo.

When individuals "believe" changes take place in the body, the self-healing process is initiated. Sir William Osler felt many years ago that "far more important than what the physician does is the physician's belief and the patient's belief in what the physician does." The vast majority of drugs have less effect than placebos. That is, even in average studies, placebos have a 35% effectiveness but many drugs have only a 40-50% effectiveness, which means that they can add only 5-15% increased effectiveness over placebos and they often have adverse "side effects" in 25% of individuals. Even after a coronary bypass procedure, 60% of those who can be demonstrated on angiogram to have had the bypass *closed and thus are not having any increased flow*, are symptomatically improved because they "believe" that the operation has been of benefit.

Placebo effects have been found in every disease from rheumatoid arthritis to cancer. Even in cancer, the amount of morphine used or needed is markedly reduced with the use of placebos. Also a skin response to tuberculin, the test for exposure to tuberculosis, can be altered by one's belief system. Those who expected their reaction to a tuberculin test to be negative had a higher incidence of negative reaction than those who did not. At least thirty double-blind studies have demonstrated that Valium is no more effective than a placebo in treating anxiety, and yet Valium is the most commonly prescribed drug for that problem. In nine double-blind studies in which both doctor and patient knew what was being done, drugs were 80% effective.

When the drugs were given in a controlled, double-blind study, effectiveness was reduced to 35 or 40%. As belief in a new drug fades, so does its potential to serve as an active placebo. Placebos can enhance, diminish or totally wipe out the active ingredients in drugs. Skeptical, critical, analytic modes of thinking (the scientific method) will attenuate or negate placebo responding. Rather than having been overestimated, the placebo's potential therapeutic effects have probably been underestimated. In the long run, we have to assume that there is nothing unscientific about a treatment that is effective in 35% of patients suffering from a variety of conditions. Interestingly, there is also no reason to believe that patients would lose their faith in a given procedure even if they are adequately informed of its efficacy.

Not only are there positive placebos, but there are negative placebos. A pessimistic view of both patients and physicians may increase the feelings of helplessness and the ultimate course of many illnesses. Even under anesthesia, patients who hear negative comments in the operating room have the potential for a variety of complications and depression after surgery. With both marijuana and alcohol, individuals who "expect" to become high are more likely to do so than those who do not. Morphine, one of our best narcotics, is effective in only 70% of pain problems, whereas a placebo, if reinforced by the belief system of the physician and nurse, can be 50% or more effective. Even in such serious instances as cancer pain, gunshot wounds and the pain of heart attacks, patients respond favorably to placebos. In one study, at least 90% of the patients with cancer pain had a significant decrease in their pain when they were given a placebo on at least one occasion.

One interesting clinical use of non-drug placebo is the example of having patients monitor their blood pressure. When told that doing it on a regular basis lowers the blood pressure, the patients who believed this seemed to have an enhanced sense of self-control and experienced a beneficial effect upon their blood pressure. Anything that seems to give individuals some increased feeling of personal control, whether it is love, faith or just plain positive cognitive attitudes, seems to increase self-healing. Individuals who believe that they can handle their problems,. even those including arthritis, have improved immune systems, less painful and fewer swollen joints, and a better T-cell response. Even in a severe congenital disorder such as ichthyosis, a congenital disease in which the skin looks as if the person has the scales of a fish, hypnosis led to a 60-70% improvement. Under hypnosis, patients showed a marked increase in immune functioning with enhancement of T-cell reactivity. Faith and belief, as well as hypnosis, all enhance the immune system, even though an individual who is a good hypnotic subject does not necessarily have a naturally positive attitude.

Of course, it has been known since the beginning of the century that the autonomic nervous system, which controls the immune system as well as the internal homeostasis of balance of the autonomic nervous system, is under the control of imagination or imagery. It has, in fact, been called the "imaginative" nervous system. Individuals who respond to placebos actually increase their level of beta endorphins. You can think yourself into a state of enhanced "narcosis."

In one study in *The American Family Physician*, 1980, Vogel, Goodwin and Goodwin reported that even when patients were told that they were receiving placebos, the placebo had a beneficial effect! Thus, "it is possible to use a placebo such as a sugar pill as an effective therapeutic device while disclosing its precise contents to the patient."

The probability that what one believes to be true actually influences what *becomes* true is the remarkable lesson that we learn from placebos. Individuals have come to believe that taking a pill spells relief and they have little specific concern for the actual pharmacological aspects of the pill. Thus, a great deal of the response of every drug is not the effect of the "active" principle in the drug but the effect on the patient's belief system. Reaction time and strength are sensitive to placebos, as are pulse rate, blood pressure, pain, short-term rote memory and relaxation. Placebos, then, represent a powerful treatment possibility for a wide variety of both psychological and physiological problems.

Interestingly, "side effects" from placebos are very similar to those of the active drug. Patients report symptoms ranging from drowsiness to headaches, nervousness, insomnia, nausea and constipation, even when the inactive placebo is given. There is even evidence that ward rounds conducted by the chief of surgery may lead to heart complications, including sudden death.

Some individuals claim that "the placebo phenomenon has been the dominant mode of healing throughout the history of human medicine. Simply put, belief sickens; belief kills; belief heals." The idea that beliefs and expectations both sicken and kill is adequately demonstrated in many publications. Similarly, attitude has the power to heal.

One of the most dramatic placebo studies of all time is that done in 1958 when Diamond, Kettle and Crockett did a placebo surgical operation, one of the few surgical procedures with a true double-blind placebo approach. In randomly selected patients, they simply opened the skin and closed it, and compared it with those patients who had an operation then in vogue, that of ligating the internal mammary artery, which feeds the breast but has no effect on the heart. They found that "100% of the control, non-ligated, patients and only 76% of the ligated patients reported decreased need for nitroglycerine and increased exercise tolerance." Those patients treated with the placebo operation remained improved for at least six to eight months. Here again is an indication of the enthusiasm of the physician combined with the patient's belief system, creating a response that is not equaled by any drug!

Some people believe that placebos should be used as the treatment of choice "where active medication is contraindicated, or where the active medication is too slow in working." Of course, the most important information from placebo studies is that the patient who receives a significant, even though perhaps transient, relief has a tremendous potential for controlling the symptom with some form of mental, self-regulation training. A positive response to placebos indicates that in that particular patient, expectancy, hope, faith and belief are the most important ingredients and this indicates that the patient has the *inner* resources to control the problem without risky intervention. It is essential to recognize the considerable value of the placebo so that it might become more widely used.

Interestingly, the majority of treatments that have passed into general medical acceptance throughout the last one hundred and fifty years have generally been relegated to this category of placebo after adequate trial. Most of the drugs currently dispensed are minimally pharmaceutically effective but quite commonly have harmful or dangerous "side effects." Indeed, even our FDA estimates that at least 35% of all drugs currently on the market have no proven response above placebos. In 1952, Dunlop, Anderson and Evans reviewed seventeen thousand medical prescriptions and concluded that at least 30% were placebos, even though they were standard, doctor-prescribed drugs. Perhaps one of the most striking reports is by Boleloucky who showed that one patient had had chronic dependence upon a placebo with severe withdrawal symptoms when the patient believed that he had been receiving morphine. It is of some interest, too, that the color of the placebo is important. Red and pink are better than blue; multicolored, large brown-green, small reddish-orange or pink pills have a greater effectiveness than other color combinations. The least effective is a small white tablet. Brand-name aspirin gives a better result than identical aspirin labeled generically. One author even believes "it is unlikely that belief in the healing power of large doses of arsenic would transform this chemical into a healing agent; yet I submit, though I will not attempt to prove it, that such a belief would retard its poisonous effects."

In summary, we are what we think. Our belief system and our basic attitude seem to be the most important factors affecting our health. Knowing all the facts, we can choose an attitude that leads to disease or to health. Let us choose wisely.

CHAPTER THIRTEEN

Self-Testing

(S h e a l y   a n d   M y s s)

Our minds, bodies and spirits are continually communicating information to us. The impulses that are transmitted through our intuitive channels are Nature's way of providing data on our well-being, on our physical, emotional and spiritual health.

Learning to hear and interpret these signals is perhaps the finest form of enhanced health care that a person can practice. The body will signal when it is in distress, when it has become overly toxic or when it cannot cope with the substances that are being ingested.

Likewise, our emotions have a feedback system that indicates when we are out of balance or contaminated with too much negativity. We feel these impulses through changes in our moods, attitudes and levels of vibrancy. While we may interpret these shifts as the "blahs," for instance, they are actually indicators that we are on negativity-overload. Moreover, these indicators suggest that a conscious response of a positive nature is needed.

The six self-evaluations contained in this chapter are meant to help you develop the habit of learning to evaluate your health habits, stress levels and inner processes on a regular basis. They are not meant to be used only once, but rather they are structured so that you will want to refer to these examinations on a regular basis as part of your overall, ongoing process of self-health care.

We recommend that you write your answers on a separate piece of paper rather than use the pages of the book itself, partly because your answers will be highly personal and also because you will want to take the exams again at a later date.

If your scores indicate that you are overly stressed or indulging in eating and lifestyle habits that do not promote health, *create a positive change that decreases stress and increases health.**

THE POWER/RESPONSIBILITY/WISDOM/LOVE INVENTORY

This self-evaluation questionnaire is designed to encourage you to be introspective, to ask questions and seek intuitive answers regarding the quality of your attitudes, beliefs and self-image. These questions relate to the greatest areas of human stress: issues of power, responsibility, wisdom and love. They are meant to cause you to think differently (and very honestly) about the personal motivations and attitudes that you bring into the activity of creating the quality of the experiences, relationships and events that fill your life.

We encourage you to approach this self-evaluation with the realization that your answers are personal and, therefore, it is in *your best interest* to answer these questions as honestly as you can. In other words, do not answer them from the per-

---

*The Power/Responsibility/Wisdom/Love Inventory was developed by C. Norman Shealy, Md., Ph.D. and Caroline M. Myss, M.A. The remaining self tests, the Human Potential Attitude Inventory©, Human Potential Development Scale©, Sexual Attitude Inventory©, Personal Stress Assessment© and Symptom Index© were created by C. Norman Shealy, M.D. Ph.D.

spective of what you want people to think about you, but rather from the deeper perspective of what genuinely is at work within your inner motivations.

As part of this first self-evaluation questionnaire, we will review the definitions of power, responsibility, love and wisdom as we have presented them in this book. You are asked to do a preparatory self-review of responses on a sheet of paper that you can refer to as you do the questionnaire.

POWER

Power has many facets. Its external manifestations are money, sex, political influence, authority and social prestige, physical strength and control of other people. Internal power, or authentic power as we have described it, is rooted in the qualities of the human spirit, such as compassion, love, honesty, integrity and self-esteem.

Pause for a moment and reflect on the meaning of power in your life. Write down your definition of power, meaning the definition that *you live by and that motivates your actions*. List every object, situation and belief that significantly influences your perception of power. Spend at least ten minutes completing your list.

Now list which objects, relationships or situations cause you to feel powerless, insecure, intimidated, frightened, worried or out of control.

RESPONSIBILITY

The concept of responsibility exceeds that of paying bills or keeping schedules and commitments. A self-actualized individual accepts responsibility for the quality of attitudes, thoughts, actions, beliefs, relationships, health and all other aspects of his or her life.

Accepting responsibility for the full scope of one's life is not easy. In fact, it is everything *but* easy. It is far more convenient, and at times it even seems reasonable, to blame, deny or avoid taking responsibility. Nevertheless, in the final analysis, the only person responsible for your thoughts or responses to outside events or people is you. The quality of your life is greatly determined by your ability to learn to respond in a health-enhancing way, even though you may have initial reactions of anger, rage and hurt.

As a beginning to this part of the questionnaire, think about and write down your comments as they relate to being alone. Then answer these questions: Do you blame others, fate, life, luck or God for the challenges in your life? Do you feel you can change what you are dissatisfied with? What are your greatest fears in terms of taking charge of your own life?

WISDOM

The nature of wisdom is beautifully described in the well-known prayer by Reinhold Neibuhr: "God grant me the serenity to accept the things I cannot change; courage to change the things I can; and wisdom to know the difference."

A major source of many diseases is the inability to accept the process of change as it unfolds in one's life. Equally stressful is the inability to accept oneself or to recognize the greater purpose underlying one's personal challenges.

Take a few minutes to review how well you accept yourself as you are—physically, intellectually, emotionally, sexually and spiritually. Also, assess how well you accept the quality of your life in relation to finances, material security, personal relationships, success, health and physical strength. Note in particular the areas of your life in which self-acceptance is not present.

LOVE

Loving and being loved is the heart and soul of the human experience. Without love, it is impossible to be healthy. A vast majority of illnesses are brought about by stress related to issues of love, such as acceptance, rejection, attention, compassion, loneliness, bitterness and all negative emotions.

In addition to interpersonal and intimate matters of love related to spouses, partners, parents, friends and family members, there are also aspects of love relating to life itself. By this, we are referring to attitudes held toward animals, nature and the planet.

Pause and reflect upon the meaning of love for you, as well as the aspects of love that consume your attention. For instance, do you manipulate others in order to receive their attention? Do you compromise your ideals in order to have a relationship? How much compassion do you have for others? Are you a forgiving person? Can you forgive others *and* yourself?

Review your answers and then proceed with the questionnaire. Some of the questions may seem similar, but there is a reason for that repetition. In grading yourself, use the numbers 0-10. Zero means that you do not feel that the issue presented by the question relates to you in any way. The number ten indicates that you strongly relate to the question.

POWER-RESPONSIBILITY-WISDOM-LOVE INVENTORY

SECTION I

1. _____ I usually feel physically strong.
2. _____ I usually understand well how physical objects function.
3. _____ I am almost always able to provide myself and/or my family with the necessities of life.
4. _____ I usually understand the complexity of physical mechanisms.
5. _____ I feel that the external world is safe.
6. _____ I am usually able to stand up for myself.
7. _____ I am usually able to protect myself.
8. _____ I feel my legal rights are well protected.
9. _____ I usually feel at home anywhere.
10. _____ I feel I have a great support system.
11. _____ I feel that I am usually supported emotionally/ financially by others.
12. _____ I feel I have at least as many human rights as people of other social classes or races.

13. ____ I feel my ability to achieve my goals is unlimited.
14. ____ I feel my ability to manifest my ideas is unlimited.
15. ____ I feel that many people take my side.

S E C T I O N   I I

16. ____ I usually feel I have control over what happens to me sexually.
17. ____ I have never been abused sexually.
18. ____ I rarely feel that I am being or have been manipulated and controlled by other people.
19. ____ In most circumstances, I feel that I control my choices.
20. ____ I usually feel adequate sexually.
21. ____ I usually enjoy sexual activity.
22. ____ I usually feel sexually equal to my spouse/partner.
23. ____ I feel no guilt about my sexuality.
24. ____ I feel no guilt about my sexual preferences.
25. ____ I consider childbirth a safe, happy experience.
26. ____ I feel comfortable about the way in which I have parented.
27. ____ I felt financially secure during my childhood.
28. ____ I felt safe in relation to my childhood home.
29. ____ I feel comfortable over financial matters.
30. ____ I never feel resentment over being controlled financially by others.
31. ____ I never feel inadequate if I do not experience social prestige.
32. ____ I never feel inadequate if I do not have money.
33. ____ I never feel victimized by my circumstances (race, color, sex, etc.).
34. ____ I never manipulate others in order to feel secure.
35. ____ I do not compromise my values for the sake of financial gain.
36. ____ I do not compromise my values for the sake of social prestige.

37. _____ I do not compromise my values for the sake of sexual gratification.
38. _____ I do not compromise my values in order to maintain friendships.
39. _____ I do not fear poverty.
40. _____ I do not fear never having enough.

SECTION III

41. _____ I never develop unequal relationships because I feel intimidated.
42. I do not fear accepting responsibility for:
    _____ my attitudes toward myself.
    _____ my needs.
    _____ my commitments.
    _____ my finances.
    _____ my thoughts.
    _____ my attitudes.
    _____ my temper.
    _____ my personal actions.
    _____ my behavior.
43. I do not resent assuming responsibility for someone else's:
    _____ mistakes.
    _____ moods.
    _____ actions.
    _____ behavior.
    _____ financial security.
    _____ commitments.
    _____ healing.
    _____ addictions.
    _____ success.
    _____ failure.
44. _____ I freely challenge others to assume their own responsibility.
45. _____ I am almost always capable of making decisions.

46. I do not allow others to:
    _____ limit my choices forcefully.
    _____ violate my self-esteem.
47. I am rarely upset because others:
    _____ neglect me.
    _____ overlook me.
    _____ criticize me.
    _____ fail to acknowledge my contributions and/or opin-
    ions.
    _____ fail to acknowledge my creativity.
    _____ fail to acknowledge my self-worth.
48. _____ I rarely worry about being criticized.
49. _____ I rarely feel controlled by the expectations of
    others.
50. _____ I do not criticize others in order to be empowered.
51. _____ I am rarely angry or frustrated because I am un-
    able to break free from the expectations of others.
52. _____ I almost never express my anger toward weaker
    individuals because I lack the ability to confront
    the real source of my anger which may be:
    a. another person.
    b. family members.
    c. myself.
53. _____ I almost never express anger toward others
    because I am upset and don't want to control my
    temper.
54. _____ I almost never feel that I am a failure.
55. _____ I rarely struggle with feelings of inadequacy.
56. _____ I express my ideas freely.
57. I value my own:
    _____ ideas.
    _____ creativity.
    _____ self.
58. _____ I usually challenge my own fears.
59. _____ I usually take charge and change the unsatisfactory
    conditions in my life.

SECTION IV

60. _____ I rarely fear not being loved.
61. _____ I usually believe I am worthy of being loved.
62. _____ I usually find it easy to express love.
63. It rarely makes me feel guilty because:
_____ I have rejected others.
_____ I have mistreated others.
_____ I have hurt others emotionally.
_____ I have attacked someone's self-esteem.
64. I rarely resent seeing others receive:
_____ more attention than I receive.
_____ more love than I receive.
65. _____ I rarely fear showing affection.
66. _____ I rarely fear sharing affection.
67. I rarely feel guilty over using anger as a substitute for:
_____ love.
_____ hostility.
_____ criticism.
68. _____ I rarely feel lonely.
69. _____ I usually feel supported by others.
70. _____ I never feel emotionally paralyzed by loneliness.
71. I rarely judge negatively the value of:
_____ other people.
_____ other races.
_____ the opposite sex.
_____ my same sex.
_____ other countries.
_____ other forms of life (animal, vegetable).
_____ the inanimate kingdom.
_____ other religions.
_____ other political viewpoints.
_____ other people's habits.
_____ other people's intelligence.
_____ other people's sexuality.

72. I rarely hold on to:
    _____ old hurts.
    _____ past resentments.
    _____ anger.
    _____ grudges.
73. _____ I rarely lack joy.
74. _____ I rarely lack the courage to express joy.
75. _____ I rarely cannot forgive.
76. I rarely attract relationships that are:
    _____ unfulfilling.
    _____ abusive.
    _____ stressful.
77. _____ I rarely feel guilty because I feel I have not successfully fulfilled my emotional commitments.
78. _____ I rarely have angry/negative/hostile thoughts.
79. My thoughts are rarely:
    _____ revengeful.
    _____ unforgiving.
    _____ concerned with getting even.

S E C T I O N V

80. _____ I rarely fear self-assertion.
81. _____ I rarely avoid self-assertion.
82. _____ I rarely feel victimized by others because I don't speak up.
83. _____ I rarely allow others to speak for me and later resent it.
84. I rarely fear expressing my emotional:
    _____ needs.
    _____ feelings.
    _____ opinions.
85. I only occasionally fear expressing my emotional:
    _____ needs.
    _____ feelings.
    _____ opinions.

86. My fears of expression rarely block my:
    _____ creativity.
    _____ advancement in life.
87. _____ Opportunities rarely slip by because I fail to speak up on my own behalf.
88. I almost never distort facts to cover up:
    _____ my feelings.
    _____ my responsibility for personal behavior.
    _____ my responsibility for personal thoughts.
    _____ my responsibility for personal actions.
    _____ my responsibility for my emotions.
89. I rarely exert my will to:
    _____ control others.
    _____ influence others to my own advantage.
90. I rarely am unable to say:
    _____ I'm sorry.
    _____ I love you.
    _____ I forgive you.
91. I rarely am angry because of my inability to say:
    _____ I'm sorry.
    _____ I love you.
    _____ I forgive you.
92. I am always able to express:
    _____ grief.
    _____ hurt.
    _____ sorrow.
93. _____ I am usually able to cry.
94. _____ I am not embarrassed if I show that I have been hurt.
95. _____ I rarely have regrets that I have missed opportunities because I was unable to speak up for myself.
96. _____ I have strong willpower.
97. _____ I rarely allow others to make decisions for me.
98. _____ I rarely gossip.
99. _____ I rarely exaggerate.
100. _____ I rarely embellish the truth.

SECTION VI

101. I rarely fear:
    _____ self-examination.
    _____ introspection.
    _____ challenging my ideas.
    _____ challenging my ideas of reality.
102. _____ I rarely fear challenging ideas of reality.
103. _____ I rarely fear introspection.
104. _____ I almost never avoid introspection.
105. _____ I enjoy thinking about the meaning of life.
106. _____ I enjoy thinking about the meaning of events.
107. _____ I usually trust my intuition.
108. I honor my intellect by participating in helpful/ positive:
    _____ actions.
    _____ behaviors.
    _____ creation.
    _____ words.
    _____ deception.
    _____ laziness.
    _____ neglect.
109. _____ I rarely deny emotional responses.
110. _____ I almost never block emotional responses.
111. _____ I almost never deny the truth.
112. _____ I face the truth easily in times of emotional stress.
113. _____ I almost never feel intellectually inadequate.
114. _____ I almost never feed myself negative comments about myself.
115. _____ I almost never feel jealous of the creative abilities of other persons.
116. _____ I rarely feel insecure because of the creative abilities of other persons.
117. _____ I usually am open to the ideas of others.

118. _____ I almost never fear being open to the ideas of others.
119. _____ I usually am willing to learn from life's experiences.
120. _____ I accept responsibility for events that go wrong in my life.
121. I believe that I helped create the larger problems in my life as related to:
    _____ finances.
    _____ marriage.
    _____ relationships.
    _____ illnesses.
    _____ failure.
122. I usually learn how to avoid further painful/ stressful:
    _____ situations.
    _____ relationships.
    _____ problems.
    _____ learning situations.
123. _____ I assume people or forces in the world are on my side.
124. _____ I usually feel anxious because I feel unsure of myself.
125. _____ I usually feel anxious because I don't feel that I know myself.
126. _____ I feel my life is meaningful.
127. _____ I feel I have a purpose in life.
128. _____ I feel I am leading a meaningful life.
129. _____ I feel there is a purpose in my difficult struggles.

SECTION VII

130. _____ I often feel that life in general is meaningful.
131. _____ I feel there is a God.
132. _____ I have strong faith.

133. _____ I find my faith is easy to maintain.
134. _____ I have a strong sense of hope.
135. _____ I feel that I can trust life's ability to work out.
136. _____ I usually have adequate courage.
137. _____ I usually have faith in myself.
138. _____ I am usually so positive that I attract
      opportunities.
139. _____ I enjoy self-development.
140. _____ I enjoy looking at my spiritual purpose for
      existence.
141. I often behave positively because:
      _____ I think beyond my needs.
      _____ I reason effectively.
142. _____ I am willing to grow or change.
143. _____ I am willing to grow or change in order to accept
      the next phase of life.
144. _____ I am willing to accept the natural cycles of life.
145. _____ I almost never get stuck in the past because I
      regret the past.
146. I usually am able to let go of cycles that have been com-
      pleted such as:
      _____ caring for my children.
      _____ my own growing up.
      _____ relationships with my parents.
      _____ relationships with a spouse.
      _____ relationships with friends.
      _____ relationships with acquaintances.
      _____ aging.
      _____ retirement.
147. _____ I see a large picture at work in my life.
148. _____ I have the courage to face life.
149. I have the courage to:
      _____ face change.
      _____ face problems.

SUMMARY AND EVALUATION REMARKS

You will have noted that this questionnaire is divided into seven sections. Each section corresponds to a chakra center; that is, Section I corresponds to the first chakra, Section II corresponds to the second chakra and so on.

In scoring your answers to each section, pay special attention to those sections in which your score indicates the presence of serious or extreme stress. Then refer to the areas of the body in which you experience the most stress and determine the issues that are at the root of the physical disturbances that are being generated in your body.

THE HUMAN POTENTIAL ATTITUDE INVENTORY AND THE HUMAN POTENTIAL DEVELOPMENT SCALE

These tests do not have a right or wrong answer. They are designed to help you to think about your expressions of certain human attitudes, attributes and potentials.

The Human Potential Development Scale is taken first in a totally conscious way, just taking the first thought that comes into your mind regarding how fully developed you are. Then, after you go into a deep state of relaxation, the questions should be asked again because you may find yourself giving very different responses.

On the Human Potential Inventory, you have an opportunity to ask more specific questions in relation to qualities of forgiveness and tolerance: Just how tolerant am I to other people's belief systems? Am I willing to allow individuals to have a totally different religion without feeling threatened by their difference? Am I willing to be tolerant of individuals who have a markedly different political view from me? How threatening is this to me?

In answering questions from minus 2 to plus 2, you will have an opportunity to decide just how evolved you are in expressing these human attributes.

Your answers to both of these tests should provide you

with insight in terms of what attitudes you hold that **generate** negativity and judgmentalism, as well as what attitudes you **hold** that generate health. Realize that negative attitudes *can and should be challenged*. In learning that our attitudes and beliefs are the tools we use to create the physical health of our bodies, as well as the quality of the other areas of our lives, none of us can afford to maintain a negative attitude because it harms us far more than anyone or anything outside of ourselves.

HUMAN POTENTIAL ATTITUDE INVENTORY

As you read each of the following items to yourself, get a sense of whether your emotional response is agreement or disagreement. If you get strong agreement, mark + +. If you get mild agreement, mark +. If you get no response at all, mark it 0 for neutral response. If you get a mild argument, mark−. If you are aware of strong disagreement, mark− −.

It sometimes happens that people are in agreement in general (which would be a +) and are simultaneously aware of an uneasy feeling that argues, or their brain shows them a single exception. In such a case, it is permissible to answer + − to reflect this conflict; this would be preferable to marking 0 if you really are getting a mixed response.

_____ I have forgiven everyone who has wronged me.
_____ I forgive those who unintentionally wrong me.
_____ I forgive those who purposefully wrong me.
_____ When I tell those who have wronged me what they have done, I expect them to apologize or repent.
_____ I have sometimes wronged or harmed others.
_____ I apologize when I wrong others.
_____ I expect others to forgive me when I apologize.
_____ I helped someone else within the last week.
_____ I walked and talked with someone I love during the last week.
_____ I attend church regularly.

_____ I believe that my attitude each day is more important than attending church.

_____ I believe my affliction(s) was given me by God for his honor and glory as part of a divine plan.

_____ I believe God is wrathful and punishes sinners.

_____ I have lots of friends and see/visit them often.

_____ I pray regularly for myself and others.

_____ I believe the most important goal of life is service to God or others.

_____ I prayed for someone else yesterday or today.

_____ I often (more than once a week) watch sunset and sunrise with a feeling of reverence.

_____ I read the Bible or inspirational materials at least once a week.

_____ I attend a fun event or listen to good music at least once a week.

_____ I meditate, pray or think about the beauty of life regularly.

_____ Everyone is born a sinner.

_____ Mankind is basically bad.

_____ I believe hypnosis is the work of the Devil.

_____ I believe everyone has a right to his or her beliefs.

_____ I believe that those who do not share my religious beliefs are sinners and are likely to go to Hell.

_____ God does not forgive sinners unless the debts of sins are paid.

_____ If your beliefs are different from mine, you cannot help me.

My spiritual/religious beliefs are:

_____ a. strong

_____ b. correct and right

_____ I feel calm and serene most of the time.

_____ When I become frustrated, I pause and calm myself.

_____ I feel compassion for all other human beings.

_____ I go out of my way to help other persons.

_____ I know I can attain my goals.

_____ I believe I can accomplish anything to which I apply myself adequately.

_____ I will apply myself enough to accomplish my goals.

_____ I feel great joy in my life.

_____ I can face whatever life offers.

_____ I believe I learn from my problems.

_____ I willingly or lovingly contribute to help others less fortunate than I.

_____ I believe tomorrow will be a better day.

_____ I believe in a benevolent God.

_____ I believe in life after death.

_____ I believe I have a soul that survives death.

_____ I believe one dies and goes to Heaven or Hell.

_____ I believe in reincarnation.

_____ Reincarnation is an evil concept.

_____ I have the willpower to accomplish my goals.

_____ I am wise enough to make the right choices.

_____ I make rational, reasonable choices.

_____ I feel love for all other human beings.

_____ I bless all other human beings.

_____ I bless all who have wronged me.

_____ I bless all who have helped me.

_____ My life is meaningful.

HUMAN POTENTIAL DEVELOPMENT SCALE

Throughout history, philosophers and religious leaders have emphasized that there are certain characteristics that represent the highest potential for service to and interaction with humanity. There is no test that we know of that measures this development, although the Human Potential Attitude Inventory gives you some hints. We'd like to offer you an opportunity to measure your feelings of your own development at this point in time. We suggest you take the following test in your ordinary state of consciousness, just by reading it. Then get into a deep state of relaxation, ask yourself the same questions and rate yourself from that point of view. One means total lack of the quality; 10 implies the maximum any person could possibly achieve.

Love	1	2	3	4	5	6	7	8	9	10
Reason	1	2	3	4	5	6	7	8	9	10
Wisdom	1	2	3	4	5	6	7	8	9	10
Will	1	2	3	4	5	6	7	8	9	10
Faith	1	2	3	4	5	6	7	8	9	10
Hope	1	2	3	4	5	6	7	8	9	10
Charity	1	2	3	4	5	6	7	8	9	10
Courage	1	2	3	4	5	6	7	8	9	10
Joy	1	2	3	4	5	6	7	8	9	10
Motivation	1	2	3	4	5	6	7	8	9	10
Confidence	1	2	3	4	5	6	7	8	9	10
Compassion	1	2	3	4	5	6	7	8	9	10
Serenity	1	2	3	4	5	6	7	8	9	10
Tolerance	1	2	3	4	5	6	7	8	9	10
Forgiveness	1	2	3	4	5	6	7	8	9	10

THE SEXUAL ATTITUDE INVENTORY

The Sexual Attitude Inventory is intended as a tool for personal reflection and insight into one's beliefs about sex and sexual behavior. It gives you an opportunity to decide what areas of sexuality may represent enough of a psychological/emotional concern that stress is created.

SEXUAL ATTITUDE INVENTORY

Sexual attitudes vary tremendously within the U.S. and throughout the world. Psychiatrists and psychologists have emphasized for the past one hundred years that sexual attitudes influence health and interpersonal relations. Even if there were no right or wrong per se, one's *belief* about right and wrong influences one's health. Kinsey, in his monumental work published a quarter of a century ago, recognized the breadth of sexual preferences and graded these on a scale of 0-6. *Most people do not score a 0 (strictly heterosexual) or a 6 (strictly homosexual), but somewhere in between.* For statistical purposes, the inventory that follows uses a scale of −5 to +5; it is designed to help you examine your sexual belief system. If you *totally disagree*, grade yourself −5; if you *totally agree*, grade yourself +5. You may grade −5, −4, −3, −2, −1, 0, +1, +2, +3, +4 or +5. Zero means neutral or no opinion. A few questions require only a true/false answer.

1. _____ Sexual intercourse is acceptable only within marriage.
2. I would consider divorce almost inevitable if my spouse had, outside the marriage, a sexual relationship:
   _____ a. with someone of the opposite sex.
   _____ b. with someone of the same sex.
3. _____ I personally have had sexual fantasies involving someone other than my spouse. (True or False)
4. _____ I personally have had sexual relationships outside marriage.
5. _____ At times, masturbation is a desirable sexual outlet.
6. _____ Sexual intercourse with animals is acceptable.
7. _____ Sexual activity among three or more persons at the same time is acceptable.
8. _____ Healthy male-male friendship may be sexual.
9. _____ Healthy female-female friendship may be sexual.
10. _____ Healthy male-female friendship may be sexual.
11. _____ Bisexuality may be healthy.
12. The vagina:
    _____ a. is able to accommodate penises up to 9 inches.
    _____ b. cannot accommodate a penis over 6 1/2 inches.
13. _____ Cunnilingus (oral manipulation of female genitals) is acceptable.

14. ____ Fellatio (oral manipulation of the penis) is acceptable.
15. ____ Anal intercourse is acceptable.
16. Sexual intercourse or masturbation is most satisfactory if it
lasts:
____ a. 5 minutes or less.
____ b. 10 minutes or less.
____ c. 15 minutes or less.
____ d. 20 minutes or more.
____ e. 30 minutes or more.
17. If my spouse and I were incompatible, I would:
____ a. divorce.
____ b. masturbate.
____ c. have an affair with someone of the opposite sex.
____ d. have an affair with someone of the same sex.
____ e. insist upon marital and/or sexual counseling.
18. ____ I believe being the sex I am is more desirable.
19. ____ I believe being the opposite sex would be more desirable.
20. ____ Dressing in clothes of the opposite sex is acceptable.
21. ____ My personal sex life is satisfactory.
22. ____ Marriage without sex is acceptable.
23. ____ Celibacy is desirable.
24. ____ Sexual interests and activity can be totally and
healthfully sublimated (diverted to other energy/
activity).
25. ____ Overall, my sex life is acceptable.
26. ____ It is possible to be affectionate without any sexual
connotation.
27. The average erect penis length is (choose only one):
____ a. 5 inches long.
____ b. 6.25 inches long.
____ c. 8 inches long.
____ d. 9 to 10 inches long.

28. I feel society's attitude toward infidelity is:
    _____ a. hypocritical.
    _____ b. permissive.
    _____ c. not permissive enough.
29. _____ A man should be head of the household.
30. _____ The most common cause of divorce is sexual infidelity.
31. The frequency with which I would most like to have sex is (check only one):
    _____ a. 1-3 times/week.
    _____ b. 3-5 times/week.
    _____ c. 6-10 times/week.
    _____ d. less than once a week.
32. I have sex with my partner (check only one):
    _____ a. 1-3 times/week.
    _____ b. 3-5 times/week.
    _____ c. 6-10 times/week.
    _____ d. less than once a week.
33. I masturbate (check only one):
    _____ a. 1-3 times/week.
    _____ b. 3-5 times/week.
    _____ c. 6-10 times/week.
    _____ d. less than once a week.
34. I feel I would be more sexually active if:
    _____ a. I were married.
    _____ b. I were not married.
35. I fantasize (check only one):
    _____ a. often.
    _____ b. sometimes.
    _____ c. never.
36. My fantasies involve:
    _____ a. women I know.
    _____ b. women I don't know.
    _____ c. men I know.
    _____ d. men I don't know.

37. _____ I have sexual intercourse as often as I like. (True or False only)
38. _____ Sexual experiences are spiritual.
39. _____ Sex with someone is wrong unless you love that person.
40. _____ Forcing sex on someone is wrong.
41. If I were not married or attached, I would enjoy having sex with (choose only one):
_____ a. no one.
_____ b. 1 partner.
_____ c. 2-3 partners.
_____ d. more than 3 partners.
42. I would be more able to experience my sexual fantasies if I were (choose only one):
_____ a. married.
_____ b. unmarried.
43. _____ I had sexual relationships before marriage. (True or False)
44. _____ I have had a sexual activity (play, experiences) with someone of my own sex. (True or False)
45. I would enjoy sex more if:
_____ a. I had more foreplay.
_____ b. the experiences lasted longer.
_____ c. no changes needed.
46. I enjoy these sexual activities:
_____ a. masturbation.
_____ b. receiving oral sex.
_____ c. giving oral sex.
_____ d. vaginal intercourse.
_____ e. anal intercourse.
_____ f. other (specify).
47. I feel my spouse/partner enjoys these sexual activities:
_____ a. masturbation.
_____ b. receiving oral sex.
_____ c. giving oral sex.

_____ d. vaginal intercourse.

_____ e. anal intercourse.

_____ f. other (specify).

48. The greatest drawback(s) to my sexual fulfillment is (are):

_____ a. my fears.

_____ b. my fantasies.

_____ c. my partner.

_____ d. my ability.

_____ e. my religion.

_____ f. my children.

_____ g. my health.

49. If I could change my sexuality, I would:

_____ a. have more orgasms.

_____ b. have stronger orgasms.

_____ c. have more lubrication.

_____ d. increase the duration of sex.

_____ e. increase my staying power.

_____ f. increase my frequency of sex activity.

_____ g. increase my number of partners.

_____ h. enjoy being more playful.

50. _____ My ability to achieve orgasm is satisfactory.

51. I feel I have been sexually exploited (abused):

_____ a. as an adult.

_____ b. as a child/teenager.

_____ c. heterosexually.

_____ d. homosexually.

52. On a scale of 0-6 as defined by Kinsey (0—capable of sexual arousal only by someone of the opposite sex to 6—capable of sexual arousal only by someone of the same sex), I consider myself:

_____ 0—purely, exclusively heterosexual (capable of sexual arousal/interest only in someone of the opposite sex).

_____ 1

_____ 2

_____ 3—bisexual.

_____ 4

_____ 5

_____ 6—purely, exclusively homosexual (capable of sexual arousal/interest only in someone of my own sex).

53. _____ In my personal business dealings, I am comfortable with a person who is homosexual.

54. For Males Only:

_____ My ability to have erections is satisfactory.

55. For Males Only:

If I could change my sexuality, I would:

_____ a. enlarge my penis.

_____ b. increase my erection strength.

Your Sex _____

Your Age _____

PERSONAL STRESS ASSESSMENT AND SYMPTOM INDEX

The Personal Stress Assessment (The Total Life Stress Test) measures, as comprehensively as we can at this time, the chemical, physical and emotional-social stress present in a person's life. It is based upon statistics related to studies of individual health habits and, when known, increases in adrenalin associated with those habits. That is, you essentially double your adrenalin level when one cigarette is smoked.

We use this test in two ways, not just in determining the total stress in a person's life. We find that people who have more than fifty points of total stress are likely to have twenty or more symptoms when it's used either with the Cornell Medical Index or the Symptom Index, which is included following this test.

When individuals have seventy-five or more points of total life stress, they are likely to have thirty or more symptoms. These figures apply particularly to individuals over the age of thirty. Individuals who have more than thirty symptoms on the Index are generally considered to be either "seriously ill" or "seriously emotionally disturbed."

We think that instead of considering individuals with high symptom levels as seriously disturbed, they should be considered as seriously *stressed*, with generalized dysautonomia as a result thereof.

The advantage to the Personal Stress Assessment is that it's fairly easy to see how stress can be reduced. We go through each page and circle those items that have the greatest number of points, subtract those from the total score, and see if we can get individuals down to a score of twenty-five points or less. It allows individuals the option of choosing the most important stressors to reduce. They can then choose to focus their energy on reducing these specific stressors immediately.

The Symptom Index in an excellent evaluation tool that can alert you to physical responses indicating the need for a physical checkup. *Symptoms* often precede illness and are a better warning of the effect of stress than *longevity* predictions. The Symptom Index measures *current* symptoms. When individuals *decrease* stress points, their *symptoms* also decrease.

PERSONAL STRESS ASSESSMENT
Total Life Stress Test

Record your stress points on the lines in the right-hand margin, and indicate subtotals in the boxes at the end of each section. Then add your subtotals to determine your total score.

A. DIETARY STRESS

Average Daily Sugar Consumption

Sugar added to food or drink	1 point per 5 tsps.	_____
Sweet roll, piece of pie/ cake, brownie, other dessert	1 point each	_____

Coke or can of soda, candy bar	2 points each	_____
Banana split, commercial milk shake, sundae, etc.	5 points each	_____
White flour (white bread, spaghetti, etc.)	5 points	_____

Average Daily Salt Consumption

Little or no "added" salt	0 points	_____
Few salty foods (pretzels, potato chips, etc.)	0 points	_____
Moderate "added" salt and/or salty foods at least once per day	3 points	_____
Heavy salt use, regularly (use of "table salt" and/or salty foods at least twice per day)	10 points	_____

Average Daily Caffeine Consumption

Coffee	1/2 point each cup	_____
Tea	1/2 point each cup	_____
Cola drink or Mountain Dew	1 point each cup	_____
2 Anacin or APC tabs	1/2 point per dose	_____
Caffeine Benzoate tablets (NoDoz, Vivarin, etc.)	2 points each	_____

Average Weekly Eating Out

2-4 times per week	3 points	_____
5-10 times per week	6 points	_____
More than 10 times per week	10 points	_____

DIETARY SUBTOTAL _____

B. ENVIRONMENTAL STRESS

Drinking Water

Chlorinated only	1 point	____
Chlorinated and fluori-dated	2 points	____

Soil and Air Pollution

Live within 10 miles of city of 500,000 or more	10 points	____
Live within 10 miles of city of 250,000 or more	5 points	____
Live within 10 miles of city of 50,000 or more	2 points	____
Live in the country but use pesticides, herbicides and/or chemical fertilizer	10 points	____
Exposed to cigarette smoke of someone else more than 1 hour per day	5 points	____

ENVIRONMENTAL SUBTOTAL   ____

C. CHEMICAL STRESS

Drugs (any amount of usage)

Antidepressants	1 point	____
Tranquilizers	3 points	____
Sleeping pills	3 points	____
Narcotics	5 points	____
Other pain relievers	3 points	____

Nicotine

3-10 cigarettes per day	5 points	____
11-20 cigarettes per day	15 points	____

21-30 cigarettes per day	20 points	_____
31-40 cigarettes per day	35 points	_____
Over 40 cigarettes per day	40 points	_____
Cigar(s) per day	1 point each	_____
Pipeful(s) of tobacco per day	1 point each	_____
Chewing tobacco— "chews" per day	1 point each	_____

Average Daily Alcohol Consumption

1 oz. whiskey, gin, vodka, etc.	2 points each	_____
8 oz. beer	2 points each	_____
4-6 oz. glass of wine	2 points each	_____
CHEMICAL SUBTOTAL		_____

D. PHYSICAL STRESS

Weight

Underweight more than 10 lbs.	5 points	_____
10 to 15 lbs. overweight	5 points	_____
16 to 25 lbs. overweight	10 points	_____
26 to 40 lbs. overweight	25 points	_____
More than 40 lbs. overweight	40 points	_____

Activity

Adequate exercise*, 3 days or more per week	0 points	_____
Some physical exercise, 1 or 2 days per week	15 points	_____
No regular exercise	40 points	_____

*Adequate means doubling heartbeat and/or sweating minimum of 30 minutes per time.

Work Stress

Sit most of the day	3 points	_____
Industrial/factory worker	3 points	_____
Overnight travel more than once a week	5 points	_____
Work more than 50 hours per week	2 points per hour over 50	_____
Work varying shifts	10 points	_____
Work night shift	5 points	_____

PHYSICAL SUBTOTAL   _____

E. HOLMES-RAHE SOCIAL READJUSTMENT RATING

(Circle the mean values that correspond with life events listed below that you have experienced during the past 12 months.)

Death of spouse	100
Divorce	73
Marital separation	65
Jail term	63
Death of close family member	63
Personal injury or illness	53
Marriage	50
Fired at work	47
Marital reconciliation	45
Retirement	45
Change in health of family member	44
Pregnancy	40
Sexual difficulties	39
Gain new family member	39

Business readjustment	39
Change in financial state	38
Death of close friend	37
Change to different line of work	36
Change in number of arguments with spouse	35
Mortgage or loan over $20,000	31
Foreclosure of mortgage or loan	30
Change in responsibilities at work	29
Son or daughter leaving home	29
Trouble with in-laws	29
Outstanding personal achievement	28
Spouse begins or stops work	26
Begin or end school	25
Change in living conditions	24
Revision of personal habits	23
Trouble with boss	20
Change in work hours or conditions	20
Change in residence	20
Change in schools	19
Change in recreation	19
Change in church activities	18
Change in social activities	17
Mortgage or loan less than $20,000	16
Change in sleeping habits	15

Change in eating habits	15
Vacation, especially if away from home	13
Christmas, or other major holiday stress	**12**
Minor violations of the law	11

TOTAL MEAN VALUE SCORE ____

This is your Holmes-Rahe total. Refer to the conversion table to determine your number of points. This will be your Holmes-Rahe Social Readjustment Rating.

Holmes-Rahe Conversion Table

Less than	60	110	160	170	180	190	200	210	220	230
Your number of points	0	1	2	3	4	5	6	7	8	9
Less than	240	250	260	265	270	275	280	285	290	295
Your number of points	10	11	12	13	14	15	16	17	18	19
Less than	300	305	310	315	320	325	330	335	340	345
Your number of points	20	21	22	23	24	25	26	27	28	29
Less than	350									
Your number of points	30									

Anything over 351 = 40+

Holmes-Rahe Social Readjustment Rating (Converted) _____

F. EMOTIONAL STRESS

Sleep

Less than 7 hours per night	3 points
Usually 7 or 8 hours per night	0 points
More than 8 hours per night	2 points

Relaxation

Relax only during sleep	10 points
Relax or meditate at least 20 minutes per day	0 points

Frustration at work

Enjoy work	0 points
Mildly frustrated by job	1 point
Moderately frustrated by job	3 points
Very frustrated by job	5 points

Marital Status

Married, happily	0 points
Married, moderately unhappy	2 points
Married, very unhappy	5 points
Unmarried man over 30	5 points
Unmarried woman over 30	2 points

Usual Mood

Happy, well adjusted   0 points

Moderately angry, de-   10 points
pressed or frustrated

Very angry, depressed or   20 points
frustrated

Television For each hour   2 points
over 1 per day

Any other major stress not
mentioned above, you
judge intensity (Specify):

_____   10 to 40 points

EMOTIONAL SUBTOTAL

Sum of subtotals = Your Personal Stress Assessment Score

A ____
B ____
C ____
D ____
E ____
F ____
____ = Personal Stress Assessment Score

If your score exceeds 25 points, you probably will feel better if
you reduce your stress; greater than 50 points, you definitely
need to eliminate stress in your life. Circle your stressor with
the highest number of points and work first to eliminate it;
then circle your next greatest stressor, and overcome it; and
so on.

SYMPTOM INDEX

For the following questions, please indicate YES or NO. Yes means *now or in the past year*. Answer all questions. Be sure to check only those now or in the *past year*.

YES NO

—— —— 1. Do you have headaches more than once a week?

—— —— 2. Does twisting your neck quickly cause pain?

—— —— 3. Have you had either lumps or swelling in your neck?

—— —— 4. Do you wear glasses?

—— —— 5. Does your eyesight ever blur?

—— —— 6. Is your eyesight getting worse?

—— —— 7. Do you ever see double?

—— —— 8. Do you ever see colored halos around lights?

—— —— 9. Do you have either pains or itching in or around your eyes?

—— —— 10. Do your eyes either blink or water most of the time?

—— —— 11. Have you had any trouble with your eyes in the last two years?

—— —— 12. Have you ever experienced loss of vision?

—— —— 13. Have you had difficulty hearing?

—— —— 14. Have you had any earaches lately?

—— —— 15. Have you been troubled by running ears lately?

—— —— 16. Do you have either a repeated buzzing or other noise in your ears?

—— —— 17. Do you get motion sickness riding in either a car or plane?

—— —— 18. Do you have any problems with your teeth?

—— —— 19. Do you have any sore swellings on either your gums or jaws?

—— —— 20. Is your tongue either sore or sensitive?

—— —— 21. Have your taste senses changed lately?

___ ___ 22. Do you wear dentures?

___ ___ 23. Is your nose stuffed up when you don't have a cold?

___ ___ 24. Does your nose run when you don't have a cold?

___ ___ 25. Do you ever have sneezing spells?

___ ___ 26. Do you ever have two or more colds in a row?

___ ___ 27. Does your nose ever bleed for no reason at all?

___ ___ 28. Is your throat ever sore when you don't have a cold?

___ ___ 29. Has a doctor told you that your tonsils have been enlarged?

___ ___ 30. Has your voice ever been hoarse when you didn't have a cold?

___ ___ 31. Is it either difficult or painful for you to swallow?

___ ___ 32. Do you either wheeze or have to gasp to breathe?

___ ___ 33. Are you bothered by coughing spells?

___ ___ 34. Do you cough up a lot of phlegm (thick spit)?

___ ___ 35. Have you ever coughed up blood?

___ ___ 36. Do you get chest colds more than once a month?

___ ___ 37. Have you been told that you had high blood pressure?

___ ___ 38. Have you been told that you have low blood pressure?

___ ___ 39. Have you been told you have heart trouble?

___ ___ 40. Have you been bothered by either a thumping or racing heart?

___ ___ 41. Do you ever get pains or tightness in your chest?

___ ___ 42. Do you get out of breath easily?

___ ___ 43. Do you awaken at night short of breath?

___ ___ 44. Do you get short of breath just sitting?

—— —— 45. Have you ever been told that you have a heart murmur?

—— —— 46. Are you troubled by heartburn?

—— —— 47. Do you feel bloated after eating?

—— —— 48. Are you troubled by belching?

—— —— 49. Do you suffer discomfort in the pit of your stomach?

—— —— 50. Do you easily become nauseated (feel like vomiting)?

—— —— 51. Have you ever vomited blood?

—— —— 52. Have you ever had an ulcer?

—— —— 53. Have you either gained or lost much weight recently?

—— —— 54. Have you lost your interest in eating lately?

—— —— 55. Do you always seem to be hungry?

—— —— 56. Do you frequently get up at night to urinate?

—— —— 57. Do you urinate more than five or six times a day?

—— —— 58. Do you either wet your pants or wet your bed?

—— —— 59. Have you ever had either burning or pains when you urinate?

—— —— 60. Has your urine ever been either brown, black or bloody?

—— —— 61. Do you have any difficulty starting your urine?

—— —— 62. Do you have a constant feeling that you have to urinate?

—— —— 63. Are you constipated more than twice a month?

—— —— 64. Are you troubled by diarrhea?

—— —— 65. Are your bowel movements ever either black or bloody?

—— —— 66. Are your bowel movements ever grey in color?

—— —— 67. Do you suffer pains when you move your bowels?

___ ___ 68. Have you had any bleeding from your rectum?

___ ___ 69. Do severe stomach pains double you up?

___ ___ 70. Do you have frequent stomach trouble?

___ ___ 71. Have you had intestinal worms?

___ ___ 72. Has a diagnosis of hemorrhoids (piles) been made?

___ ___ 73. Have you had jaundice (yellow eyes and skin)?

___ ___ 74. Do you bite your nails?

___ ___ 75. Are you troubled by stuttering or stammering?

___ ___ 76. Are you a sleep walker?

___ ___ 77. Have you had any serious problem with your genitals (privates)?

___ ___ 78. Have you had a hernia (rupture)?

___ ___ 79. Do you have either kidney or bladder disease?

___ ___ 80. Do you suffer from nervous exhaustion?

___ ___ 81. Are you frequently ill?

___ ___ 82. Are you frequently confined to bed by illness?

___ ___ 83. Are you a sickly person?

___ ___ 84. Are you troubled with either stiff or painful muscles?

___ ___ 85. Are your joints ever swollen?

___ ___ 86. Are you troubled with either stiff or painful joints?

___ ___ 87. Are your feet often painful?

___ ___ 88. Are there any swellings in either your armpits or groin?

___ ___ 89. Do you have trouble with swollen feet or ankles?

___ ___ 90 Are you getting cramps in your legs either at night or upon walking?

___ ___ 91. Does your skin either itch or burn?

___ ___ 92. Do you have trouble stopping even a small cut from bleeding?

___ ___ 93. Do you bruise easily?

___ ___ 94. Do you have trouble with either dizziness or lightheadedness?

—— —— 95. Do you ever either faint or feel faint?

—— —— 96. Is any part of your body always numb?

—— —— 97. Do you have either cold hands and/or feet even in hot weather?

—— —— 98. Has any part of your body been paralyzed?

—— —— 99. Have you blacked out?

—— —— 100. Have you ever had either fits or convulsions?

—— —— 101. Has your handwriting changed lately?

—— —— 102. Do you have a tendency to either shake or tremble?

—— —— 103. Do you have a tendency to be either too hot or too cold?

—— —— 104. Are you sweating more than usual?

—— —— 105. Do you have hot flashes?

—— —— 106. Does every little effort leave you short of breath?

—— —— 107. Do you seem to feel exhausted or fatigued most of the time?

—— —— 108. Do you have difficulty either falling or staying asleep?

—— —— 109. Do you fail to get the exercise you should?

—— —— 110. Are you definitely overweight?

—— —— 111. Are you definitely underweight?

—— —— 112. Have you lost more than half your teeth?

—— —— 113. Do you have bleeding gums?

—— —— 114. Is your tongue often badly coated?

—— —— 115. Do you usually eat between meals (sweets and other foods)?

—— —— 116. Do you often have small accidents or injuries?

—— —— 117. Do you have varicose veins (swollen veins) in your legs?

—— —— 118. Is it usually hard for you to make up your mind?

—— —— 119. Are you usually either unhappy or depressed?

—— —— 120. Do you cry often?

___ ___ 121. Does life look entirely hopeless?

___ ___ 122. Does worrying often get you down?

___ ___ 123. Are you either extremely shy or sensitive?

___ ___ 124. Does criticism usually upset you?

___ ___ 125. Do little annoyances either get on your nerves or make you angry?

___ ___ 126. Do you flare up in anger if you can't have what you want right away?

___ ___ 127. Are you nervous around strangers?

___ ___ 128. Do you find it hard to make decisions?

___ ___ 129. Do you find it hard to either concentrate or remember?

___ ___ 130. Do you often feel lonely?

___ ___ 131. Do you have difficulty relaxing?

___ ___ 132. Are you troubled by either frightening dreams or frightening thoughts?

___ ___ 133. Have you ever considered committing suicide?

___ ___ 134. Are you disturbed by either work or family problems?

___ ___ 135. Have you ever desired psychiatric help?

___ ___ 136. Are you often or usually tense and uptight?

___ ___ 137. Are you often nervous or jittery?

___ ___ 138. Are you easily upset?

___ ___ 139. Are you in low spirits most of the time?

___ ___ 140. Are you often in *very* low spirits?

___ ___ 141. Do you believe that your life is out of your hands and controlled by external factors?

___ ___ 142. Is your life empty, filled only with despair?

___ ___ 143. In your life, do you have no goals or aims at all?

___ ___ 144. Have you completely failed to progress toward your life goals?

___ ___ 145. Concerning your freedom to make your own choices, do you believe you are completely bound by limitations of heredity and environment?

FOR MEN ONLY

__ __ 146. Is your urine stream either very weak or very slow?

__ __ 147. Has a doctor ever told you that you have prostate trouble?

__ __ 148. Have you had either burning or any unusual discharge from your penis?

__ __ 149. Do your testicles get painful?

__ __ 150. Do you have trouble having erections (getting a hard-on)?

FOR WOMEN ONLY

__ __ 151. Are you having trouble with your menstrual periods?

__ __ 152. Have you ever had bleeding between your periods?

__ __ 153. Do you have heavy bleeding with your periods?

__ __ 154. Do you feel either bloated or irritable before your periods?

__ __ 155. Have you ever taken any birth control pills?

__ __ 156. Have you had any lumps in your breasts?

__ __ 157. Have you had any excessive discharges from your vagina?

__ __ 158. Are you often either weak or sick with your periods?

__ __ 159. Do you often have to lie down when your period starts?

__ __ 160. Are you usually tense and jumpy with your periods?

__ __ 161. Do you have constant severe hot flashes and sweats?

Now add your total symptoms. If you have 20 or more, look at your Total Life Stress Test and decide which stressors you are able and willing to avoid.

MYERS-BRIGGS TYPE INVENTORY TEST

You might also want to take a Myers-Briggs Type Inventory Test, available through most psychologists. Because this test is such a valuable tool, it is worth mentioning in this section of the book.

Isabelle Myers-Briggs developed the Myers-Briggs Type Inventory Questionnaire based upon Jungian concepts of personality. An individual is either an introvert or an extrovert; a sensor or an intuitive; a feeler or a thinker; a perceiver or a judger.

The words, rather common with Jung, do not mean what we usually think of them as meaning. An introvert is an individual who bases decisions almost totally upon inner-dialogue. An extrovert certainly may make decisions quite independently, but tends to like a great deal of input from the other people before making decisions.

A sensor, or sensing individual, is one who prefers to work with known facts. An intuitive likes to look at all the various options and possibilities or at the broad picture. The shortcoming of an intuitive is that he or she may miss some of the smaller details, and the shortcoming of a sensor is that the greater potentials could be ignored because of a need for facts.

A feeling individual makes a decision based upon inner values, whereas a thinker makes decisions based upon logic. A perceiver is an individual who likes to hang loose and not have life too well organized. A judger prefers life to be as organized as possible.

With each of these different personality types, there are relative expressions of their characteristics, from very slight to very extreme. With eight different characteristics one is classified into one of sixteen basic personality types.

When one reads the descriptions of these various personality types, they are remarkably accurate reflections of the way in which individuals think and process information. We find this test to be one of the most useful for understanding how a person will relate to other individuals.

There are no rights or wrongs with the Myers-Briggs

Test. No one personality "type" is better or worse than another. There is no psychopathology associated with it. It is just the way you are.

If you are interested in this evaluation, I would encourage you to look into obtaining the test through a psychologist who may do it, or get the book, *Please Understand Me*, written by David Keirsey and Marilyn Bates.

SELF-TESTING SUMMARY

What do you do with the results of these tests? We suggest if you feel that the results indicate the need for changes in lifestyle or attitudes, or the need for a physical examination, that you act on these signals immediately. We also recommend that you refer to these tests as a reference point for reevaluating your ongoing growth and personal development processes.

CREATING HEALTH

CHAPTER FOURTEEN

Creating Health and Staying Healthy

(Shealy)

Once one has been born and is *healthy* at the time of birth, as are approximately 95% of people in the United States, it appears that nutrition, physical exercise and mental attitude are the major determinants of how that state of health continues. Obviously it is mental attitude that ultimately determines not only what we eat but whether or not we exercise and whether or not we smoke, drink excessively or maintain our weight within a normal range. It has been found that the average life expectancy of individuals could be increased an average of twelve years if they had only seven basic health habits. These are:

1. Eating three meals a day.
2. Eating breakfast every day.
3. Sleeping seven or eight hours every day.

4. Exercising at least three times a week (one hour each time).

5. Avoiding smoking.

6. Keeping the weight within 10% of the ideal.

7. Minimizing alcohol (maximum ten drinks per week).

The Surgeon General has emphasized, in order of importance, that disease is the result of:

1. Cigarette smoking.

2. Excess alcohol consumption.

3. Obesity.

4. Excess consumption of fat, salt and sugar.

5. Inadequate physical exercise.

6. Failure to use seat belts or observe the speed limit.

Note the similarity of these two lists. Note that all of these factors are attitudinally controlled.

In the Winter 1977 issue of *Daedalus*, Dr. John Knowles, President of the Rockefeller Foundation, wrote about the "Responsibility of the Individual." Essentially he indicated that technical medicine had reached almost as far as we could expect it to in improving health, and he emphasized that the overwhelming majority of illnesses today are the result of personal choices and health habits. He went on to suggest that a minimum of 80% of cancer is created by health habits (smoking and high fat diet, etc.); that high blood pressure, obesity, diabetes and most of the diseases that plague Americans at this point in time can be overcome not through drugs, surgery or further "miracles," but by changes in lifestyle. As late as 1988, only 54% of Americans even try "to avoid eating too much fat." This percentage represents a drop of 2% from the year before.

Dr. James Michael McGinnis, Director of the Office of Disease and Prevention and Health Promotion, has emphasized the need to "redouble our efforts to convince Americans that health promotion ideas are not a fad." Thomas Dybdahl of *Prevention Magazine*, which has been doing an annual poll since 1984, has stated that "in key areas such as diet, exercise, and weight control, there is still much room for improvement."

In 1976 Dr. Thomas McKeown, in his magnificent book, *The Role of Medicine: Dream, Mirage, or Nemesis*, wrote that 92% of the improvement in life expectancy in this century is the result of improvement in sanitation, such as sewage disposal, chlorination of water and pasteurization of milk, as well as adequate supplies of food. Only 8% is due to the "miracles" of modern medicine and science. Dr. McKeown also stated that "most of those who are born well will remain well, apart from minor morbidity, at least until late life, if they have enough to eat, if they are not exposed to serious hazards, and if they do not injure themselves by unwise behavior, particularly departing radically from the fundamental conditions under which man evolved." He also stated, "the treatment of established disease, although important for patients, does not usually restore them to a life of normal duration and quality and the modern improvement in health was due to prevention of disease rather than treatment after it occurred." He emphasized that "both health and quality of life are improved by taking exercise, avoiding tobacco and other drugs, and limiting the consumption of alcohol and food." He also stressed that reducing fat consumption, increasing exercise, and replacing refined flour by whole meal could do more than any anticipated change in medicine could. I would remind you that even these very simple changes toward a healthy lifestyle require an attitude of health.

Dr. McKeown also emphasized that "it should be recognized that disease problems are rarely solved by therapeutic intervention, that new methods of investigation and treatment are often ineffective and are sometimes unsafe, and that laboratory evidence, however exhaustive, is not a sufficient basis for judgement of the effects of a procedure when applied to man." And finally, "my own impression, for what it is worth, is that if the term medicine is taken to include the whole enterprise—nutritional, hygienic, and behavioral as well as therapeutic—there is little doubt that the balance is strongly in medicine's favor." Unfortunately, medicine has virtually ignored nutrition, has in recent years paid minimal attention to behavior, and has even minimized emphasis upon good hygiene in the last few decades.

Dr. George Solomon of the University of California, who coined the term psychoneuroimmunology, has stated that all disease is the result of interaction among many factors—genetic, endocrine, nervous, immune and behavioral-emotional. "Such a frame of reference has been championed by such pioneers as George Engel and Jonas Salk. It has also been sensed by wise clinicians since ancient time—from practitioners of Ayurvedic Medicine in India, of two millennium ago to Hippocrates, Galen, and Osler."

NUTRITION

Americans probably spend more time, energy and money on nutrition and nutritional programs than on all other efforts to enhance personal health. And more claims are made for diets and nutritional supplements than P. T. Barnum could have imagined.

The average American diet consists of 45% fat, 12% protein, 18% sugar, 18% white flour (processed starch) and only 7% real carbohydrates. The ideal is 10 to 20% fat, 10% protein and 70 to 80% real carbohydrate. A variety of low fat and other alternative diets are pushed by promoters and followers, with very little scientific evidence of efficacy. Indeed, I cannot find any competent nutritionist who is able to recommend even an adequate *study* to *determine* an optimal diet. We simply don't know what measurements are essential to prove whether a diet is excellent or poor.

Some of the more widely touted plans that I believe are good are the following.

THE MACROBIOTIC DIET

The macrobiotic diet consists of at least 50% (of every meal) of cooked, whole cereal grains, including short and medium grain brown rice, millet, barley, corn, whole oats, wheat berries, rye or buckwheat. Occasional use (once or twice a week) can include sweet or long grain brown rice, whole wheat noodles, buckwheat noodles, unleavened whole wheat, whole grain breads, rice cakes, cracked wheat, bulgur, rolled oats, cornmeal, grits, rye flakes, couscous, seitan and fu.

Approximately 5% of the daily diet may be soup (one or two cups) in the form of miso or tamari broth with a wide variety of vegetables added to these soup bases.

About 25 to 30% of each macrobiotic meal should consist of vegetables, about two-thirds of which can be sauteed, steamed, boiled or baked. The other one-third of the vegetables may be eaten uncooked.

About 5 to 10% of the daily diet should consist of cooked beans and sea vegetables. The most suitable beans are azuki, chick-peas and green lentil, with other beans being eaten on occasion for variety.

A maximum of 5 to 10% of the diet should consist of fruits, nuts, beverages and natural "sweeteners." Individuals are advised to eat wakame sea vegetables every day and are encouraged to use umeboshi plum, sea vegetable powders, roasted sesame seeds, sea salt and tekka.

Beverages recommended for this diet are roasted bancha or kukicha twig tea, roasted brown rice tea, toasted barley tea, dandelion tea and cereal grain coffee; but no caffeine is allowed.

Dark sesame oil is allowed for cooking.

The recommended water is well water or fresh spring water.

A small amount of white fish is allowed about once a week.

THE PRITIKIN DIET

The Pritikin Diet emphasizes complex carbohydrates and fiber with de-emphasis on fats, animal proteins, salt and simple carbohydrates, such as sugar. Essentially, the Pritikin diet totally forbids red meat, oils, sugar, salt and egg yolks. The diet allows most fruits and vegetables in relatively unlimited quantities, most beans and whole grain pastas, whole wheat flour, arrowroot flour and cornstarch, corn flour or rice flour, tapioca flour, non-fat dry milk and Grape Nuts cereal (the nuggets, not the flakes). It also allows dry cottage cheese, non-fat yogurt and non-fat or skimmed milk, popcorn, corn tortillas, and fish that is baked or broiled. On the stricter version of the diet (for those with severe heart disease), only 1½ oz. of fish are allowed per week. Except on the strict diet, small amounts of fish, up to 3 oz. or so per day, and about the same amount of chicken breast, are allowed. No cooking oils of any type, no butter and no "spreads" are used.

THE McDOUGALL PLAN

This is the only one of these specialized diets that is backed by a physician. Dr. McDougall is an internist on the faculty of the Medical College at the University of Hawaii. His diet is strictly a vegan vegetarian diet, which means no red meat, no poultry, no fish, no dairy products and no eggs. It significantly limits "simple sugars." Ideally, not more than 5% of total calories should come from fat in the McDougall plan except for "very active healthy adults or pregnant or lactating women who may increase that to 15%." High fat vegetable foods include tempeh, wheat germ, soy beans, tofu, sunflower seeds, peanut butter, almonds, coconut, olives and vegetable oil. Obviously all of the animal and dairy products are loaded with fat. Dr. McDougall emphasizes that all types of fat affect hormones, in particular the levels of prolactin, estrogen and testosterone, partly because diets high in animal fats encourage the growth of hormone-producing bacteria in the large intestine and because obesity also affects this level. Menopause occurs about four years later on a high fat diet; menstrual periods are further apart, longer, heavier and more painful when the fat intake is high; and there is a marked increase in breast cancer and colon cancer as the fat content in the diet increases.

THE HAAS DIET—EAT TO WIN

Dr. Haas, a nutritionist, proposes a diet that consists of complex carbohydrates or starches, which should comprise 60 to 80% of the daily calories; simple carbohydrates or sweets are 5 to 10% of daily calories; protein, both animal and vegetable, is a total of 10 to 15% of daily calories; and fat, both animal and vegetable, is somewhere between 5 and 20%.

This diet consists largely of potatoes, topped with Butter Buds or dry cottage cheese, or low fat or not-fat yogurt, chives, pepper or granulated vegetable seasonings; whole grains of any kind; whole grain pasta; very low amounts of dry cottage cheese and low-fat yogurt; up to one cup of legumes per day; up to four egg whites per day with no yolks; about 2½ oz. of salmon, mackerel, lobster, turkey or chicken per day; fresh fruits up to two per day; grated parmesan or romano cheese up to three teaspoons per day; unlimited raw or steamed vegetables except for avocado, hearts of palm, seeds, nuts and olives; up to one 3½ oz. glass of wine or 12 oz. of light beer or 1½ oz. of hard liquor; and once you have gotten to ideal weight and performance, increases in daily intake of chicken, fish or turkey to 4 oz. He then also allows beef, pork or veal on one day per week, instead of fish or chicken.

FOOD SUPPLEMENTS

When it comes to food supplements, the water is even murkier. It seems obvious that most foods are deficient in minerals because our soil has been radically depleted. And with stress of any kind (smog, smoking, social, etc.), we need more vitamins and minerals. But how much of what?

If 45% fat is excessive, what *is* ideal? And if there is a range, how does an individual choose?

If 18% sugar (35 to 42 teaspoons per day) is bad, how much is "safe"?

If 18% white flour is bad, how much is "safe"?

There is relatively little difference in the four diets summarized here and those diets are really ideal for most people. As a result of that, I have tried to integrate them into what I call the No Added Fat Diet.

THE NO ADDED FAT DIET
(Created by C. Norman Shealy, M.D., Ph.D.)

Principles:

1. No added fat, butter, margarine or oil.
2. *Minimize* high fat foods such as:
   Peanut butter
   Cheese
   Dairy products
   Eggs
   Meats and fish of all kinds (Beef, pork, chicken, etc.)
3. Plan an entire *day's* food to contain a *maximum* of 20 grams of fat from the high fat foods. Examples:

2 oz. lean beef	13.5 grams
1 oz. cheddar cheese	9.5 grams
8 oz. of 2% milk	4.0 grams
8 oz. of 1% milk	2.0 grams
1 egg	7.0 grams
4 oz. chicken (without skin)	4.0 grams
4 oz. dry cottage cheese	1.0 grams
4 oz. salmon	7.0 grams
1 oz. ricotta cheese	3.0 grams

   If in doubt, look it up!
4. *Avoid*

Bacon	Luncheon meats
Ham	Processed meats

5. *Emphasize Real Starch (Complex Carbohydrates)*

Oats	Potatoes
Wheat	Sweet potatoes
Rice	Winter squash

Corn	Pastas, especially whole
Couscous	grain, including
Bulgur	corn, rice, soy,
Millet	semolina and spinach
Buckwheat	
Rye	

6. Learn to season with herbs, spices, Butter Buds and no-fat sauces.

ANOPSON DIET

The Anopson diet consists of only raw food in its original state which is chosen by "instinct," that is, by smell and taste. Theoretically, one is supposed to have huge varieties of raw foods available, to scratch and smell each of them, and to eat that which smells best and continue eating that particular food until it changes in flavor from luscious to unpleasant. This diet consists very largely of raw, whole fruits with whatever vegetables one finds palatable, raw eggs, raw nuts and seeds, and raw meat of any kind ranging through fish, fowl and various red meats. The proponents do not recommend eating raw pork until one has been on the diet for three months, after which they claim that the immune system is so strong that one is virtually resistant to all infections and parasitic infestations. None of the food may be blenderized, dried, cooked or ground in any way. You don't have to eat the banana peelings or the orange peelings, but in general most of the food is eaten *au naturel*.

When immune competence is most impaired, I believe that the Anopson Diet is the ideal. However, it might be better to convert first to one of the other diets, either Macrobiotic or the No Added Fat Diet, and after a month or two on that, then try a period of four to six weeks on the Anopson Diet. The simple basis of the Anopson Diet is to eat as many ripe, tasty fruits as possible, as many vegetables as one is willing to eat and to supplement that with organically raised raw eggs, raw fish (Pacific red snapper and ocean fish are quite delicious eaten raw and probably are quite safe, but I can't be as certain about any other "meat"), raw nuts and seeds, especially cashews and almonds. These are adequate for completing the Anopson Diet, and I think most individuals, if they eat enough of the fish and nuts and seeds, will thrive on that type of diet. But if their systems are too "toxic" from cumulative bad habits, smoking and an inadequate diet, they may have many more symptoms and, thus, I would probably choose one of the other abovementioned nutritional programs.

THE FIT FOR LIFE DIET

This nutritional program created by Harvey and Marilyn Diamond has been one of the most popular in the history of this country. Three million copies of their book have been sold. It comes closer to the Anopson Diet than any of the others but is even more restrictive in food combining. According to these authors, you should eat nothing but fresh fruit or fresh fruit juices from the time you wake up until noon. During the time from noon until evening, you can have essentially unlimited vegetables, raw as much as possible, or if you really want to go ape, you can have for lunch a "properly combined sandwich," which consists of whole grain bread with various vegetables and sprouts. For dinner you are allowed either starches of any kind, including potatoes, rice, etc., plus vegetables, or meat, particularly chicken or fish plus vegetables, but never combining meat with starch. Great claims are made for losing weight on this diet and for increased energy.

Alcohol is an important consideration. In general, it is certainly not healthy for anyone and individuals should minimize their intake of alcohol; that means a maximum of ten drinks per week. If you have any kind of illness, no amount of alcohol can be considered safe or reasonable.

As a rule, not more than two cups of any kind of caffeinated beverage should be taken by anyone per day. Soda and "soft drinks" should also be avoided. Finally, good quality water should be drunk at the rate of one-half one's body weight in pounds, but converted to ounces. That is, a 150-pound person should drink 75 ounces of water per day.

Finally, in nutrition we have the question of food supplements. Theoretically, if one eats a really excellent diet and is not exposed to a great deal of environmental pollution or other stress, no vitamin supplements are necessary. Unfortunately, most people live in polluted cities, drink polluted water, are exposed to cigarette smoke, diesel fumes and other petroleum products and probably get food that is significantly deficient in vitamin, and especially in mineral, content. I personally take a very comprehensive multivitamin mineral complex that includes: Vitamin A, Beta-Carotene, Xanthophyll Complex, Vitamin B_1, Vitamin B_2, Vitamin B_3, Vitamin B_5, Vitamin B_6, Vitamin B_{12}, PABA, Folic Acid, Biotin, Vitamin C, Ascorbyl Palmitate, Sodium Selenate, Seleno-Methionine, Vitamin E, Calcium Orotate, Calcium Aspartate, Vitamin D_3, Magnesium Orotate, Magnesium Aspartate, Potassium Orotate, L-Cysteine, L-Methionine, L-Glutathione, Choline Bitartrate, Phosphatidul Choline, DMAE, Inositol, Luteolin Complex, Robinetin Complex, Myricetin Complex, Hesperidan Complex, Co-enzyme Q_{10}, Dilaurylthiodipropionate, Thiodipropionic Acid, Bromelain, Freeze Dried Cabbage Conc., Zinc Orotate, Zinc Chelate, Chromium Sulfate, Molybdenum, Manganese and Iodine. In addition, I take at least eight to ten grams a day of either a 50% mixture of salmon oil and evening primrose oil, or just plain salmon oil.

PHYSICAL EXERCISE

Limbering (calesthentics or hatha yoga), strengthening (muscle-building, weight-lifting), and cardiovascular strengthening (aerobic) exercise are all useful and healthful. All three forms of exercise make you feel good physically and mentally. They increase Beta-endorphin production (the natural narcotics). All three forms provide significant stress reduction. Aerobic exercise has been researched extensively, and increased aerobic activity leads to improved physiologic functioning: decreased resting heart rate, increased HDL cholesterol, decreased cholesterol, decreased fasting blood sugar, lower blood pressure, etc. Similar studies have not been done as comprehensively with limbering and strengthening exercise. There is good evidence that aerobic exercise decreases the risk of heart attack and some evidence that it improves health, longevity and sense of well-being. Whether physical exercise is *essential* to health and longevity in virtually everyone is unknown. That is, if you have superb attitude, eat well and/or have good genes (choose your parents well), will exercise create better health or a longer life? From a health/ longevity point of view, can you substitute limbering or strengthening exercise for aerobics? Probably *any* exercise is better than none, and it makes you *feel* better.

Physical Exercise—Limbering

Physical inactivity is stressful, and our society increasingly discourages physical activity. Automobiles, escalators, elevators and even "moving sidewalks" in airports are signs of "progress." Our first suggestions for physical fitness are:

1. Walk whenever possible, especially if your destination is less than a mile. If more, consider a bicycle.

2. Walk up and down stairs whenever possible. If you work up to it gradually, you will easily be able to walk up at least ten flights of stairs. In many buildings it will save time, too!

Walking and stair-climbing are partly limbering and partly cardiovascular strengthening. But even when intensely used, they are not adequate for keeping the body flexible. Each joint, muscle and tendon needs a full range of motion daily. The following simple exercises can be done in ten or fifteen minutes. Start with one repetition; each week add another repetition; build up to ten of each. Breathe slowly and deeply, exhaling during the most strenuous part of the exercise.

> *NECK*—roll head *slowly* in all directions, clockwise and counter-clockwise, stretching (but not straining) to limits.

SHOULDERS AND ARMS—Shrug shoulders up and back in a smooth, easy motion, then relax. Raise arms over head, swing out to shoulder level and make circles with hands and arms, first in one direction, then in the opposite direction.

TRUNK—Stand erect and bend to either side. Return to an upright position. Keeping feet flat and straight ahead, turn as far to either side as possible. Straighten. Let your head and body drop gently forward, stretching as far as you can loosely go. Go further each day or week.

LEGS AND HIPS

a. Lying on your back, with one knee bent, raise your other leg straight up as far as it will go; lower to floor; repeat with opposite leg.

b. Pull one knee up to your chest; then turn knee out to the side; hold foot in crotch as you stretch knee to side; gradually straighten leg; repeat with other side.

SPINE

a. Lying on your back, bend knees with feet flat on floor; raise buttocks as high as they will go; lower slowly.

b. Get on all fours; arch your back up while you bend your head forward; raise your head up and back while you arch your back down (buttocks up).

Physical Exercise—Strengthening The Heart

Earlier in this century, most individuals did physical work; today even farmers rarely get adequate exercise. But exercise can and should be fun. The minimum requirements for adequate heart exercise follow. In general, it is best to do one exercise regularly, but various groups can be interchanged. *In any case, start very slowly* and build up gradually to the final recommended amount; take at least *sixteen weeks* to build up to maximum; if you're over forty and haven't exercised regularly, take twenty-four to thirty-two weeks to build up.

WALKING

Start with ¼ mile at your own pace.
Work up (over 16 to 20 weeks) to 4 miles in 59 minutes, 5 times per week.

STANDING JOGGING

Use either a jogging trampoline (start with 1 minute) or a mattress on the floor.
Start with 1 minute at your own pace. Work up slowly to 20 minutes, 5 days a week, jogging at least 180 steps/minute.

BICYCLING

Start with 2 miles at your own leisurely pace.
Work up slowly to 10 miles in 50 minutes, 5 days a week (take 20 weeks to work up).

RACQUETBALL, SQUASH OR HANDBALL

Start only if you can walk comfortably (and have built up slowly) to 4 miles in 59 minutes.
Start with 30 minutes 3 times a week. Build up slowly to 60 minutes 5 times/week.

STAIRS

Start with one flight at your own pace. Build up to 50 flights up and down, as rapidly as you can go, 5 days per week. Build up over 20 weeks.

SWIMMING

Start with 100 yards at a leisurely pace. Build up to 1,000 yards in 30 minutes, 5 times a week. Take at least 16 weeks to build up.

BOUNCING

Stand erect; bend your knees about 1/4 to 1/2 toward a squat, while you swing your arms forward; bounce up and down, slowly building up speed. Start with 1 minute daily. Build up slowly to 20 minutes, 5 times a week, of bouncing as rapidly as comfortable. Take at least 15 weeks to build up.

Mental Self-Regulation

Some form of mental self-regulation training is integral to all major religions or societies. Meditation is as much a part of Christianity as it is of Judaism or Buddhism. Self-hypnosis and relaxation training are similarly universal. Modern American society seems to have abandoned these techniques more than any other society in history.

For over eighty years, very extensive scientific study has confirmed this ageless wisdom. Virtually every physiologic function is improved with many forms of self-regulation training. At least 80% of all illnesses respond well to self-regulation, far better than to drugs or surgery; and it is safer than any other known therapy. Biofeedback training has, in the past two decades, led to some acceptance of self-regulation techniques. Skin temperature, a reflection of circulation, is one of the easiest functions to regulate. It speeds up learning to control migraine headaches and high blood pressure. EEG (brain wave activity measurement) feedback is especially helpful for persons with obsessive thinking and for those who suffer from epilepsy. EMG (muscle tension measurement) feedback is particularly helpful in overcoming torticollis (wry neck) and other forms of muscle tension. But biofeedback is only a reinforcer of sensory awareness or internal feedback. It is the regular practice of autogenic training (such as used in Biogenics) that is essential for self-regulation training to be successful.

For health enhancement, health restitution and disease treatment, physically, mentally and emotionally, there is no other approach that comes near the value of self-regulation training.

For basic relaxation, just assume a comfortable position, close your eyes and breathe slowly, repeating with each breath, "I am relaxed."

Memorize the following phrases and, with eyes closed, repeat each phrase slowly 12 to 15 times:

My arms and legs are heavy and warm.
My heartbeat is calm and regular.
My breathing is free and easy.
My abdomen is warm.
My forehead is cool.
My mind is quiet and still.

Done over a six-month period, this type of "autogenic therapy" provides a remarkable sense of balance and stability.

Dealing With Fear—Balancing Emotions

There is only one really negative emotion: that is *fear*. As Franklin D. Roosevelt stated so eloquently, "The only thing we have to fear is fear itself." Anger is one of the reactions to fear. When a person or an event threatens you and you become afraid of losing body, life, money, love, or sense a moral injustice; you may react with anger. The next time you are angry, just ask yourself what you are *afraid of losing*.

Whatever the situation, however, you have only four possible ways of reacting to emotional distress:

1. Continue to be upset or angry, which is committing suicide in a socially acceptable way.
2. Assert yourself to try to bring about a positive solution.
3. Divorce the person or situation with joy. If you don't divorce with joy, you are still upset and have not gained anything by the separation.
4. Accept and forgive. Sometimes we need to recognize that we're not perfect and other individuals are not perfect either, but that the value of continuing the relationship far outweighs the shortcomings or negative aspects of the relationship. Learning truly to accept and forgive, without resentment, is a mark of great maturity.

Most individuals in our society believe that social stress is the greatest problem in American health. As we've emphasized in other writings, nutrition and physical exercise are equally important in balancing emotions. Good nutrition, in which one avoids sugar, white flour and other processed foods and eats a wide variety of natural foods helps to prevent unreasonable fear and anger. Similarly, active physical exercise helps to stimulate the body's normal homeostatic or balancing mechanism and decreases the tendency to become upset over relatively minor problems.

There is, however, a place for righteous indignation. In situations like those, one has a right and, in fact, a responsibility to state that one is offended or upset, and to assert oneself and request that the other individual change. If that is not possible, then get into a quiet state, close your eyes, relax, balance the feelings within your body, and then ask yourself: Is the situation or problem so great that I cannot tolerate it or accept it any way, so that I must get away from it? If so, then divorce it with joy because of your ability to make this intelligent decision.

If such a separation does not seem necessary or possible, then ask yourself: Can I really accept and forgive the other individual's shortcomings, because, overall, I value continuing the relationship? If the answer is yes, then *truly* forgive and your anger will be *released*.

Guilt is another reaction to fear. Whenever we become angry enough to want to harm someone else, or when we fear we have not lived up to our "expectations," we may feel guilty. You never *need* to feel guilty if you always do the best you can. Whatever is past cannot be changed, but recognize that *you* can change your reaction, attitude and behavior. As long as you do your best to be productive and loving, you need not be guilty. (We often give our patients "Not Guilty" buttons.)

Depression is an overwhelming reaction to fear in which we allow ourselves to feel unworthy or so afraid that we give in to what Freud called the "death wish."

Anxiety is either unfocused fear or fear of one or more relatively minor concerns. Regular practice of good nutrition, adequate physical exercise and self-regulation exercises is the best way to deal with depression and anxiety.

SPIRITUAL ATTUNEMENT

Once emotions are balanced, you are ready for attunement with your inner ideals—your personal attunement with The Golden Rule. This is a time for focus upon forgiveness, tolerance, compassion, joy, faith, hope and love, invoking these principles into all aspects of your life, to acknowledge the wisdom of your soul or spirit, and the loving power of God.

CREATING A SACRED PLACE

A major symbolic contribution to mental self-regulation is having personal space that is unpolluted. Even if it is only a small corner of a room, it is wise to have your own area in which no one but you enters where you can keep religious symbols or any other personal objects that, to you, radiate a sense of security. In this space, you may wish to sit in the lotus position or on a small, firm pillow with your spine erect and practice mental self-regulation exercises. Although it is impossible to keep outside sounds out of this space, it is nice to have in it a source of good, calming music and to be certain that the air is as clean as possible. If necessary, use an air purifier and be certain that no one smokes in this environment. It is satisfactory to burn incense or candles to enhance the feeling of your sacred space. Creating a space like this where you can go and really be alone is an ideal adjunct to mental health.

OTHER ALTERNATIVES FOR HEALTH
MAINTENANCE

KINESIOLOGY—This system uses muscle strength, tested by the examiner, to evaluate the effect of thoughts, foods, supplements and drugs. Kinesiology enthusiasts claim that *anything* can be tested this way. If it's good for you, muscles are stronger; if bad, muscles are weaker. There is minimal quantifiable, scientific evaluation to confirm claims made by enthusiasts. Effects usually are very transient (a minute or so).

ACUPUNCTURE—Well over four thousand years old, acupuncture is based upon a concept of circulating body energy, which is pragmatic, practical and functional. In the past twenty years, extensive scientific evaluation of acupuncture has consistently demonstrated statistically significant effects upon a wide variety of physiological parameters. Having practiced acupuncture for twenty years, I consider it the most comprehensive and useful alternative to allopathic medicine. It is useful in at least 85% of disorders, but of limited value in the 15% of individuals who are seriously physically ill when they seek medical care. For infections, major trauma, cancer and most surgically correctable problems, acupuncture has little to offer. For stress illnesses and those still creating only electrical or chemical changes, acupuncture is probably the treatment of choice. It is unsurpassed, for instance, in treating male infertility.

ROLFING—Ida Rolf created a concept of dysfunction resulting from failure of the connective tissue between muscles to glide smoothly. Very deep and sometimes painful massage is used to correct these problems. I suspect its major use is in assisting some individuals with repressed emotions to release their hang-ups.

FELDENKRAIS—Moshe Feldenkrais developed a concept of neuromuscular integration that involves abnormal postural reflexes as major aspects of pathology. The theory is brilliant. In practice, it appears to me to be most helpful in disorders of the brain and spinal cord that led to spasticity and incoordination.

HERBS—Clearly, some herbs are of value and some have led to discoveries of active principles that become drugs. Digitalis, for instance, comes from foxglove. Most of the claims made in popular publications have no scientific study to support them. Undoubtedly, many more active drugs will someday be discovered if herbs are studied adequately.

CHIROPRACTIC AND OSTEOPATHIC MANIPULATION—Osteopathy, begun almost one hundred years ago by an M.D., Andrew Taylor Still, was rejected by allopathic medicine from the very beginning. Although manipulation of joints, muscles and tendons has been used for thousands of years, osteopathy has provided a much more organized and scientific approach that is of great use in spinal problems. I would not want to practice without good osteopathic consultation.

Chiropractic medicine was initiated by an untrained fish-

monger who spent about two weeks as a patient of Still and
then "discovered" chiropractic. Chiropractic has improved its
educational programs over the years and is legal now. But its
practitioners sometimes make claims that are not documented,
and chiropractic remains one of those practices most rejected by
the A.M.A. and M.D.'s in general, not because of manipulation
but because of the claim that all illness results from pressure on
spinal nerves.

RADIONICS—Basically a mantric or psychic device, this
allows some practitioners a tool for divining suggestions for
diagnosis and treatment. No scientific studies have been done
and the approach is generally regarded by science as quackery.
If the practitioner has good intuition it probably works.

IRIDOLOGY—Only one scientific study has been done and
it reported no efficacy of iridology. The thesis of iridologists is
that they can see discolorations and other gross changes in the
iris that allow a specific diagnosis. My suspicion is that any
good iridologist—if there's one who is accurate—is a good intuitive.

SYNTHETIC FIBERS AND ELECTROMAGNETIC INFLU-
ENCES—John Ott and others have significant scientific evidence
of an *adverse* effect of many synthetic vibrations upon health.
These include fluorescent lights, most 60-cycle electrical appli-
ances, TV, microwaves, etc. And Ott shows equally bad effects
of synthetic fibers, such as polyester, acrylic, etc., even showing
that some cases of sexual impotency are created by synthetic
fibers in bed clothes and nightwear. Finally, there are many
claims for the adverse effects of ELF (extra-low frequency) waves
supposedly beamed at the U.S.A. by a hostile Russia.

What is missing are double-blind studies and percentages
of persons affected. In other words, are all of us more or less
equally adversely affected by these relatively *subtle* aspects of
vibration? If so, how far should we go in protecting ourselves?
Should a truly health-conscious individual *avoid* totally, or nearly
so, television, synthetic materials and microwaves?

COLORS AND MINERALS—Rampant in folklore are claims

of health effects of various colors, crystals and stones of many types. Scientific studies have suggested that color does indeed affect *mood*. Beyond that there is no evidence for or against such claims. Just how much does *color* influence mood and/or health? Can crystals *really* affect our health?

(M y s s) The fact that colors have been proven to affect our moods does suggest a connection to our quality of health since our moods so strongly influence our health. Color therapy, like sound therapy, belongs to the dimension of energy medicine. As we learn more about our subtle natures and our auric fields, we will no doubt come to learn more and appreciate the healing influence of the use of light (colors) and sound.

ASTROLOGY—Astrological influences have been part of folklore for thousands of years. There is some evidence for influences of sun signs, rising signs and moon signs upon our personalities. Partly related to biorhythm (the lunar month coincides with one of the cycles), astrological influences may not be as influential as your parents, but what is their role in health?

(M y s s) For me, astrological influences are authentic, but not as commonly thought of by people who assume that astrology is a form of fortune telling. It is not. It is the study of the influences of the energies of the planets on the entire system of life, including human life. That we are part of a whole is a given. That individual parts of that whole radiate certain qualities is natural. Astrological influences do not control one's life; they merely indicate potentials and possibilities.

I personally have read the charts of people whose astrological influences indicated that they had potential weaknesses in certain parts of their bodies. This means that if they were to ignore the proper needs of their bodies, minds and spirits, illness would most probably occur in those parts of their bodies. This does not mean illness is meant to occur in those parts of their bodies.

We always have the power to make choices. Properly understood, astrology is an excellent tool for understanding the properties of the energies influencing your life.

CREATING HEALTH

In summary, creating health is easy. It requires a very simple, safe set of health habits:

Physical Reality

1. Avoid smoking and tobacco.
2. Avoid or minimize alcohol consumption (maximum ten drinks per week).
3. Eat a wide variety of real food (minimize fat, salt, sugar and caffeine).
4. Eat breakfast every day.
5. Eat three meals a day.
6. Exercise adequately.
7. Keep your weight within 10% of the ideal for your height and build.

Energy Reality

8. Resolve your anger, guilt, depression, anxiety and fear daily. Never go to bed with a grudge.
9. Practice relaxation and mental physiological balancing thirty minutes daily (Biogenics).
10. Train yourself to resolve all emotional conflict.
11. Have a positive attitude.
12. Create a sacred space in which to practice spiritual attunement.

CHAPTER FIFTEEN

The Way of the Elegant Spirit

(Myss)

T hat we create the quality of our health is a reality. Even if some people can accept that premise only as it relates to creating the common cold or a tension headache, nevertheless, it is a beginning toward understanding how one's emotions affect one's physical body. More importantly, this acceptance is a crucial first step in shifting one's consciousness toward an understanding of the interdependency of all systems of life.

For those who can and already do accept this premise, it, too, is only a first step. Indeed, the direction we are all headed in is potentially much grander than the basic recognition of personal responsibility regarding the creation of health. What we are now learning in terms of the creative power of our emotions and thoughts represents a *fundamental shift* taking place in our collective conceptual framework of reality itself, and it extends well beyond our individual lives.

Through the study of how our inner processes affect our physical form, we are learning that we do indeed create what we call physical reality. We influence events, weather, ecology, geography and politics. We influence the quality of opportunities that come our way and we create our personal financial circumstances. We influence, in other words, individually and collectively, all that we experience.

Those who are able to understand that they are in charge of their realities considerably increase their capacity to heal any illness because they can no longer be victimized by the idea that the illness occurred randomly, without just cause. They are able to understand that if they have participated in the creation of their illnesses, they can participate in the re-creation of their health. And when they heal, these individuals retain an instinctive recognition about the process of creation itself—namely, if they create the substance that is their physical body, they also create the substance of their environment and therefore, of the whole force field of life. In other words, the teaching that "what is in one is in the whole" becomes a living, breathing truth because they have experienced it personally through re-creating the "earth" that is their body.

Illness is not the only path to this realization. The fact is that every person's life is being touched, somehow, by a crisis that is unsolvable through "ordinary thinking," meaning the use of a previous effective solution applied to new problems. Clearly, the crises of today are far more intense that what we have had to cope with in former decades.

The breakdown of the family unit and long-term personal relationships, the massive increase in drug addiction and alcoholism, the rise in adolescent traumas (such as substance abuse, teenage pregnancies, sexual abuse, child abuse, increasing levels of illiteracy) and the increase of serious diseases coupled with the high cost of treatment, to list just a few of our present dilemmas, are all indications that "ordinary thinking" no longer produces effective resolutions.

Our thinking processes, steeped in familiar and well-worn

patterns of reasoning, have become exhausted and obsolete. No longer capable of responding to the stresses of our world, we are producing long-term solutions to problems (such as pollution and species extinction) that desperately require more immediate and more effective responses. Whether the area of crisis is a health epidemic, such as AIDS, or a tense political situation, the ordinary thinking of traditional medicine or of global politics is no longer expansive enough to grapple with these challenges.

When ordinary thinking can no longer accommodate the demands of the times, new paradigms of conceptual thinking must be sought in relation to the nature and spectrum of the crises. We clearly need to grasp the fact that all crises are now global in proportion and no longer limited to national boundaries. Thus, we must create a paradigm of conceptual thinking that is inclusive of the whole of the globe rather than just selective nations. This is identical to the transition of perception that occurs between traditional medicine (viewing the parts of the body as separate) and the holistic model, which embraces treatment of the whole human being.

The premise that we create our own realities as individual parts of an interconnective force field of life represents a higher order of reasoning that is capable of producing solutions to the challenges of our world. That all systems are interdependent is a perception that is now filtering into our world through every possible channel: health, science, ecology, economics, world government, as well as international movements on behalf of saving the planet from nuclear and ecological disasters.

These insights have enough potency to transform the way we live and the manner in which we understand reality. They are so powerful, in fact, that one must consider why these perceptions are now simultaneously penetrating into every level of life. Like a foundation being laid to house an entirely new species, we must ask, "Who is the architect of this design and for what purpose is this happening? Is it possible that we are being directed by Divine Guidance to enter into a process of transformation in order to insure the survival of life on this planet?"

THE TENUOUS PASSAGE INTO
THE THIRD MILLENNIUM

As the year 2,000 approaches, one cannot help but become absorbed into the wonderment of what it means to enter a new millenium. Many have begun to call the Twenty-first century the New Age, one destined to be a time of enlightenment and advanced spiritual understanding. Predictions state that diseases will be understood fully as energy imbalances, and healing will then be a much gentler process of delicately manipulating the etheric body through the use of crystals, sound and color.

Others anticipate the coming years in far more pragmatic terms. They believe that the coming years, particularly the next two decades, will be a time of great and dramatic transition, literally a time of cleansing. Some of the predictions include catastrophic earth changes, droughts, famine, plagues, the collapse of the international banking system and the probability of nuclear disasters.

Which scenario is the more probable? Or do both have an element of possibility to them? While it may not be realistic actually to *predict* what tomorrow will bring, it is possible to assess the areas of crisis and *project likely outcomes*, since we are indeed creating our future through how we are currently responding to our present challenges.

A GLANCE FORWARD

The history of our planet is a turbulent one. All the nations and the peoples of earth, at one time or another, have known war, starvation, plagues, disease and rule by inhumane systems of government.

These conditions, as we all know, still exist. So our "ordinary thinking" process allows us to view them as unfortunate but chronic human problems. We have numbed ourselves to the fact that the destructive power behind each of these problems has increased dramatically. Where once war, plagues and epidemics were contained in or localized to specific areas of the globe, now each of these dilemmas has worldwide consequences. It is becoming all too apparent that while we may have always confronted these problems, we have so effectively increased their destructive capacity that our survival now is dependent upon removing these problems *entirely* from the human experience.

Consider that the introduction of nuclear weaponry has not only changed the face of war but elevated war to nothing less than a predictable horror resulting in global annihilation. Every area of disturbance on the planet can now potentially explode into a worldwide nuclear crisis.

The AIDS epidemic has spread to virtually every country on earth, making it the first global health crisis. Whereas previously, health crises were limited to certain areas, the mobility factor of human beings has brought this virus to the world arena.

Starvation, poverty and famine are occurring in extreme proportions due to an inability to challenge effectively the root causes of these ills.

The ecological imbalances contribute yet another major factor to the highly volatile condition of the earth, one that, like the nuclear crisis, has not been present prior to the past forty years. A very critical imbalance now exists within the natural order of life. The influence of acid rain, pollution, pesticides and other toxic substances has released vast quantities of poison into the environment, exceeding Nature's own capacity to maintain balance in the environment.

BREAKDOWN OF THE ESSENTIAL
ELEMENTS OF LIFE

Consider the status of the essential elements of life: air, water, earth and fire. The air is filled with contaminants that are so severe that living in major cities, such as Los Angeles or New York, has the same impact on the human lung as smoking one pack of cigarettes per day. The wind currents now carry nuclear pollution. The meltdown at the Chernobyl nuclear power plant brought contamination across the northern hemisphere. Radiation from that one nuclear accident was responsible for the contamination of milk from cows as far away from the site as Minnesota. Sheep in Scotland were so toxic that their meat products could not be consumed.

Our water supplies are loaded with chemicals. There is not *one* unpolluted river in the United States. The toxic substances that are dumped into the bay areas on our coasts are causing the deaths of hundreds of thousands of sea life creatures, such as is evidenced in the highly poisonous Chesapeake Bay area, noted for its extreme levels of pollution. Acid rain is yet another contributor to the toxicity levels in our drinking water.

The earth itself has reached such a highly toxic level that crop growing in several farm areas is in danger, if not already totally halted. The prolonged use of pesticides, herbicides and fertilizers has resulted in such serious damage to the earth that the crops are themselves now toxic, having absorbed the poisons from the earth.

The hole in the ozone layer has produced a breakdown in the protective atmospheric shield, making the natural life-giving rays of the sun, the element of fire, a very real health hazard. Skin cancer, associated with extreme exposure to sunlight, is now even more likely. Further, other imbalances created by the ozone depletion are inevitable.

The crises that have been created, and continue to be created by these environmental stresses, are destroying life at a rate that is, for most people, incomprehensible. Estimates from environmental groups state that one thousand species per year are becoming *extinct*. This is one tragic yardstick by which we can measure the end result of living unconsciously upon this earth.

We can no longer afford to underestimate the significance, both literally and symbolically, of the fact that all of the essential elements for life—*ALL LIFE*—have become toxic. We are made of the same ingredients. We are air, water, earth and fire. That we are now living in a very tenuous condition is a reality.

THE PATH OF SURVIVAL:
RESPONSIBLE CHOICE

Ordinary thinking processes will not produce solutions to our global crises any more than ordinary thinking results in solutions to contemporary personal challenges. Our perceptual system needs to be elevated and transformed to a higher order of reasoning, making it possible to shift our value system from the needs of the individual to the needs of the whole.

How is this to be accomplished? Certainly it is naive to assume that human beings are going to awaken suddenly en masse and change their lifestyles and values to reflect an entirely different set of priorities based upon responsibility toward the greater spectrum of life. And yet, from another perspective entirely, there is a type of natural selection process occurring that might well be aimed at accomplishing just such an awakening.

In recent years, a vast number of people have united their energies in response to global concerns. To list just a few examples: Aid to Africa—an international response to the massive starvation occurring in Ethiopia; Greenpeace and Save the Whales—international organizations formed to protect the "right to life" of the planet and its creatures; PETA—People for the Ethical Treatment of Animals; Planetary Citizens—an organization aimed at uniting all of the peoples of the planet into one human network; The Rain Forest Action Network—an organization formed to raise the consciousness about the tragic effects of the destruction of the rain forests of this earth.

The list of such organizations, which are based upon concerns over the quality of life, could fill a book. What they represent is a signficant movement taking place at the grass roots level of life to take more responsibility for the well-being of life on this planet.

An equally impressive movement is occurring within the field of health care. Scientific research aimed at curing cancer has spun off a remarkable amount of data indicating what food and chemical products are carcinogens. Likewise, research into the effects of certain food products on the heart and on high blood pressure, such as salt, sugar, cholesterol, high fat consumption and red meat, has resulted in raising the consciousness levels of millions of people in terms of understanding the contribution that diet makes to health. And this research, incidentally, comes from the *traditional* medical and scientific communities.

Coupled with the research emerging from the holistic arena, which points to the effects of attitudes and beliefs on the quality of health, the result of this massive wave of research is what we are now experiencing as an explosion of health-conscious, health-oriented individuals in our society. Even commercials advertising breakfast cereals now have people "jogging" before eating a healthy breakfast of bran or granola (with reduced salt and sugar content also available).

Running marathons has become common in this country, as evidenced by the overwhelming increase in the design and productivity of athletic clothing, shoes and other specialty items. Health centers have sprung up in almost every city and town in the country. Smoking has been banned from airplane flights under two hours and from most places of business entirely.

In other words, *health consciousness is here to stay*. People have begun to take dramatic steps toward living, thinking, breathing and eating more responsibly. This is not a temporary fad brought about through the advent of holistic thinking. These changes represent the shift of fundamental human priorities in which responsible personal choice has become a value.

Can changes such as these impact the crises we face politically or socially? How much must a person change in order to make a difference?

ONE MAN'S JOURNEY

There is probably no way of truly measuring the effects our choices have in terms of the overall quality of our lives or of the lives of those around us. And yet, it is intriguing to follow a type of cause-and-effect chain reaction as it unfolds in one person's life.

I met John at a conference four years ago. He was obviously a body builder. He was also a runner. And a vegetarian. He was involved in several planetary organizations and he was a central networker who seemed to know everyone in the New Age field. Moreover, he was a successful businessman, having earned a substantial fortune in real estate. In short, he was impressive. But more impressive was his personal story, primarily because of its simplicity and his gradual process of awakening.

While a real estate tycoon, John was a heavy smoker and a hearty drinker. He battled high blood pressure and a slight weight problem. He admitted to having absolutely no interest in anything other than money and power. Certainly, he never attended conferences that were aimed at raising the awareness levels of humanity.

His fortieth birthday, as he recalls, took him by surprise. As he looked at himself in the mirror, he saw a man who had seemingly aged overnight. He didn't much like what he saw and so, right then and there, he decided to take up running.

That very day he purchased his first pair of running shoes and "huffed and puffed," as he described it, for exactly five blocks. He knew that if he were to succeed at any level of running effectively, he would have to quit smoking. And so he did.

After about two months of consistent running, John was jogging almost three miles per day. His body was gaining in tone and stamina, and he was beginning to feel more vibrant and alive than he had felt in a long time. He then began to become conscious of his diet. He became interested in a more balanced nutritional program and, thus, he stopped his consumption of red meat, chemical products, sugar, fats and all alcohol.

Within four months of that decision, John became a committed vegetarian. His interest in nutrition led him to start reading more about balanced eating regimens. While in a bookstore, he picked up a magazine called *Vegetarian Times*, thinking that it was a recipe magazine.

For the first time in his life, John read about alternative

lifestyles and was introduced to a quality of spiritual thinking that he had not previously encountered. He had long ago abandoned religion and did not feel that "God-stuff" had any place in anyone's life, "in particular", he added, "if they were interested in money, which I was."

What captured John's attention more than he thought possible was the idea of meditation. As he described it, he decided to try it simply because the article said that meditation was a good way to minimize the effects of stress in the body. There was one problem, though, and that was that John did not know how to meditate, nor did he know anyone who did.

He went back to the bookstore, bought five books on meditation and, as the clerk was writing up his order, John asked in a whisper, "Do you know anyone who teaches this stuff?" The clerk produced a newsletter that included advertisements of local therapists and teachers of various alternative practices. That night he called someone listed as a meditation teacher and, thus, he began to walk his spiritual path.

John has since shifted all of the concerns of his life to reflect his spiritual beliefs. His investments of time, energy and money are dedicated to making a difference in the quality of life on this planet.

John's story is actually far more typical than it is extraordinary. It only takes *one* conscious action to start the energy of transformation in motion, like the decision to start running. It's not even important that one make the decision from a position of consciousness. John's decision to start running was motivated by the desire to retard the aging process, not to become a spiritual force on the planet.

But any decision in which the individual is taking more responsibility for the quality of his or her life *inevitably will lead to a heightening of that person's awareness*. The process of cause and effect has an intelligence of its own, leading a person continually toward greater dimensions of personal choice and self-empowerment.

This process is at work in millions of people's lives. Each

person who has done even one simple thing, such as releasing sugar from a daily diet or quitting smoking, has placed himself or herself on a path of greater awareness. Though we do not all move at the same pace, the path we are on is identical. Inevitably, once you take even the slightest degree of personal responsibility for yourself, you cannot move backwards. The thought form of personal responsibility becomes firmly planted in your consciousness and, from that moment on, it will call to you at every possible opportunity.

This is the way that change is unfolding on this planet—person by person, choice by choice. Dramatic change is not brought about through visions from the heavens. It is gradual, but the effects are indeed dramatic.

WHERE IS THIS ALL HEADED AND
WILL IT PRODUCE PEACE?

Each person who awakens to a stronger degree of personal responsibility becomes another voice for peace on this planet, even if that voice is never raised in public. The effects of becoming a health-conscious person will result in creating a peace-conscious person automatically. The reason this is so is because *it is impossible to be hostile and completely healthy simultaneously*. Like John, even if your interest is to halt the aging process of your physical form, inevitably you will be led to discover your inner self.

And then, it is only a matter of time before you realize that your emotions affect your body. All the running you can do, and all the healthy foods you can consume will not counterbalance the effects of a hostile, contaminated emotional nature. Thus, the payoff to becoming peaceful and peace-minded is a healthy body and a healthy, peaceful planet. Peace, in other words, is built into the awakening of becoming fully healthy and self-empowered.

There is yet another benefit to becoming awakened, and that is that in all likelihood, it represents the only guarantee of immunization against the viruses now raging on the planet. Like a global, natural process of selection, all of the crises loom over-

head as opportunities to take more responsibilty for the quality
of life on the planet.

Whether one responds by increasing personal health, or
whether one directs his or her energy toward saving the rain
forests of South America is irrelevant. What is at stake is the
fact that each of us must respond in some form to assist the
healing of the earth. Each response contributes an act of positive
energy that heals the whole of life—including the essential elements of life—our air, water, earth and fire.

It represents, in my opinion, a global effort to heal the
earth's immune system. And in so responding, each person who
takes more responsibility for the quality of life, either at the
individual level or at the group level, has accomplished self-
immunization.

Ultimately, what is being formed out of this global response
to crises is a unified spirituality that recognizes and honors the
sacredness of all that has life. Through our need to unite as
human beings in order to survive as a species, we are creating
a spirituality based upon universal principles and the realization
that we create our realities, personal and global.

Our thoughts are real. They have energy and this energy
creates. It creates the matter that is our bodies and it creates the
matter that forms our experiences and our planet. Living according to this truth requires a spirituality unlike that which has
been practiced by the masses ever before on this planet. We
have reached the moment of our evolution in which we must
*humanize the sacred and lessen the distance between nonphysical and
physical intelligence.* This is the way of the elegant spirit.

BECOMING AN ELEGANT SPIRIT

The principle of healing—of that which creates and maintains
health and life—is spirituality in motion. That we create our
own realities is the activity of spirituality in motion.

Even if a person cannot accept the existence of a God or
of some form of Divine Intelligence, nevertheless, the evidence
illustrating the connection between human emotions and the

condition of the physical body stands as tangible proof that the energy of our consciousness is real. And more than real, it is a creative force.

What does this information have to offer us in terms of how we live our lives? At the very least, it suggests that to live unconsciously, that is, unaware of what we are thinking, feeling and thus creating, is threatening to our health, not to mention the other areas of our lives. It is simply not productive to deny one's own power. It is, in fact, self-defeating.

The other option, the higher one, is to learn to live consciously, developing skills of awareness and insight that release a person from having to feel victimized or controlled by life's challenges ever again. This quality of personal power transforms ordinary human consciousness into a force that radiates elegance and grace.

The presence of a person whose spirit is truly "elegant" is unmistakable. These individuals project an energy which communicates that "visitors passing through their energy fields" are welcome and safe. The usual barriers created through human insecurities are absent.

This quality of consciousness is fertile ground for the seeds of unconditional love, an attitude of nonjudgmentalism and acceptance of all that has life. That is what it means to be an elegant spirit—an individual who has awakened to the realization that he or she is a creator and, therefore, acts to honor that power through living with love, wisdom and compassion. This person is an example of what Abraham Maslow calls "self-actualized." These are the peace-makers, and they will indeed "inherit the earth."

PRINCIPLES FOR LIVING THE WAY
OF THE ELEGANT SPIRIT

Becoming an aware human being is a full-time job. At times, you might regret your ever having stepped foot on this path because awareness does not necessarily make your life easier. In fact, it will most certainly bring you challenges that seem to be monumental. To see clearly, to have the inner vision clear enough to penetrate the illusions other people still maintain, can be very discouraging.

Likewise, to choose a path of awareness is not an intellectual exercise. It is a living, breathing, constant discipline. If you choose to believe that you create your own reality, that perception does not include any vacation time. You must always live in that perception, no matter what the situation, no matter what the challenge. Indeed, your intellect will not be your opponent on this path—your challenges will come from your emotions. It is your emotional warehouse that holds your fears, insecurities and lesser qualities. Healing these inner limitations will be your challenge, again and again.

A word of caution is also required here. Spiritual power is not earned casually. Regardless of what information you may pour into your brain, and how well you may intellectually understand Buddhism, Zen or the Christian mystical traditions, the intellect is no match for the soul. Your life will most certainly change if you direct it toward spiritual awakening. The wisdom of your soul will take over the driver's seat of your life, and your lesser needs, those coming from fear or illusion, will ride along like hitchhikers until you are ready to drop them off.

And finally, there is no turning back. Once you accept the journey to become whole, to become an elegant spirit, you cannot go backwards. You cannot become "unaware" ever again. You can take a detour or two, but you cannot release awareness once it is your own. It is yours for all eternity.

It is inevitable that every human being will become an "elegant spirit." As the *Course in Miracles* so beautifully says, "It is not a matter of *if*, it is a matter of *when*."

We offer the following suggestions for those on the path to becoming *ELEGANT SPIRITS*.

- Personal values must be based upon the truth of your origin. You are spirit. You command energy to take form according to your thoughts, feelings and words, and you are responsible for the quality of that which you contribute to the creation of life. It is, therefore, in your own best interest as well as that of others to create with love and wisdom. Keep your words, thoughts and emotions clear and honest.

- Universal Principles serve as guidelines for creation: cause and effect, what is in one is in the whole, manifestation is the result of intention. These, and all other Universal Principles, are your power tools. The more you know and understand Universal Principles, the more empowered you become.

- Each person who enters into your life is a reflection of some aspect of your own being. Likewise, you are a reflection for each person also. Whether you are drawn to their positive qualities, or repelled by their negative traits, you are only seeing yourself. This reflection is often difficult to see clearly because the depth of the reflection is usually disguised by the personality of the individual. If you can look beyond the personality traits, you will see yourself in the depths of a person's motivations, fears, strengths and compassion. Blaming others, therefore, serves no purpose.

- All artificial barriers that separate the essential oneness of life should be disregarded. Boundaries between nations which maintain that certain people are different than others are obsolete, meaningless and serve only to separate people from one another. Allegiance belongs to life itself. Life has no boundaries. It thrives anywhere there is love.

- Likewise, the boundaries that are now present among all of the other kingdoms of life—animal, mineral and plant—are also artificial barriers that prevent respect, interspecies communication and emotional bonding. All life has consciousness.

- What is in one is in the whole. Apply this teaching to your life and all that you create, realizing that every positive and negative action you put into motion affects the whole of life.

- Time and space are nonexistent in the dimension of

thought. Thoughts travel in an instant. Therefore, learn to think in terms of your thoughts as a multi-level communications system in which such activity as healing at a distance can be accomplished.

- Because thoughts are power, develop a quality-control checkup on yourself on a regular basis. When you feel that too much negativity is present in your system, do something to heal yourself immediately. Pay attention to the law of cause and effect, and study the consequences of your actions, words and thoughts, realizing at all times that *you* are the creator behind that which you are studying.

- Heal your own addiction to violence in any and every form: actions, attitudes, words, habits and thoughts. Our violent natures create our violent politics, weapons, and all violent human actions and interactions. We all have violence in us. Our world is a violent world, and these proclivities have entered into us through the very air we breathe. Remember that violence breeds disease and destroys the human emotional system.

- Study those desires in your life that control you, and strive to release yourself from anything artificial that exerts power over you: drugs, alcohol, negative habits, fears—anything that causes you to lose power.

- Remember at all times that you are constantly healing. The process of healing is a *verb and not a noun*. Your body is reacting every second to your thoughts, feelings, emotions and experiences. Health is not a permanent condition unless you create it so each day.

- When you must take time to heal, do it gently. Healing through force of will alone, through determination without self-compassion, is a form of self-inflicted violence. Don't resent your body for breaking down; learn from the experience so that it does not have to be repeated. Trust the process of healing. It has an intelligence of its own. Learn to listen to what your body needs and to what your spirit needs. Above all, value your health and your well-being as your first priority. Honor thyself.

- Clearly define in your heart your spiritual principles. Know and be clear about what you believe. Do not accept beliefs without question. Keep your focus on yourself and not on others.
- Set time aside each day for your spiritual practice. Meditation and prayer are essential. Learn to be still and hear the inner voice of your soul.
- Above all, practice loving. Unconditional love requires the ultimate of efforts and it reaps the ultimate of rewards.

Teilhard de Chardin said that when we discover how to be truly loving, we will have discovered the power of fire for the second time.

The decision to become *spiritually elegant* is worth the effort required. One reaps the rewards of health, wisdom and compassion and becomes an instrument of peace. Many times in our history, we have been blessed with people of vision, people who could clearly see that the massive amount of suffering and destruction in our world is unnecessary. If we could only see through eyes not blinded by fear, we would discover solutions to all of our global problems. We would discover how to be global beings, sharing one planet, sharing one way of life.

May we all discover the power of fire for the second time and, in doing so, heal ourselves, heal our planet and enter into the twenty-first century as a global community of *elegant spirits*.

Recommended Reading

AIDS: PASSAGEWAY TO TRANSFORMATION by C. Norman Shealy, M.D., Ph.D. and Caroline M. Myss, M.A., Stillpoint International, 1988.

THE MALE MACHINE by Marc F. Fasteau, Delta Books, New York, 1975.

SOCIOLOGY FOR THE SOUTH by George Fitzburgh, 1854.

MALE SEXUALITY by Bernie Zilbergeld, Bantam, New York, 1978.

THE PSYCHOLOGY OF POWER by Ronald V. Sampson, Pantheon, New York, 1966.

MASCULINE/FEMININE edited by Betty Roszak and Theodore Roszak, Harper and Row, New York, 1969.

SEXUAL BEHAVIOR IN THE HUMAN MALE by Alfred C. Kinsey, Wardell B. Pomeroy and Clyde E. Martin, W. B. Saunders, Philadelphia, 1948.

SEX AND HUMAN LOVING by William H. Masters, Virginia E. Johnson and Robert C. Kolodny, Little, Brown, Boston, 1986.

HOW BIG IS BIG? by Dr. Zven Wanderer and Dr. David Radell, Bell Publishing, New York, 1982.

FROM EDEN TO EROS: ORIGINS OF THE PUT DOWN OF WOMEN by Richard Roberts, Vernal Equinox Press, San Anselmo, California, 1985.

AN EXPERIENCE OF WOMEN by Priscilla Robertson, Temple University Press, Philadelphia, 1982.

"Perspectives on Psychic Diagnosis" by C. Norman Shealy, M.D., THE A.R.E. Journal, pp 208–217, 1976.

WOMEN'S REALITY by Anne Wilson Schaef, Winston Press, Inc., Minneapolis, MN, 1981.

"Science, Intuition and Medical Practices" by Irvin H. Page, POSTGRADUATE MEDICINE, pp 217–221, Nov. 1978.

"From Intuition to Computation. Development of Problems of Medical Diagnosis" by R. Gross, INFORMATION IN MEDICINE, pp 35–39, 1966.

THE WAY TO HEALTH by Robert R. Leichtman, M.D. and Carl Japikse, Ariel Press, 1970.

HEAL THYSELF by Edward Back, M.D., C. W. Daniel Company Ltd., Keats Publishing Co., New Canaan, CT, 1986.

IRRITATION, THE DESTRUCTIVE FIRE by Torkom Saraydarian, Aquarian Educational Group, Sedona, AZ, 1983.

WHO GETS SICK: THINKING AND HEALTH by Blair Justice, Peak Press, Houston, 1987.

MIND AS HEALER, MIND AS SLAYER by Kenneth R. Pelletier, Delta Press, 1977.

"Psychoneuroimmunology: Interactions Between Central Nervous System and Immune System" by G. F. Solomon, JOURNAL OF NEUROSCIENCE RESEARCH 18:1–9, 1987.

PLEASE UNDERSTAND ME by David Keirsey and Marilyn Bates, Gnosology Books Ltd., Del Mar, CA, 1984.

"Religious Involvement and the Health of the Elderly: Some Hypotheses and an Initial Test" by Ellen L. Idler. SOCIAL FORCES 66:227–238, 1987.

"Natural Killer Cell Activity and MMPI Scores of a Cohort of College Students" by J. Stephen Heisel, et al, AM. JOURNAL OF PSYCHIATRY 143:11, pp 1382–1386, 1986.

"Suspiciousness, Health, and Mortality: A Follow-up Study of 500 Older Adults" by John C. Barefoot, et al, PSYCHOSOMATIC MEDICINE 49:450–457, 1987.

"A Psychoneuroimmunologic Perspective on AIDS Research: Questions, Preliminary Findings, and Suggestions" by George F. Solomon, et al, JOURNAL OF APPLIED SOCIAL PSYCHOLOGY 17:286–308, 1987.

"Endorphins: A Link Between Personality, Stress, Emotions, Immunity, and Disease?" by George F. Solomon, et al, EN-KEPHALINS AND ENDORPHINS, Plenum Publishing Company, 1986.

FIT FOR LIFE by Harvey and Marilyn Diamond, Warner Books, New York, 1985.

SPEEDY GOURMET by C. Norman Shealy, M.D., Ph.D., Brindabella Books, Fair Grove, MO, 1984.

INSTINCTIVE NUTRITION by Severen L. Schaeffer, Celestial Arts, Berkeley, CA, 1988.

90 DAYS TO SELF-HEALTH by C. Norman Shealy, M.D., Ph.D., Brindabella Books, Fair Grove, MO, 2nd edition 1987.

THE AEROBICS WAY by Kenneth H. Cooper, M.D., Bantam Books, New York, 1981.

MACROBIOTICS by Michio Kushi, Japan Publications, Tokyo, Japan, 1977.

THE ART OF LIVING by Carl Japikse and Robert Leichtman, M.D., Ariel Press, Columbus, OH, 1986.

MEDICAL NEMESIS by Ivan Illich, Calder and Boyars, Ltd., London, 1975.

MATTERS OF LIFE AND DEATH: RISKS VERSUS BENEFITS OF MEDICAL CARE by Eugene D. Robin, W. H. Freeman, New York, 1984.

MEDICINE ON TRIAL by Dannie Abse, Crown Publishers, Inc., New York, 1976.

TO PARENT OR NOT by C. Norman Shealy and Mary-Charlotte Shealy, Donning Company, Virginia Beach, 1981.

EDGAR CAYCE ENCYCLOPEDIA OF HEALING by Reba and Karp, Warner Books, 1986.

THE ROLE OF MEDICINE: DREAM, MIRAGE OR NEMESIS by Thomas McKeown, Nuffield Provincial Hospitals Trust, London, 1976.